Community Informatics

T0174038

Community groups, social support networks, voluntary agencies and government organisations are all actively exploring the potential of the new information and communications technologies to bring about democratic development and renewal. A rich variety of social experiments in what has become known as Community Informatics is now beginning to provide useful research findings and exciting examples of innovative applications. This book sets down some of the defining features of a Community Informatics approach and some of the common themes which are emerging. In particular it considers the following issues:

- sustainability
- employment
- community management
- public service provision
- partnerships of stakeholders
- local learning
- social support and networks.

This edited collection brings together leading exponents of Community Informatics from around the world and critically evaluates their experiences.

Leigh Keeble and **Brian D. Loader** are both at the Community Informatics Research and Applications Unit (CIRA) based at the University of Teesside.

Community Informatics

Shaping computer-mediated
social relations

Edited by Leigh Keeble and
Brian D. Loader

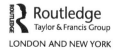
Routledge
Taylor & Francis Group

LONDON AND NEW YORK

First published 2001
by Routledge
2 Park Square, Milton Park, Abingdon, Oxon OX14 4RN

Simultaneously published in the USA and Canada
by Routledge
711 Third Avenue, New York, NY 10017

Routledge is an imprint of the Taylor & Francis Group
© 2001 Selection and editorial matter,
Leigh Keeble and Brian D. Loader;
individual chapters, the contributors

Chapter 3 by Barry Wellman previously printed in *The
International Journal of Urban and Regional Relations*, June 2001,
Vol. 25.2. Permission for reprint and copyright holder is Blackwell
Publishers and the editors of IJURR.

Chapter 17 by Doug Schuler. An earlier version of this chapter
appeared in *Information Communication and Society*, Vol. 4, No. 2,
2001 http://www.T&F.co.uk/journals/. Permission for publication
given by Taylor & Francis Ltd. and the editors of *Information
Communication and Society*.

Typeset in Times by Steven Gardiner Ltd, Cambridge

British Library Cataloguing in Publication Data
A catalogue reference has been requested

Library of Congress Cataloging in Publication Data
Community informatics: shaping computer-mediated social relations/
edited by Leigh Keeble and Brian D. Loader.
   p.   cm
Includes bibliographical references and index.
1. Social groups – Computer network resources.
2. Social interaction – Computer network resources.
3. Community organization – Community network resources.
I. Keeble, Leigh. II. Loader, Brian, 1958–
HM176.C64   2002
302.23 – dc21   2001034795

ISBN 978 0 415 23112 1 (pbk)
ISBN 978 0 415 23111 4 (hbk)

Dedicated in memory of
Denis John Noble (1938–1985)

Contents

PART IV
Policy implications of community informatics

Contributors

Abdul Alkalimat is Professor of Africana Studies and Sociology and Director of the Africana Studies programme at the University of Toledo, Ohio, where he has engineered the only known Internet-based course taught from Africa to students in the US. He moderates the largest African-American Studies discussion list H-Afro-Am and created and edits *Malcolm X: A Research Site* as well as *eBlack Studies*. He served as cyberorganiser for the 1998 Black Radical Congress held in Chicago, Illinois, and is a member of the editorial boards of *cy.Rev*, and *Black Scholar* and *Information, Communication and Society*. He is currently guest-editing an issue of *Black Scholar* devoted to cyberspace and the Black experience. Alkalimat is also co-authoring (with Kate Williams) a study of public computing in Toledo, Ohio.

Perry Bard has exhibited video and installations internationally: in New York at P.S. 1 Museum, the New Museum, the Alternative Museum; at the Southeast Museum of Photography in Florida; in France at the F.R.A.C. des Pays de La Loire; at the São Paulo Bienal in Brazil; in Spain at the Reina Sofia, Madrid; at Ostranenie Electronic Media Forum in Dessau, Germany; at Videoarchaeology International Video Art festival in Sofia, Bulgaria; in Canada at Mercer Union, Toronto, and the J. Yahouda Meir Gallery in Montreal. She has done temporary Public Art projects for Petrosino Park, Snug Harbor and the Staten Island Ferry Terminal Building in New York. Her work has been reviewed in *Artforum*, *Art in America*, *Arts Magazine*, *Flash Art*, *Vie des Arts*, *New Art Examiner* and *Lapiz*, and is in the collections of the Canada Arts Council, V Tape and Groupe Intervention Video, Canada, the Frac des Pays de la Loire and the Southeast Museum of Photography. She has been awarded grants by the National Endowment for the Arts and the Canada Arts Council.

Roger Burrows is Assistant Director of the Centre for Housing Policy at the University of York. A sociologist and a statistician by background, he has published extensively on issues relating to: housing; health; work and employment; and technology. Some recent books include the co-edited

Cyberspace/Cyberbodies/Cyberpunk (Sage, 1996) and *Homelessness and Social Policy* (Routledge, 1997). He recently led a research team examining the emergence of 'virtual community care' as a part of the ESRC's 'Virtual Society?' programme and is currently working on a Joseph Rowntree Foundation research project called 'wired for independence'.

Giovanni Casapulla has worked for over fifteen years in the field of networking technologies and virtual communities. He was very young when, in the 1980s, he promoted several bulletin board systems on the Fidonet-like technology. In 1994 he became one of the founders of the Milano Community Network (RCM) at the Computer and Information Science Department of the Milano State University. After more than five years as System administrator of RCM, in January 2000 he became responsible for IrisCube of the 'Business Community' branch, which develops community-based solutions within enterprise portals.

Peter Day is a lecturer at the University of Brighton's School of Information Management, teaching across a wide range of Information Society related subjects. He combines this teaching with a Community Informatics research focus. Peter is a co-author of the IBM-CDF sponsored COMMIT report *Down-to-Earth Vision: Community Based IT Initiatives and Social Inclusion* and has recently completed his Ph.D. thesis entitled *The Networked Community: Policies for a Participative Information Society*. He is a Steering Group member of the Brighton & Hove Community Information Network initiative and has actively participated in a number of Community Informatics related workshops and conferences. These include co-ordinating the 'Broadening our Understanding: Community Networks and other forms of Computer Supported Community Work' workshop at the ECSCW99 conference and the 'Community Informatics: participatory tools for social inclusion and active citizenship' at PDC2000 conference as well as participating in the 'Designing Across Borders: The Community Design of Community Networks' workshop at the PDC98 and CSCW98 conferences. He was also a Programme Committee member of the PDC2000 conference and Programme Chair of the DIAC-00, 'Shaping the Network Society: The Future of the Public Sphere in Cyberspace' conference held in Seattle in May 2000.

Fiorella de Cindio is Associate Professor of Programming Languages at the Computer and Information Science Department of the State University of Milan. Her research interests include Petri nets as concurrency theory, programming languages (namely, object-oriented and distributed programming languages) and the applications of information and communications technologies to support life and work within social and office systems. In this field, during the 1980s she undertook action research and education on workers' participation in system design. Fiorella was also a member of the team which conceived and developed one of the first CSCW prototypes (CHAOS, Commitment Handling Active Office System). In 1994, she promoted the Civic Informatics Laboratory, for which she is now responsible, and, in that role, set up the Milano Community Network (RCM) which is a Participatory Foundation.

Eileen Green is Professor of Sociology and Director of the Centre for Social and Policy Research (CSPR) at the University of Teesside. She is co-author of *Women's Leisure What Leisure?* (Macmillan, 1990) (with Sandra Hebron and Diana Woodward), and has co-edited *Gendered by Design? Information Technology and Office Systems* (Taylor & Francis, 1993) (with Jenny Owen and Den Pain), *Women, Work and Computerization: Breaking Old Boundaries Building New Forms* (North-Holland, Elsevier) (with Alison Adam, Judy Emms and Jenny Owen) and *Virtual Gender, Technology, Consumption and Identity* (Routledge, 2001) (with Alison Adam). She has also guest-edited 'Gender, Society and ICTs', a special issue of *Information, Communication and Society*, Vol. 2, No. 4 (with Alison Adam). She is currently grant holder of the ESRC research seminar series 'Equal Opportunities on Line, Gender and IT' and is an invited member of the international experts group attached to the Netherlands Research programme 'Society and the Electronic Highway'.

Michael Gurstein, Ph.D., completed a B.A. at the University of Saskatchewan and a Ph.D. in Sociology at the University of Cambridge. Dr Gurstein has published widely in both scholarly and more popular journals. His publications include editing *Community Informatics: Enabling Communities with Information and Communication Technologies* (Idea Group Publishers, 2000), *Burying Coal: Research and Development in a Marginal Community,* (Collective Press, 2000). *The Net Working Locally: Information and Communications Technology in Support of Local Economic Development* is currently under review by several publishers. Dr Gurstein is currently an Associate Professor in the Management and Technology Program of the Technical University of British Columbia and the Director of the Centre for Community Informatics at TechBC.

Ed Hollander, Ph.D., is Senior Associate Professor at the Department of Communication, and Director of Studies at the University of Nijmegen, the Netherlands. His research interests include policy studies and theoretical and empirical research on local and regional media and digital online communities. For the past three decades he has been involved in (early) studies of local cable television experiments in the Netherlands and has done research on development communication, community press, community radio and television and digital community networks. He has published both theoretical and empirical studies on these media. In the early 1980s he was commissioned by the Dutch government to investigate the emergence of local and regional media in western Europe. The research for his dissertation, *Local Communication and the Local Public Sphere* (1988), provided the groundwork for translating Habermas's notion of public sphere to community media. Hollander is an associate editor of *Gazette, the International Journal for Communication Studies*, and member of the Intergovernmental Council of the International Program for Development Communication of UNESCO.

John Hood is a lecturer in Risk Management at Glasgow Caledonian University. His main teaching and research interests lie in the area of public sector risk management. He has recently completed a Ph.D. into the impact of compulsory competitive tendering on occupational health and safety. At present, he is involved in the evaluation of the first major residential CCTV system in Scotland, which has been installed in the Easterhouse housing scheme in Glasgow.

Birgit Jæger has a Master's degree in Technological and Social-economic Planning and a Ph.D., both from Roskilde University. From 1997 Birgit Jæger has been Associate Professor at Roskilde University, Department of Social Sciences. She is affiliated to the Center for Local Institutional Research and is a member of a research group working with technology and innovation. Primarily concerned with the Social Studies of Technology she has evaluated experiments with information technology in local communities; studied the Danish development of multimedia in a local as well as an international context and she is now studying the use of information technology in the public sector in Denmark. She has just finished working on the EU-funded project 'Social Learning In Multimedia' (SLIM) and is about to start working on a research project funded by the Danish Research Council.

Nicholas W. Jankowski is Associate Professor, Department of Communication, University of Nijmegen. He has been involved in investigations of community media since the mid-1970s when experiments with community television were initiated in the Netherlands. In addition to small-scale electronic media, Jankowski has studied the introduction of cable and network-based services providing interactive facilities for users. Some of his publications in this area include *The People's Voice: Local Radio and Television in Europe* (co-editor) and *The Coming of Interactive Media* (co-editor). He has also been concerned with methodological issues for investigating small-scale media (co-editor of *A Handbook of Qualitative Methodologies for Mass Communication Research*) and is currently working on a methodology textbook for new media research. Jankowski is currently Chair of the Community Communication Section of the International Association of Media and Communication Research (IAMCR) and co-editor of the journal *New Media & Society*.

Leigh Keeble is a Research Fellow in the Community Informatics Research & Applications Unit (CIRA), University of Teesside. She has been involved in a range of projects including the evaluation of community informatics projects and the role of such projects in combating information exclusion and researching the impact of technology in the voluntary sector. She is currently engaged in research involving topics such as young people and ICTs and the gendered use of technology.

Brian D. Loader is Co-Director of the Community Informatics Research & Applications Unit (CIRA) based at the University of Teesside. He is also General Editor of the international journal *Information, Communication & Society* (www.infosoc.co.uk) and is editor of *The Governance of Cyberspace* (Routledge, 1997), *Cyberspace Divide* (Routledge, 1998) (co-editor), *Digital Democracy* (Routledge, 1999) (co-editor), *Cybercrime* (Routledge, 1999) (with Nichole Ellison, Nicholas Pleace and Doug Schuler) and *Key Concepts in Cyberculture* (Routledge, 2002).

Sonia Liff is a Senior Lecturer at Warwick Business School, Warwick University. Earlier research and writing focused on the impact of technical change at work for jobs, skills and gender-based occupational segregation. She also has more recent publications on workplace equality policies and their operation in practice. Currently the principal investigator on a project entitled 'Gateways to the Virtual Society: Innovation for Social Inclusion' which is part of the ESRC's 'Virtual Society?' programme.

Steve Muncer is a Lecturer in Applied Psychology at University College Stockton, University of Durham, UK.

Sarah Nettleton is a Senior Lecturer in Social Policy at the University of York, UK.

Margaret Page is an independent researcher and organisation consultant and visiting Fellow at the School for Policy Studies, Bristol University. She specialises in facilitating learning and exchange between individual managers and change agents in organisations, networks and partnerships. She co-designed and is now an external consultant to Women Connect. Through her consultancy and research she supports women's equality and social values and initiatives to use ICTs to strengthen voluntary and community organisations.

Nicholas Pleace has worked in social policy research for the last decade. He is based in the Centre for Housing Policy at the University of York; much of his research has been focused on housing and community care, homelessness, rough sleeping and social housing management. More recently, he has become interested in the use of ICTs for health and social care, pursuing a particular interest in the use of CMC for self-help and social support through his work with Roger Burrows, Brian Loader, Steven Muncer and

Sarah Nettleton on 'Virtual Community Care' funded by the ESRC. Nicholas is a member of the editorial board of *Information, Communication and Society* and also edits the journal's website at http://www. infosoc.co.uk/. He is about to commence work on the use of ICTs by social services and supported housing social landlords for the Joseph Rowntree Foundation.

Agneta Ranerup is a Lecturer in the Department of Informatics at the University of Göteborg in Sweden. She received her Ph.D. in informatics from the University of Göteborg in 1996. Her main research interest is democratic aspects of information systems development in the public sector, with a special focus on deliberative processes. Another theme in her research has been change management aspects when introducing groupware in local government in Sweden. Agneta Ranerup is a member of the Swedish Commission on Information Technology, Democracy and Citizenship.

Laura Anna Ripamonti took her degree in Engineering of Business Management and Organization at the Politecnico of Milan in 1999. Her Master's thesis was about the possibility of using civic networks as a support for the economical development of Italian industrial districts. She was then awarded a fellowship to carry out a survey on the state of the art of civic informatics in the Lombardy region, and collaborated with the Milano Community Network to design new development strategies. At the moment she is a Ph.D. student in Informatics at the Computer and Information Science Department of the Milano State University and she co-ordinates a project aimed at the development of information and communications technologies to support local communities.

Doug Schuler is a former chair of Computer Professionals for Social Responsibility (CPSR) and a founding member of the Seattle Community Network (SCN). For nearly twenty years Doug has been engaged with issues relating to society and computing as an activist and a citizen. He has worked on many CPSR projects including all seven of CPSR's symposia on the 'Directions and Implications of Advanced Computing' (DIAC) conferences, which provide a public forum for social implications of computers. A member of the faculty (part-time studies) at The Evergreen State College, Doug is currently teaching 'Community Information Systems', a year-long programme in which student teams develop Web-based applications for communities all over the world, and consulting on educational, community and democratic computing. Some of Doug Schuler's publications include: *New Community Networks: Wired for Change* (Addison-Wesley, 1996), *Participatory Design: Principles and Practices* (co-edited with Aki Namioka, Lawrence Erlbaum and Associates, 1993), *Reinventing Technology, Rediscovering Community: Critical Studies* *in Computing as a Social Practice* (co-edited with Philip Agre, Ablex Publishing Co., 1997).

Anne Scott is a lecturer in Sociology at the University of Canterbury, New Zealand. She is currently writing an introductory book on feminist debates relating to science and technology, and is researching process issues in women's uses of the information and communication technologies.

Tamara Seabrook is a research assistant in CSPR and a part-time lecturer at the University of Teesside. She is currently working on a Single-Regeneration-funded project on Empowering Young Parents, and an action research project involving young people on Teesside in the design of a virtual reality model of their local youth centre.

Sergei Stafeev is a director of a Russian NGO 'Gardarika' based in St Petersburg. 'Gardarika' is a computer-design studio pioneering the use of Internet resources for Russian 'third'-sector development. He is also one of the founders of the Institute of Research on Problems of Non-Profits in Newly Independent States (IRPN). Stafeev's research interests are focused on using ICTs for NGOs and community development and community informatics. Sergei is currently engaged (as chief of the Russian team) in a joint British–Russian long-time research project involved in creating an experimental model of NGO's information network in north-west Russia.

Fred Steward is Reader in Innovation and Director of the Innovation Research Centre at Aston Business School, Birmingham, UK. He has conducted a variety of research projects on the management of techno-logical innovation and associated social changes. He recently completed a study in the UK Economic and Social Research Council 'Virtual Society' programme on Innovation for Social Inclusion which investigated the role of new e-gateways in challenging the digital divide. This project was in collaboration with Dr Sonia Liff at Warwick Business School and involved fieldwork in Finland and California as well as the UK. He is a member of the editorial board of the *International Journal of Innovation Management* and of the journal *Technology Analysis and Strategic Management* and has been chair of the ESRC postgraduate subject area panel on science, technology and innovation studies. He has contributed to a range of academic journals including *Organization, Nature, International Journal of Innovation Management, Journal of Applied Management Studies* and *International Journal of Technology Management.* He teaches courses on innovation and entrepreneurship.

Erik Stolterman is an Associate Professor at the Department of Informatics, Umeå University, Sweden. Stolterman's research interest is focused on the philosophy of design and design theory, especially in relation to the practice of design, design skill and design ability. The result of this work together with Dr Harold Nelson will be published in a forthcoming book, *Creating a Design Culture*. Stolterman also works with issues related to information technology and its influence on the society at large.

Martine van Selm is Associate Professor at the Department of Communication, University of Nijmegen, the Netherlands, and earned her Ph.D. at the Department of Psychogerontology of the same university. She has published on meaninglessness in the second half of life, portrayal of the elderly in the media, elderly readers of women's magazines, online newspapers, and on (older) users of information and communication technologies in organisational and other settings. She is currently writing a textbook about new media research methods with Nicholas Jankowski.

Louise Wattis is a postgraduate student based in the Centre for Social and Policy Research at the University of Teesside working on a funded research project 'Campus Safety Matters', which is concerned with investigating staff and students' attitudes towards safety and experiences of victimisation at the University of Teesside. In addition to this project she is also undertaking her own doctoral research relating to the gendered fear of public space and leisure.

C. William R. Webster is a lecturer in Public Management at the University of Stirling. He has been researching the policy processes surrounding the uptake of closed-circuit television (CCTV) surveillance systems since 1995 and has presented and published a number of times in this area. William is a nominated UK representative in the 'Government and Democracy in the Information Age' (GaDIA) Research Action (No. 14) of the European Union Co-operation in the Field of Science and Technological (COST) research programme and a member of the European Group of Public Administration (EGPA) Permanent Study Group on 'Informatization in Public Administration'.

Barry Wellman learned to keypunch in 1965 when he was a Harvard graduate student. He joined his first computer network in 1976 and has been connected ever since. Professor Wellman is a sociologist at the University of Toronto. He founded the International Network for Social Network Analysis in 1976. He is currently chair-emeritus of the Community and Urban Sociology section of the American Sociological Association, and Virtual Community adviser for the Association for Computing Machinery's Special Interest Group on Group Processes. Wellman recently published the updated edition of *Social Structures: A Network Approach* (JAI Press, 1997) and *Networks in the Global Village* (Westview, 1999), and has just co-edited *The Internet in Everyday Life* (*American Behavioral Scientist*, 2001 with an expanded book being published by Blackwells, 2002).

Kate Williams is a doctoral student at the University of Michigan School of Information and research assistant with the Alliance for Community Technology, a partnership launched by the University of Michigan with the W. K. Kellogg Foundation. Her research focuses on the public sphere in cyberspace and the adoption and use of technology by low-income communities. She has published a survey of Ohio libraries providing dial-up Internet service, 'Libraries as ISPs', in *Ohio Libraries* (spring/summer 2000) as well as an online report 'Literacy and computer literacy: the Cuban experience'. She also has academic degrees from MIT and the University of Chicago.

Foreword

Communities and communication technologies have shaped each other for millennia, but people have only recently begun to understand how that co-evolutionary process works. We might now have an opportunity to take more conscious control over something that has repeatedly, radically transformed the way people live for the past ten thousand years. This recent glimmering of understanding of the social consequences of communication media provokes a moral question. If our uses of alphabets, printing presses or Internets shape the way we live, what can we do about that shaping?

Before we can act, we must know. In what ways must the effects of the Internet be studied as social phenomena? What can we learn about the ways communities are changed by the way we use the Net?

Decades ago, at the beginning of the creation of the ARPAnet, the US Defense Department sponsored project that grew into the Internet, the project's first directors foresaw the emergence of online communities and forecast some of the social questions these phenomena would raise, including the 'digital divide'.

> For society, the impact will be good or bad, depending mainly on one question: Will 'to be on-line' be a privilege or a right? If only a favored segment of the population gets a chance to enjoy the advantage of 'intelligence amplification', the network may exaggerate the discontinuity in the spectrum of intellectual opportunity.
>
> On the other hand, if the network idea should prove to do for education what a few have envisioned in hope, if not in concrete detailed plan, and if all minds should prove to be responsive, surely the boon to humankind would be beyond measure.
>
> J. C. R. Licklider, Robert Taylor and E. Herbert,
> 'The Computer as a Communication Device',
> *International Science and Technology*, April 1978

Public discussion of the ways Internet-enabled media affect society has gone through a number of stages, from the utopian to the severely critical to an insanely accelerated boom and bust cycle. Mass-media journalism utterly failed in its duty to inform citizens about the meaning of events that affect life and liberty. We've been through ten years and several different flavours of obfuscation.

In the early 1990s, the fervour of the early Internet evangelists, the premature hopes of the first waves of enthusiasts, utopian expectations, and misplaced technological determinism coloured the earliest depictions of the social potential of many-to-many communication. In some cases, I've been personally guilty of abetting overheated rhetoric around the subject of 'electronic democracy'. Criticism and experience led me and others to change our minds about the likelihood that the new technologies' humanistic potentials would be realised. As we who observed social cyberspaces gained more years of experience, we came to understand more about the relationship between technological potential and human foibles. In the mid 1990s, Internet use grew explosively among the mainstream population, with the emergence of the Web. Then in the late 1990s, an enormous tidal wave of dotcom cash washed ashore, and just as quickly washed out again. First the Net was something highly technical, for nerds only. Then it was utopia. Then it was a gold mine. Then a failed business model.

At the same time that the more spectacular events reported in the media were occurring, less publicised but perhaps more significant experiments were under way. For close to a decade, people such as those represented in this volume have been acting online and in their geographic communities to adopt technology to their own purposes. Authors such as those contributing to this volume have observed what people have done and tried to do. I would like to think that *Community Informatics* marks the beginning of a new era, neither naively utopian nor paralytically critical, based on actual findings by people who have tried to use online media in service of community, then reported on their results. In the absence of such systematic observation and reporting by serious practitioners, public discussion will continue to oscillate between ideological extremes, in a never-ending battle of anecdotal evidence and theoretical rhetoric.

Although the mass media never seem to deviate from the most sensational stories about cyberporn and dotcom zillionaires, a few books have established the foundation of a necessarily cross-disciplinary field of social cyberspace studies, for example Smith and Kollock, *Communities in Cyberspace*, Routledge, 1999; Steven G. Jones, *Virtual Culture*, SAGE, 1997; Mowbray and Werry, *Online Communities*, Prentice Hall, 2001). Doug Schuler's *New Community Networks* (Addison Wesley, 1996) brought community networking to public attention. And *Community Informatics* reports internationally, across a range of social issues, on how successful – or not – people have been in creating community networks.

Among the most important points made in this book are:

- Citizens can use technologies in ways that can help increase social capital, but this result won't happen automatically. It is a function of human action, not of the technology. Know-how, planning, support, and above all, cooperation are required.
- The Net empowers citizens and it also empowers those who would control and influence citizens. The Net is also a trap. Surveillance and mind-control are the shadows of many-to-many publishing and access to knowledge.
- The market is powerful, but not all-powerful. It is only one manifestation of human cooperation, and cannot produce all the public goods necessary for sustainable and democratic societies.
- 'Civic intelligence' and 'citizen technology', two terms emphasised in *Community Informatics*, are not necessarily going to govern the majority decision-making – unless a large number of people put the words into action. Therefore, it is worth trying.

In 1985, when I created the Mind conference on the Well, I chose as the logout message 'What it is → is → up to us'. I've used the phrase as an email signature for a decade. Although I've learned to look a great deal more critically at the odds against democratic outcomes in a market-dominated milieu, I still believe the future can be influenced by informed populations. If that wasn't true, we wouldn't have the degree of democracy we have. If a sufficient people know enough about what to do – by reading books like *Community Informatics* – unlikely outcomes become possible.

Howard Rheingold
Mill Valley, California, 2001

Preface

This book is the outcome of an international conference which was organised by the Community Informatics Research and Applications Unit (CIRA) based at the University of Teesside, UK, in April 2000.

It was an event which brought together a number of leading practitioners, academics and community activists who share a common desire to understand and use the potentially transforming qualities of information and communications technologies (ICTs) for developing stronger community relationships.

The vision and energy of community informatics practitioners is now beginning to provide us with some exciting examples of innovative applications and a growing source of lay experience and academic research outputs upon which to gain a clearer understanding of these developments and their potential consequences for community relations. The chapters in this book provide a wide coverage of the lessons which are beginning to be learnt from many of these social experiments. They sometimes identify a significant divergence between the rhetoric of enthusiasts and the actual experience on the ground. Moreover, we cannot even be sure that they do not represent a transitory set of well-intentioned projects and that the torches of the early community-network pioneers will not be extinguished by greater social and economic forces. Yet they may also give us an insight into the potential of people to shape the new media in ways which are emancipatory, creative, educational and socially supportive. As such they could provide some valuable early lessons to inform future policy choices.

We hope that some sense of the generosity and desire to share and help others, which was such a prominent aspect of the conference, is conveyed within the pages of this book. We would like to thank all the authors and participants for their encouraging and stimulating contributions. For the supportive environment and efficient organisation which enabled us to enjoy the experience we are grateful to June Ions, Irene Versluijs, Mathilde Gorte, Heike Van Steensel and Vicky Rushin. For the digital arts section of the conference, we would like to thank Perry Bard, Jen Southern from IDEA, Rupert Francis, Ling Wong, the young people from the *M@RC* project and the young people from Macmillan College, Middlesbrough, who all gave their time freely to make this such a success. Lastly, we would like to thank all of our colleagues at CIRA for their perpetual inspiration and for their support during the conference, and Claire Taylor whose responsibility it has been to pull this collection together.

Finally, we would like to thank John Keeble and Kim Loader for their forbearance and for the usual unsolicited help from William and Christopher Loader.

Leigh Keeble   Brian D. Loader
Darlington 2001   Swainby 2001

Chapter 1

Community informatics
Themes and issues

Leigh Keeble and Brian D. Loader

A human being has roots by virtue of his [*sic*] real, active and natural participation in the life of a community which preserves in living shape certain particular treasures of the past and certain particular expectations for the future.

(Weil 1952: 41)

Introduction

Throughout the world in recent years there has been a dramatic surge of activity by hundreds of community groups, social support networks, voluntary agencies and government organisations dedicated to exploring the transforming qualities of the new information and communications technologies (ICTs) such as the Internet for the development, economic regeneration and democratic stimulation of communities. A rich variety of social experiments in what we term *community informatics* (CI) are giving community activists, policy-makers and citizens a new set of possibilities for fostering social cohesion, strengthening neighbourhood ties, overcoming cultural isolation and combating social exclusion and deprivation. For some commentators the new media offer us the prospect of resuscitating community life from its torpid condition in the modern world (Rheingold 1994, Schuler 1996). Computer-mediated social relations are depicted as the conduit through which new forms of community structures and culture can evolve through spontaneous electronic interaction.

The rapid convergence of new media such as the Internet, digital television, cell phones and other ICTs is providing a powerful set of tools with which to challenge many aspects of our social and economic behaviour. In the home, at work and in our public spaces these technologies are beginning to facilitate new patterns of social interaction and exchange. By enabling communication between people to be conducted across the world at any time they begin to challenge traditional distinctions of time and place. News of human rights violations, environmental catastrophes or military aggression can no longer be easily suppressed by nation states (Hick *et al.* 2000). Medical advice and social support can be shared across national boundaries (Burrows *et al.* 2000). Remote locations can offer the ideal prospect of employment opportunities for tele-working and local economic sustainability. In addition, e-commerce provides the potential for producers to access wider markets to sell their goods and services and also for greater price responsiveness to customer demands.

For many commentators the transforming capabilities of the new digital media are providing the conditions for an economic and social revolution leading to the collapse of the industrial society and its replacement by the Information Age (Castells 1996). At the heart of this transition is the creation of a 'global knowledge economy' where the communication of information, knowledge and other symbolic goods rather than material goods becomes the primary motor for economic development. As a consequence governments and policy-makers around the world are urgently extolling the need to put their populations *online* by sponsoring awareness-raising programmes and computer-literacy courses, and by connecting schools, libraries and other public amenities to the Internet (Cabinet Office 2000, HM Treasury 2000, NTIA 2000). To be without access to the *Web* in the Information Age, it seems, is to run the risk of losing competitive advantage in the race for economic prosperity.

Yet information, knowledge and its communication are not simply economic variables, they are also cultural assets. They enable us to create our identities, develop a shared sense of community and gain an understanding of communities which are different from ourselves. The transforming force of the information revolution is not therefore primarily technical but rather social and cultural in nature (Loader *et al.* 2002). New forms of computer-mediated communication (CMC) are challenging our self-perceptions and the communities within which we interact. But they are also in turn being shaped by social and cultural forces. The technologies are not inert. They are not independent of the social and cultural conditions from which they have emerged. Rather they are the product of imaginations which are themselves formed within complex and dynamic cultural, economic and political relations. The social crucible of technological development is therefore both a highly contested space as well as a creative one. Competing desires and unequal access to human resources ensure that the factors shaping the development and diffusion of community informatics are highly unpredictable and not easily determined by those who deign to prophesy them.

Few can now doubt the enormous potential of new information and communications technologies such as the Internet for facilitating social and economic change. But are the impressive transforming capabilities of this new media likely to regenerate community social relations during this century or are they the harbinger of the breakdown of locally based social interaction? Can the Internet, for example, strengthen bonds between neighbours, provide job opportunities, improve local access to public and commercial services, stimulate cultural activities and facilitate the creation and communication of information between local residents? Or conversely, does online connectivity lead to the replacement of face-to-face interaction by an incorporeal communication network? (Kraut *et al.* 1998). Does remote computer-mediated communication lead to remoteness between individuals who share the same geographical community space? (Haywood 1998).

These questions are the primary focus of this book. Whilst somewhat exaggerated in their starkness, they represent significant concerns which human societies are currently grappling with as a consequence of an uneasy alliance with the new ICTs. This ambivalence is played out through a number of dichotomies which arise from the catalytic qualities of the new technologies. For example, its capacity to facilitate the development of a 'global informational economy' (Castells 1996) provides great opportunities for opening up worldwide economic markets but also for placing many regions into economic insecurity as a result of global competition. A global network facilitating contact between millions of people across many nations may stimulate not only greater co-operation and understanding but also a weakening of national and local cultural differences as we witness an increasing cultural homogenisation. The development of online public information services may provide the prospect of improved democratic accountability between local citizens and their elected representatives but it could also provide the tools for more sophisticated management of the population. Surveillance technologies such as CCTV may enable community members to feel safer in their streets and homes but the information such technologies procure may also threaten people's privacy and freedom from commercial or state abuse. Such competing scenarios are woven throughout the chapters contained in this book.

What is community informatics?

Community informatics is a multidisciplinary field for the investigation and development of the social and cultural factors shaping the development and diffusion of new ICTs and its effects upon community development, regeneration and sustainability. It thereby combines an interest in the potentially transforming qualities of the new media with an analysis of the importance of community social relations for human interaction. Community informatics is therefore concerned to foreground through its analyses the complex dynamic relationship between technological innovation and changing social relationships. It pursues this objective by bringing together and drawing upon the work of community activists, webmasters and Internet enthusiasts, policy-makers, digital artists, science-fiction writers, media commentators and a wide variety of academics including sociologists, computer scientists, communications theorists, information systems analysts, political scientists, psychologists and many more.

Community informatics is also a broad approach which offers, on the one hand, the opportunity to investigate the rich diversity of virtual communities which are forming between normally disparate individuals as a consequence of CMC (Smith and Kollock 1999). Typically these are communities of shared interest rather than spatially or geographically constructed. Through a variety of Internet and Web-based technologies millions of people are able to interact socially, economically and politically around the world in what is popularly known as *cyberspace*. On the other hand, community informatics, as we have noted elsewhere, also enables us

> to connect cyber-*space* to community-*place*: to investigate how ICTs can be geographically embedded and developed by community groups to support networks of people who already know and care about each other. It thereby recognises both the transforming qualities of ICTs as well as the continuing importance of community as an intermediate level of social life between the personal (individual/family) and the impersonal (institutional/global). The numerous community enthusiasts . . . who are building interactive Web sites, virtual chat rooms and electronic-lists as tools to support local communication between their members, are a striking testament to the value of a CI perspective.
>
> (Loader *et al.* 2000: 81)

Such initiatives, however, are not uniform in their spread across the globe or indeed throughout national populations (Holderness 1998, Loader 1998). At a time when the value of being 'connected to the Net' for individual life opportunities is being recognised, there is also a growing concern among policy-makers that many countries are witnessing a 'digital divide' between those members of society who have access to networked computers and the skills to use them and a large section of citizens who are excluded from such advantages. Given the perceived increasing importance of communications and information exchange for job opportunities, educational achievement, access to good-quality public services, improved independent living and economic advantage, these divisions between the information-rich and the information-deprived may become reinforced by the manner in which the new technologies are designed and dispersed. Consequently many community informatics initiatives often arise as a means to raise awareness of the importance of computer literacy to people living in deprived areas as well as providing them with communal access and training opportunities.

Yet to be effective in bridging the digital divide CI perspectives need to avoid approaches which assume that communities are 'densely-knit and tightly bound' (Wellman *et al.* 1999a). The reality for many individuals is that their 'personal communities' are 'sparsely knit and loosely bound' (*ibid.*). Within these fluid community networks the new media provides the opportunities of enabling people to span across geographical, social and cultural boundaries and constraints. The new media thus offer the potential of being used as a liberating and empowering tool by many people and, particularly more relevant here, for the disadvantaged and excluded, to 'challenge entrenched positions and structures' (Loader *et al.* 2000: 87). The Internet and World Wide Web allow individuals access to global information and potentially provides a space for participation without preconceived socially constructed identities based on gender, age, sexuality, ethnicity, disability and the like constraining meaningful interaction. Many of the community informatics initatives mentioned in this book demonstrate the potential of ICTs to support, strengthen and extend individuals 'personal communities'.

Structure of the book

The first contribution in the book is from Perry Bard, a video artist based in New York. A key component of the conference which we held in April 2000 was digital arts. We ran two different digital-arts projects over the duration of the conference. First, Perry worked with a group of young people aged 16 to 25 from a local young people's project, *M@RC*. The young people and Perry spent a couple of days with a mini-disc recorder and a digital camera. They then cut together a PowerPoint presentation with words, sounds and images which presented the issues which faced young people in Middlesbrough. The piece was presented to the conference participants on the final day of the conference.

The second digital arts project was an artslab in which young people aged 11 to 13 worked with Jen Southern and other artists from the IDEA (Innovation in Digital and Electronic Art) project based in Manchester, UK. Jen worked with the young people teaching them HTML and scanning in parts of their body and working with the digital camera. Each of the young people participating in the project produced their own web page and learnt to use photo-editing software, the scanner and the digital camera.

Our motive for including the digital arts work in the conference was our recognition that arts are potentially a powerful way of engaging people with the new technologies. In particular, we are keen to explore how young people might make use of different software and how they might use it to give themselves a voice. Our colleague Rupert Francis was fundamental in the organising and running of the digital-arts section of the conference.

The benefits of working creatively with technology are many. Over the course of our work on various projects, our colleagues have demonstrated how this work has the potential to boost confidence, expand social skills and enhance literacy and numeracy. Rupert Francis and Steve Thompson of CIRA work to promote the idea that there is a sense of empowerment in creation, in creating and in being creative. Effective examples of such work can be seen on the Tees Valley Communities Online website at www.tvco.org.uk.

The chapter by Perry Bard describes a project in which she worked with a small community to install a piece of video art into the Staten Island Ferry Terminal building. Perry describes the processes involved in realising the project and some of the problems encountered. However, despite the difficulties, the end result is a piece of work which has given the individuals involved a great deal of pleasure and which has undoubtedly taught them some new skills.

The remainder of the collection has been divided into four parts. The first part we have called 'Community Informatics as Place and Space' as the chapters which form this part explore the relationship of physical place to the engagement of individuals within cyberspace. In the first chapter in this part (Chapter 3), Barry Wellman explores how networks of community exist in physical places and how they might be moving to exist in cyberspace. The relationship of cyber-space to cyber-place is important to Wellman. He argues that online relationships and online communities have developed their own strength and dynamics. Wellman identifies that participants in online groups have strong interpersonal feelings of belonging, being wanted, obtaining important resources and having a shared identity. For Wellman, these communities are truly in cyber-place, and not just cyber-spaces. Wellman also examines the development of computer-supported community networks and how this affects access to resources. Wellman focuses on the opportunities and transformations for communities afforded by computerised communication networks.

Chapter 4 is about the design of the technology by the public. Erik Stolterman argues that, in a democratic society, a public sphere in cyberspace must be defined and designed by the people using that sphere. Stolterman suggests that technology can be deliberately and consciously designed by community groups, and in fact this happens every day. The overall message of this chapter is that technology cannot be regarded as a ready-made tool that can be used to create community.

The issue of the design of technology is picked up in Chapter 5. Eileen Green and Leigh Keeble use case studies of two women's centres from the north-east of England and describe how the women themselves are taking the new technologies and integrating them into their 'everyday' experience. The chapter addresses the issue of the everyday design of technological systems and asks questions about the potential of the women in the community groups to become involved in a user-centred process of community-based design.

Chapter 6 looks at the impact of computer-mediated social support (CMSS). Nicholas Pleace, Roger Burrows, Brian D. Loader, Sarah Nettleton and Steve Muncer examine the benefits of CMSS and acknowledge its potential to enhance the lives of some individuals by offering access to communities of interest. Such communities are potentially of particular benefit to individuals who are housebound. However, the authors do express some words of caution and remain critical of the ability of CMSS to replace 'real-life' social networks or to be the only source of information.

Part II of the collection moves on to explore some real experiences of community informatics. The first chapter by G. Casapulla, Fiorella de Cindio and L. Ripamonti (Chapter 7) begins by discussing access to the new technologies and the impact of such access on the Milan community network. The chapter then explores how access has been facilitated and extended through the design and implementation of a game, 'Cyberhunts'. The chapter describes how 'Cyberhunts' began by engaging schools but then moved on to involve other members of the wider community as word of its success spread. The game and process described by de Cindio *et al.* demonstrate how innovative software can be used in an effective way to teach people how to use the Internet in an informal and fun way.

Chapter 8 by Nicholas W. Jankowski, Martine van Selm and Ed Hollander discusses the development of a research project around two digital community networks in The Netherlands. Jankowski *et al.* do present some findings of a preliminary study conducted on one of the community networks, but the focus of this chapter is on considering theoretical perspectives and methodological issues in relation to researching community informatics projects.

The next chapter in Part II is a contribution by Sergei Stafeev. Stafeev explores the issues around developing a research programme which would support the funding of Internet connections for non-governmental organisations (NGOs) in Russia. Stafeev's main theme is that the Internet potentially offers NGOs in Russia not just access to a wide range of information but, more importantly, a networking tool which could support Russian NGOs in their work.

Birgit Jæger explores in Chapter 10 the impact of ICT projects in Europe and, more specifically, Denmark. Jæger describes the development of 'social experiments' in Denmark and discusses how such projects have been evaluated, what lessons have been learned and how these lessons have been disseminated to other projects.

The final chapter in Part II examines how to sustain community informatics projects in women's centres. Anne Scott and Margaret Page focus on the experience of the 'Women Connect' project and argue that online communities need to be built in such a way as to utilise face-to-face interaction and political will.

Part III of the collection brings together chapters which tackle the issues of empowerment and surveillance. Whilst some of the chapters in this section do present case study material, their main focus is on how technologies can be used to empower individuals or communities or how the introduction of CCTV has impacted on a local community.

The first chapter in Part III, Chapter 12, is by Abdul Alkalimat and Kate Williams, focusing on the experiences of a community technology centre based in Toledo, Ohio. The main objective of the chapter is to establish how public computer centres can play a role in sustaining the African-American freedom struggle. The chapter concludes by drawing out the implications of this research as guidelines for future research but also for the public sphere. Alkalimat and Williams argue that building a sustainable democratic equality in the Information Age means working and supporting people with information technology in those organisations which are already active.

Agneta Ranerup continues with the theme of democracy in Chapter 13. Ranerup focuses on whether local government initiatives in Sweden established to provide a virtual public space have functioned as a tool for people-centred governance. From her survey of local-government provision in Sweden, Ranerup found that simply establishing a space on a local-government website will not suddenly result in citizens starting to debate. Ranerup concludes, like Alkalimat and Williams, that without support these spaces are not sustainable.

The next two chapters in Part III examine the impact of closed-circuit television (CCTV) in different local communities. C. William, R. Webster and John Hood argue (Chapter 14) that the introduction of CCTV into an area is a community informatics initiative as it represents the provision of an electronic service to meet local demand. Drawing on evidence from a case study based on the Greater Easterhouse CCTV system, Webster and Hood suggest that whilst CCTV can be in the community, for the community and demanded by the community, it inevitably leads to increased surveillance of communities which has significant ramifications for democracy and individual privacy.

The issue of surveillance is further explored by Tamara Seabrook and Louise Wattis in Chapter 15. Seabrook and Wattis focus on the perceptions of young women to the introduction of CCTV in their local community. They argue that, although the young women in their sample viewed the cameras as providing them with greater interpersonal safety, the reality is that, when the nature of public crime is deconstructed in relation to gender, this sense of protection that CCTV offers is unfounded. Accordingly, Seabrook and Wattis suggest that CCTV represents a 'heightened manifestation of the male gaze' which legitimises men watching women.

Part IV examines the potential research and policy agenda of community informatics in both Europe and North America. Michael Gurstein opens this section (Chapter 16) by exploring the history of 'citizen technology' and discussing strategies for local development by using the new technologies. Gurstein addresses some of the outstanding research issues identified through his work and concludes by examining some of the future implications for research and sustaining community informatics projects.

Doug Schuler's chapter (Chapter 17) is designed to challenge the pessimistic and defeatist views of our capabilities to confront and overcome many of the social and environmental problems facing us. Through an evocation of earlier utopian visions of human society using scientific knowledge and technologies as a means of amelioration, Schuler presents us with a new formulation which he describes as a 'world brain'. Whilst such futuristic theorising is highly unfashionable, the author attempts to ground his idea in the work and practices of the social network movement. In particular, Schuler suggests that many of the problems confronting society can be understood and challenged by mobilising what he calls 'civic intelligence': that is, collective knowledge and its communication used as a means for collective problem-solving. Such an approach is clearly ambitious and Schuler makes no claims for it being a panacea for all our ills, but for the author it does represent a positive, evidence-based proposal for civic engagement.

The contribution by Peter Day (Chapter 18) draws on a longitudinal study of Scandinavian and UK community ICT initiatives to examine tensions between policy and some of the attempts to address social exclusion through ICT initiatives. Day describes the UK policy environment in relation to ICTs and reflects on these policies. Day concludes that despite the rhetoric of UK government policy in relation to access and involving citizens in the decision-making process, policies remain fundamentally techno-economic, that is policy-makers regard people in terms of their market potential rather than as citizens. Whilst such an approach is identifiable in government policies, Day argues that community efforts to shape information-society policy will be limited. He concludes that we must establish a framework of methodological tools that informs policy.

The closing chapter by Sonia Liff and Fred Steward (Chapter 19) stresses the importance of social networks to the successful operation of what they call 'e-gateways'. By discussing the practitioner literature on community e-gateways and studies of actual practice, the authors argue that, whilst the importance of networking is implicit in much policy advice, its full implications are not always drawn out and are actually contradicted by some funding regimes. The adoption of a network-mapping approach provides a visual representation of internal and external relationships of an organisation. The mapping is done in a way that is informed by the social scientific understanding of different types of networks and forms of learning. Liff and Steward argue that such analysis might prove useful to centres themselves in identifying areas for future development.

Conclusion

It is hoped that the contributions to this book go some way towards demonstrating the rich range of community informatics projects which are happening around the world. We also hope that, as the implications of living in a global information age become more apparent, the research which informs these contributions may help the future development and sustainability of community informatics projects.

Chapter 2

Staten Island stories – handing over the tools of video communi-creation

Perry Bard

My recent art project *The Terminal Salon* is a large-scale video projection presented in the waiting room of the Staten Island Ferry Terminal building in New York. I collaborated with local residents who did most of the video-taping and are also the subject of the work. They talk about issues that are their own and at the same time are relevant to society at large.

Staten Island is ethnically and economically diverse: the Ferry Terminal Building is a space where that diversity converges. Sixty thousand people a day pass through it commuting to and from Manhattan. By centring a project at this location I wanted to create a site for conversation, one in which fixed ideas might shift, where new social relationships might emerge. It was inspired by the idea of the town square, in less complicated times a place where people congregated to talk and get the latest news.

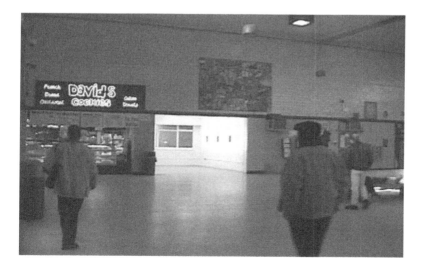

Figure 2.1 Staten Island Ferry Terminal building

Genesis of the project

I was invited by Olivia Georgia, director of the Newhouse Center for Contemporary Art on Staten Island, to collaborate with residents of Richmond Terrace Houses. The two sites are less than a mile away from each other and the relationship is one that both organisations want to develop. The art centre is part of a larger cultural institution (Snug Harbor Cultural Center) on the island. Richmond Terrace Houses has a community centre with programmes for all age groups.

I knew there was video equipment at the centre that wasn't being used and I wanted to place a video in the ferry building that involved local people. I was convinced this would happen only if members of the community did the taping and editing. Finding committed participants was difficult, but after a month of hanging out I met Joan Henry, a resident who wanted to learn about video. Joan had lived in the building for eight years. She had already raised five children and was now bringing up her granddaughter. She knew everyone in the vicinity by name – in short, she was the unofficial mayor. I taught her to use the equipment and in June we began showing young teens (age 10 to 12) how to videotape each other. They were thrilled to see themselves on camera and the activity was attracting a lot of attention.

There were complications. The director of the centre had changed and our plans were delayed three weeks. The change of personnel meant that equipment had to be inventoried before we could continue. Eric Baez, the youth programme co-ordinator, was interested in the video project and had

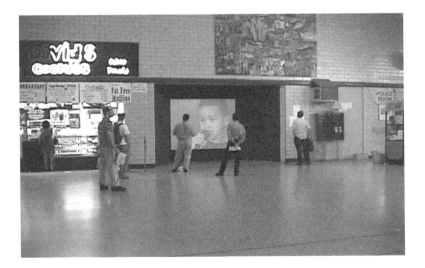

Figure 2.2 The Terminal Salon video project (i)

used the equipment to record events for the centre. During the first week in July at the height of our effort to shoot footage, Eric was transferred to another site for the duration of the summer. This was tragic; he had a close relationship with most of the young people who use the centre. The older teens stopped showing up and the younger ones were basically too young to take on the project.

We met snags at every turn. Internal politics at the community centre made it difficult to proceed: there were additional personnel changes, scheduling errors, equipment problems, access problems. Anything that could go wrong did, and always at the zero hour. Fewer than half of the events we planned occurred as scheduled. The greatest snag was with the camera. For some reason the community centre had bought professional video equipment. It was heavy, intimidating and complicated to use, and the few people allowed to touch it hadn't figured out many of its functions. It was deemed so valuable it was kept under lock and key and getting access to it was a full-time job. We tried to get the institutions involved to buy us a camcorder. It was promised but it never materialised and I got into the habit of carrying my own camera just in case. We ended up using it most of the time.

The area did have considerable problems relating to drugs and violence, as a result of which many people refused to appear on screen. Thus in retrospect, video was probably the most difficult medium I could have chosen. The only people willing to be on camera were under 6 or over 65. We were popular with the after-school programme for youth under 12 (most of whom were too small to carry the centre's camera) and with the senior citizen programme in the

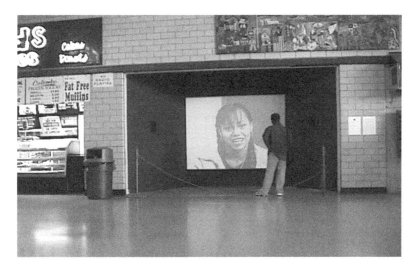

Figure 2.2 The Terminal Salon video project (ii)

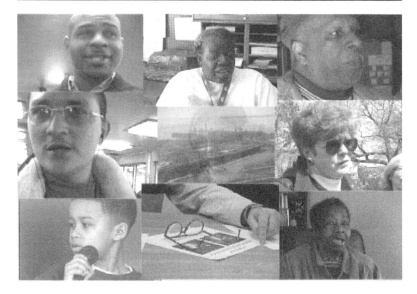

Figure 2.2 The Terminal Salon video project (iii)

morning (most of whom complained about drugs and violence but didn't want that part to be on the video).

Our goal was to videotape a cross-section of that community and then spread into adjacent neighbourhoods involving more people as we went. In February we realised that there wasn't a single teen on tape. We went to a local high school and asked Jo Scro, an English teacher who was running an after-school video club, to get his students involved. They brought new energy to the project. Taping was done at other community centres, on the street, at bars, on the ferry and in the ferry building. Because many people we talked to compared the present with the past we also collected images from the Historical Society. The resulting video is a database of faces, memories, diverse voices, diverse and shared experiences.

We installed the piece in the Ferry Terminal in June 2000. Passers-by immediately became engaged. They saw themselves, their friends and waited through an additional nine-minute cycle to see themselves again. They brought their friends. People wanted to know what they had to do to be on the video. It was never vandalised even though there was twenty-four-hour access to it.

We live in a mediated environment but we have no control over who the media represents, nor how those who are, are represented. The appeal of using digital media in the public realm is that it can address a gap in representation that mainstream media creates.

Part I

Community informatics as place and space

Chapter 3

Physical place and cyberplace
The rise of networked individualism

Barry Wellman

Introduction: a computer network is a social network – the network revolution

We find community in networks, not groups. Although people often view the world in terms of groups (Freeman 1992), they function in networks. In networked societies: boundaries are permeable, interactions are with diverse others, connections switch between multiple networks, and hierarchies can be flatter and recursive. The change from groups to networks can be seen at many levels. Trading and political blocs have lost their monolithic character in the world system. Organisations form complex networks of alliance and exchange rather than cartels, and workers report to multiple peers and superiors. Management by multiple connected network is replacing management by hierarchical tree and management by matrix (Berkowitz 1982, Wellman 1988, Castells 1996). Communities are far-flung, loosely bounded, sparsely knit, and fragmentary. Most people operate in multiple, thinly connected, partial communities as they deal with networks of kin, neighbours, friends, work-mates and organisational ties. Rather than fitting into the same group as those around them, each person has his or her own 'personal community' (Wellman and Leighton 1979, Wellman 1999a).

Eric Wright (1979) has taught us that social class is a relational phenom-enon: control over one's own labour power and that of others. Manuel Castells (1972) has taught us that class pertains to relations of production and reproduction – including communities. Hence the structure and composition of community networks affect people's control over their lives, and people's structural positions in community networks affect the kinds of resources to which they have access. In these ways, relations in cyberplaces join with relations on the ground.

Complex social networks have always existed, but recent technological developments in communication have afforded their emergence as a dominant form of social organisation. When computer-mediated communication networks link people, institutions and knowledge, they are computer-supported social networks. The technological development of computer networks and the societal transformation into social networks are now in a positive feedback loop. Just as the flexibility of less-bounded, spatially dispersed social networks creates demand for the World Wide Web and collaborative communication, the breathless development of computer networks nourishes societal transitions from little boxes to social networks.

My principal concerns in this chapter are: how networks of community exist in physical places – such as neighbourhoods and cyberplaces – such as the Internet; and how the development of computer-supported community networks affects access to resources. I define 'community' as networks of interpersonal ties that provide sociability, support, information, a sense of belonging and social identity. I do not limit my thinking about community to neighbourhoods and villages.[1] This is good advice for any epoch and especially pertinent for the twenty-first century.

The technological developments I shall describe are currently exciting the public, scholars, financiers, the media and politicians. Yet it is when technological changes become pervasive, familiar and boring that they affect societies the most. This is an old story. For example, few scholars think about the telephone now (but see Fischer 1992), yet it has thoroughly affected the spatial and social structure of communities. I do not argue technological determinism (e.g., Ogburn 1950): people and institutions often take over and reorient technological developments. Rather, I examine the 'social affordances' of technology: the possibilities that technological changes afford for social relations and social structure.[2]

I am especially interested in how affordances in computer-supported interpersonal communication affect the ways in which people connect with each other: hugely greater bandwidth for non-face-to-face communication, wireless portability of computerised communication devices, globalised ease of connecting with others and accessing information, and the personalisation of technology and knowledge-management (discussed in more detail in the companion paper to this, Wellman 2000a). The human use of these technologies is creating and sustaining community ties. Although these ties exist in cyber*space*, they have become cyber*places*, as people connect with others having shared interests, engage in supportive and sociable relationships with them and imbue their activity online with meaning, belonging and identity.

When many sociologists think about the future, they often focus on interpersonal abuses to be redressed and structural wrongs to be righted (see the various utopian statements in Risman, Tomaskovic-Devey and Dimes 2000). By contrast, I focus here on the opportunities and transformations for communities afforded by computerised communication networks. To be sure, these technologies also have negative affordances, such as interpersonal alienation, lessened privacy, increased surveillance, and machine-dependent vulnerability to computerised crime and breakdown (forecast a century ago by E. M. Forster 1909). But to address these issues would take many more pages.

The social affordances of computerised communication networks

Bandwidth

The number of bits that can be pushed through a computer network connection in a given hour has risen from 110 bits per second (bps) in the mid-1970s to routine home speeds ranging from 30,000 bps (with dial-up telephone modems) to 1 million bps (for cable modems and ADSL phone connections). It will soon rise sharply again. High-capacity bandwidth is important for its speed, so that text messages and web pages become readable without distracting delay. It affords 'instant' messaging and feedback. It also affords the exchange of complex communication, so that large documents, drawings etc. can be attached to email messages or read on web pages. Bandwidth allows the transmission of high-quality pictures, fostering 'telepresence' (Buxton 1992). One new application connects a digital picture frame to a website (www.ceiva.com) so that grandparents can see updated pictures of their grandchildren. Another transmits continuous video from a 'fly-on-the-wall' camera for parents to keep a concerned eye on frail elderly grandparents (www.camrades.com).

Although the selling point of currently new 1 million bps connections is their speed/bandwidth, our study of a leading-edge wired suburb (with 16 Mbps connections) is finding that the always-available feature is more valued than sheer speed. As high-speed connections do not block telephone calls from the family phone and do not cost any more for being on '24×7', people get in the habit of sending email or web-surfing whenever the thought strikes them, glancing frequently at the incoming email box or frequently checking to see who is currently available for instant messaging, that is email that happens in real time rather than through one-way sending and receiving. The easily available Internet – no need to boot up or connect – makes the Web a handy place to find quick information and makes email a handy way to share quick thoughts (Hampton and Wellman 2000).

Wireless portability

Although wires still carry the most bandwidth, the proliferation of wireless, mobile cell phones will soon be integrated with the multifunctional capacity of computers. The proliferation of portability will be the embracing and negation of ubiquitous globalisation. Computer-supported communication will be every*where*, but, because it is independent of place, it will be no*where*. The importance of place as a communication site will diminish even more, and the person – not the place, household or workgroup – will become even more of an autonomous communication node.

Globalised connectivity

The world of computerisation has oscillated between centralised control (computer centres) and personal control (standalone computers) (Kling and Iacono 1984). The current situation, 'networked computing', means that information (and control) flow up and down between central servers and somewhat autonomous personal computers. Despite organisational control, most people in organisations use their computers for social, community-maintaining reasons (Haythornthwaite and Wellman 1998). Computer networks are expanding as the World Wide Web is becoming more comprehensive and worthy of its name. Global portability will be afforded by the standardisation of mobile phone specifications, the spread of wireless towers to physically isolated and impoverished 'fourth-world' areas (Castells 1998) and the availability of satellite communication in very remote areas. This will mean the potential availability of 'small-world' interpersonal connectivity with all connected to all, either directly or through short chains of indirect ties.

Personalisation

The Internet has changed the nature of the continuing tension between centralisation and personalisation. The Internet's original key use, email, has been very much of a personal thing, with individuals usually managing their own address books and sending messages one-to-one. By contrast, the web affords both personalisation and centralisation. Although choice of sites viewed is usually a personal decision, the responses of the sites have been standardised at all but the most superficial level. Yet personalisation tools are developing. For example, people should soon be able to tell their communications devices whom they wish to get messages from, about what and when. They should soon be able to provide personalised responses on voicemail and email to specific individuals. Website portals such as www.excite.com are becoming more tailorable to individual preferences so that individualised news compilations are available, at the cost of reducing the populace's common awareness of current events. Personal software agents can scan online newsgroups and chat groups, collecting and organising desired information.

Collaborative filtering is developing, where people contribute to evaluations of books, restaurants (Schiesel 2000), politicians and movies (e.g., www.movielens.umn.edu/). People can use their filters and personal agents to find like-minded others and form communities of shared interest. For example, *Yenta* is an experimental matchmaker system, designed to find people with similar interests and introduce them to each other online (Foner 1997). Will they be physically available for face-to-face interactions? 'If you combine virtual community, collaborative filtering, and web-to-cellphone, you get a scenario in which you always know who in your physical vicinity at the moment shares certain affinities and willingness to be contacted' (Howard Rheingold, personal email, 11 January 2000; see also Rheingold 1993a, 2000).

Communities transcend the group and the locality

The proliferation of computer-supported social networks is fostering changes in the ways that people contact, interact and obtain resources with each other. One transition was the nineteenth/twentieth-century move from door-to-door to place-to-place community relationships. This transition was driven by revolutionary developments in both transportation and communication. It was a move away from a solitary group in a single locale to contact between people in different places and multiple social networks. Households became important centres for networking; neighbourhoods became less important. Another transition has already started. It is the communication-driven shift away from place-based inter-household ties to individualised person-to-person interactions and specialised role-to-role interactions.

Door to door

First, a brief excursion to the past to provide some grounding before travelling back to the future. All urban and community scholars 'know' that since the agricultural revolution, community has traditionally been based in itinerant bands, agrarian villages, trading towns and urban neighbourhoods. In these milieux, people walked to visit each other. The community was spatially compact and densely knit (Thébert 1985, Barthélemy and Contamine 1985, Ward 1999). If most settlements or neighbourhoods were a thousand people or less, then it is a safe guess that everyone knew each other. Even today we carry around with us a mental list of a thousand or so souls whom we know well enough to converse with (Kochen 1989).

Communities were bounded, so that most relationships happened within their gates rather than across them. They were not necessarily immobile, but, even in big cities and trading towns, much intercourse stayed within neighbourhoods. Such communities had door-to-door connectivity. When people went to visit each other, they generally walked. If they were affluent and living in post-bridle/stirrup times, they travelled on horses, in carriages and on boats. Whatever the mode of transportation, only heavily veiled and wilfully myopic elites could avoid being steeped in local context – and, if they were unlucky, avoid stepping in it. Social class was based on control over labour power and resources. It was based on position within the small community and the access to external resources afforded by the few links to outside.

This is a chapter about the future and not the past, so I do not want to belabour the details of pre-industrial connectivity. Moreover, a pastoralist nostalgia for quaint little villages can lead one to overlook the abundant evidence of pre-industrial connectivity over long distances. Hunters, gatherers, soldiers, prostitutes, artisans, pedlars and shepherds travelled between towns, regions and continents. Elite traders, scholars and the idle rich journeyed to market towns, great universities, and resorts. As Charles Tilly has pointed out, it is easy to project the near past on to the distant past and overestimate the prevalence of closed, immobile communities:

> Of the million-odd years human beings have been around, a majority have lived in settled villages for no more than four millennia. Most of the time, humans have been hunters, gatherers, and/or flock-tending nomads. The yurt is a better logo for humanity than the stone cottage. Although culturally homogeneous localities have of course existed, such crucial structures as trade diasporas, religious solidarities, lineages, and mutual aid networks have commonly cut across localities. Because states and holders of capital were pushing in the same direction, the period from 1750 to 1950 was, contrary to myths of mobility, humanity's great time of settling into legally established settled communities. Fixed capital and circumscribing states promoted immobile labour forces.
>
> (personal email, 11 February 2000)

Whether travelling with yurts or huddling in stone cottages, the important point is that people went through villages and neighbourhoods to communicate. Most people in a settlement knew each other, were limited by their feet-power in whom they could contact, and, when they visited someone, most neighbours knew who was going to see whom and what their interaction was about. The contact was essentially between households, with the sanction – or at least the awareness – of the settlement.

Such door-to-door communities contained triple inequalities. Not only did a community's inhabitants vary in the amounts of resources to which they had access; their communities and societies varied as well. The densely knit interconnectivity of such communities made it easy to control material goods and behaviour. The tight boundaries that contained interactions ensured that few resources – including knowledge – would be imported or exported. The broadly based ties of community members ensured that much feasible support could be provided, but only when the community wanted to provide it. As there was only one network, the only alternative was running away – to the military, the church or the merchant traders (Davis 1983, Wolf 1966, Wellman and Leighton 1979, Bodemann 1988).

To be sure, place-independent communities have always existed, especially among the leisure class, professional travellers and hoboes. Witness the galloping or carriaging to-and-fro of home-visiting elites in Jane Austen's novels. Yet place-independent communities needed technological help to become generally widespread. Until the nearly simultaneous proliferation of railways and telegraphs in the mid nineteenth century, communication speeds were about the same as door-to-door transportation speeds. The telegraph greatly increased the speed of communication.[3] Since then, the effective speed of transportation has increased twice from the 30 mph of early railway speed to 60 mph for automobiles, five times to 150 mph for high-speed trains, and twenty times to 600 mph for airliners.

Although the telegraph was generally only used for short, high-priority messages, it was the harbinger of communication becoming divorced from transportation. The increased speed of routine communication has been more dramatic than the increased speed of transportation. Communication has broken loose from the need to be carried somewhere by someone. Now it is being conducted at the speed of light by electrons – on wires and more recently through the 'ether'. As long-distance telephone systems proliferated and became routinely affordable, the 30-mph speed of mail carried on early trains has increased by more than fifty thousand times. A twenty-page document might take thirty-plus hours to go a thousand miles in 1850. It takes a few seconds now, with the limiting factor being the speed of personal connections to the Internet.[4] This huge increase in speed has made door-to-door communications residual, and made most communications place-to-place or person-to-person. The length of the message is a more salient limiting factor than the distance that the message has to travel.

Place to place

Community goes beyond the neighbourhood

When I was a child living in the Bronx, New York City, I took the subway several times a week to Manhattan. Along the way, we went through the predominantly African-American Harlem area. We never thought to get off there. The express train did not even stop at its stations, as it sped middle-class Bronxites to the work and fun of Times Square and Greenwich Village. We got on the train in the Bronx, got off in midtown Manhattan, and saw nothing in between except each other. Forty years later I do the same thing when travelling transcontinentally. I get on an aeroplane in Toronto and get off five hours later in Los Angeles, with only the Rockies poking through the clouds to capture my attention through the window. As in the subway, passengers rarely communicate with each other. Between visits, I telephone or, increasingly, I email. Friends send emails, asking me to look at pictures of their weddings and children on their websites.

The big change from door-to-door to place-to-place community is old news by now – apparent to all but politicians and community scholars habituated to thinking of neighbourhoods as the only possible sources of community. Contemporary communities are found only rarely in neighbourhoods, when one defines community socially and not spatially (Wellman and Leighton 1979, Wellman 1999a). This is because people usually obtain support, sociability, information and a sense of belonging from those who do not live within the same neighbourhood or even within the same metropolitan area. People maintain these community ties through phoning, writing, driving, rail-roading, transiting and flying. Although characteristics of neighbourhoods remain important – like differential real estate values between neighbour-hoods – they are not important sources of community. They have become variably safe and salubrious milieux from which people sally forth in their cars or telephone from their kitchens.

Most North Americans have little interpersonal connection with their neighbourhood; they have less connection to the social control of a neigh-bourhood group.[5] Community interactions have moved inside the private home – where most entertaining, phone-calling and emailing take place – and away from chatting with patrons in public spaces such as bars, street corners and coffee shops. Even when people do go out with others – to restaurants or movie theatres – they usually leave their neighbourhoods (Lofland 1998). For example, the percentage of Americans regularly socialising with neighbours has been steadily declining for at least twenty-five years. In 1999, only 20 per cent spent a social evening with neighbours several times per week as compared with 30 per cent in 1974. Similarly regularly socialising in pubs has declined from 11 per cent to 8 per cent (T. Smith 1999).

Although I have concentrated on spatial effects here – community ties spreading beyond neighbourhoods – social structural effects are important too, especially the predominance of networks (rather than groups) in communities.[6] Living in networks has profound implications for the nature of place-to-place communities as compared with door-to-door communities:

- an ability to connect with multiple social milieux, with limited involve-ment in each milieu
- a decreased control that each milieu can have, while decreasing the commitment of each milieu to a person's well-being
- active maintenance of people's sparsely-knit ties and fragmented networks. By contrast, it is easier for people in groups to sit back and let group dynamics and densely knit structures do the work. That is why friendship networks are less apt than kinship networks to persist in times of overload
- a shift in the proportion of interactions away from those based on 'ascriptive' characteristics people are born with – such as age, gender, race and social class – and towards those based on 'achieved' characteristics that they have adopted throughout the life course – such as lifestyles, shared norms and voluntary interests
- fostering 'cross-cutting' ties that link and integrate social milieux, instead of such groups being isolated and tightly bounded
- an increase in choices while reducing the palpable group memberships that provide a sense of belonging

- reduced identity and pressures of belonging to groups. Increased opportunity, contingency, globalisation and uncertainty through participation in social networks
- increased emphasis on structural position in different networks – such as brokerage ties that connect multiple networks – and decreased emphasis on group membership. Active networking is more important than going along with the group.

Community gets domesticated

Place-to-place community links households that are not in the same neighbourhood (Wellman and Leighton 1979; Wellman 1979, 1999a). You go from somewhere to somewhere to meet someone, usually inside their homes. Or you telephone somewhere to talk to someone. The household is what is visited, telephoned or emailed. Moreover, the community ties of married couples often involve both husbands and wives. They see their friends in common, interact with each other's families, and get support from in-laws as easily as they get support from their own kin. It is a privatised relationship that does not involve the local area. Few neighbours are known, and those known are rarely known well (Wellman 1985, Wellman and Wellman 1992). Physical closeness does not mean social closeness.

Home is now the base for relationships that are more voluntary and selective than the public communities of the past. Only a minority of community ties in the western world operate in the public contexts of neighbourhood, formal organisations or work. Community networks now contain high proportions of people who enjoy each other and low proportions of people who are forced to interact with each other because they are juxtaposed in the same neighbourhood, kinship group, organisation or workplace. Friends and relatives get together as small sets of singles or couples, but rarely as communal groups. Where once-public communities had been men's worlds, now home-based community networks bring husbands and wives together. Men's community ties are now tucked away in homes just as women's ties have usually been (Wellman 1992a, 1999a).

In place-to-place communities, married women not only participate in community, they dominate the practice of it. Women have historically been the 'kin-keepers' of western society: mothers and sisters keeping relatives connected for themselves, their husbands and their children. Women are the pre-eminent suppliers of emotional support in community networks and the major suppliers of domestic services to households (Wellman 1992b). With the privatisation and domestication of community, community-keeping has become an extension of kin-keeping, with both linked to domestic management. Husbands and wives no longer have many separate friendships. Men usually stay at home during their leisure time, and the informal ties of their wives form the basis for relations between married couples. Women define the nature of friendship and help maintain many of their husbands' friendships. Women bear more than the 'double load' of domestic work and paid work. Their 'triple load' now includes community 'network'.

Thus, the privatisation and domestication of relationships are concomitant with place-to-place community. The domesticated community ties interact in small groups in private homes rather than in larger groups in public spaces. This has made it more difficult for people to form new community ties with friends of their friends, and it has focused the concerns of relationships on dealing with household problems (Wellman 1992a). Women's ties, which have dominated place-to-place community networks, provide important support for dealing with domestic work. Community members help with daily hassles and crises; neighbours mind each other's children; sisters and friends provide emotional support for child, husband and elder care. Because women are the community-keepers and are pressed for time caring for homes and doing paid work, men have become even more cut off from male friendship groups (Wellman 1992a). In place-to-place communities, North American men have rarely used their community ties to accomplish collective projects of work, politics or leisure. Their relationships have largely become sociable ties, either as part of the relationship between two married couples or as disconnected relations with a few male 'buddies'.

The abundance of within-household interaction and the scarcity of neighbourly community means that the search for the right neighbourhood is not necessarily a search for the right set of community members. People want to live in safe areas, with good public schools for children and good medical resources for the elderly (Dear *et al.* 1996). Paradoxically, because the lack of neighbourhood community does not preserve local safety, living in a low-crime area is especially important if few neighbours know each other. The value on living in the right place may be another sign of individual and household privatisation rather than a sign of a premium on neighbourhood community.

Compared with door-to-door community, place-to-place community operates in a contextual vacuum. The most obvious manifestations of this are automobile travel (especially on expressways), telephones (since party lines became passé before the Second World War; see Fischer 1992) and email. People and places are connected. Yet there is little social or physical intersection with the intervening spaces between households. People often get on an expressway near their home and get off near their friend/kin's home with little sense of what is in between. Aeroplane travel is even more contextless, despite occasional gasps as the Rockies or the Alps are sighted beneath the clouds.

The domestication of the Internet

Despite the heralding of the Internet as the basis for McLuhan's mythical 'global village', many characteristics of the Internet reinforced place-to-place connectivity. Although an Internet account is usually for a person and not for a place, Internet communications are usually sent and received from a fixed place: home or office. Always-on, 24×7 Internet connectivity means that you have a fair bit of confidence that people will be available to read your messages or agree to an instant chat. Moreover, you usually have a good idea of the socio-physical places in which the people you know are reading your messages. If you send a message to your mother, you have a high expectancy that your father will also read it.

The Internet both provides a ramp on to the global information highway and strengthens local links within neighbourhoods and households. For all its global access, the Internet reinforces stay-at-homes. *'Glocalisation'* occurs, both because the Internet makes it easy to contact many neighbours, and because fixed, wired Internet connections root users at their home and office desks. It is to the household or workplace that Internet communications come; the Internet café in the mall is only for outsiders. Many emails are local and refer to local arrangements.

For example, Keith Hampton and I (2000) find in our study of a leading-edge wired suburb that those who are online are the most active neighbours: the wired residents of 'Netville' know twenty-five neighbours; the unwired know eight. Moreover, the ties of the wired suburbanites range further through the neighbourhood instead of just clustering on the same block. Nor is glocalisation only a leisure-hours phenomenon. While email goes to the place where a person logs on – usually home or office – it is directed to the person and not to the household. Many business emails are local. More than half (57 per cent) of all the email messages received by computer-intensive students in my Berkeley graduate course came from within Berkeley, with another 15 per cent coming from within the Bay area (Wellman 1999b). The visiting Norwegian students in the course received many long-distance messages, but almost all were from Norway.

The Internet itself is not fully connected: slow access times, poor phone lines, expensive telecommunications charges, government surveillance and limited access to computers hamper connectivity. Only the one-third of the sites at the core of the Web are interconnected and easily reachable. Twenty-two per cent of all websites are so locally isolated that they cannot be reached by or connected to the core group (Bloomberg 2000). Even when the Internet connects globally, it often functions lumpily: messages are not dispersed evenly around the world but are disproportionately exchanged with a few geographical areas, certain types of people or people in the same social networks (including 'friends of friends'). Having global access does not mean having global connectivity.

Because using the Internet was so immersive, Netville residents used it heavily at home. After the initial learning curve for 'newbies', Netville family members helped each other to use computers, shared online discoveries and replaced time spent watching television with net surfing. For example, one family has a Saturday evening ritual of gathering around the computer with the family and a bowl of popcorn. Parents have rarely complained that the time their children and spouse spend online took away from family activities (Wellman and Hampton 1999).

The Internet increases long-distance involvement as well as local involvement. When Netville residents receive high-speed connections to the Internet, their social contact and supportive exchanges with friends and relatives living more than 50 kilometres away increases substantially. There are several reasons:

- It is almost as easy to send a message to ten friends as it is to contact one.
- Group aliases allow people to contact a hundred or more friends by typing a single word.
- Email discussion groups and real-time chat groups provide specialised audiences – and some respondents – in hundreds and thousands.
- Many online ties are palpable, supportive relationships. The Internet is useful for maintaining both strong ties of intimacy and weaker ties of acquaintanceship.
- Rather than being exclusively online or in-person, many community ties are complex dances of face-to-face encounters, scheduled get-togethers, dyadic telephone calls, emails to one person or several, and broader online discussions among those sharing interests.

Controlling connections to resources

Thus the turn away from door-to-door contact and towards place-to-place contact has been a twofold turn away from both involvement in a single place and a single group. It is conceptually and practically important not to conflate these two turnings. The shift to place-to-place contact enables people to find community while not being bound up in either their physical neighbourhood (place) and their neighbourhood community (group). Yet place-to-place contact means that localities may still be important – unless friends and relatives hide inside their households – but these localities may be far from where we live. It is the intersection of what Manuel Castells (1996) has called the traditional 'space of places' and the developing 'space of flows'.

Based on inter-household networks, place-to-place connectivity creates a more fluid system for accessing resources – material, cognitive and influential. No more are people identified as members of a single group; they can switch among multiple networks. Switching and manoeuvring among networks, people can use ties to one network to bring resources to another. The very fact of their tie to another network will be a resource, creating the possibility of linkage, trade and co-operation. For example, the Italian-American 'urban villagers' studied by Herbert Gans (1962) could not prevent their door-to-door community from being destroyed by a municipal-developer alliance intent on building new high-rises. Their bounded community had no links to politically powerful coalitions outside their Boston neighbourhood. Not only do people living in insalubrious neighbourhoods suffer, those without networking resources are interpersonally adrift.

As such, place-to-place connectivity has dual resource control imperatives, as Charles Tilly (1973) pointed out when he wondered the circumstances under which communities act (see also Tilly 2000). On the one hand, the security of the household base and its surroundings are important, and neighbours are scarcely known and not knit into a strong network. This makes a household's local politics one of securing the property and area with guarded gates; getting people as neighbours with the 'right' demographics and lifestyle; encouraging a strong, responsive police presence. On the other hand, residents want high-speed, unfettered access to the Internet, expressways and airports to facilitate their links with people in other places (Hampton and Wellman 2000). Their security concerns start turning to anti-virus checkers, spam and obscenity filters, disk backups, and firewall-like protection against hacker intrusion.

Control of resources in such place-to-place systems is thus a mixture of control of property and control of networking resources. Knowing how to network (on- and offline) becomes a human capital resource, and having a supportive network becomes a social capital resource (Wellman and Wortley 1990). The cost is the loss of a palpably present and visible local community to provide a strong identity and belonging. The gain is the increased diversity of opportunity, greater scope for individual agency and the freedom from a single group's constrictive control.

The rise of networked individualism person to person

From place to person

When a close New York relative suddenly became hospitalised in February 2000, Bev Wellman and I wanted to be always 'on call' in case we suddenly had to fly to New York. Yet we had just flown to visit friends in Los Angeles, and were travelling the freeways between places. Moving around with a mobile phone made me almost completely independent of place. It was I alone who was reachable wherever I was: at a house, hotel, office, freeway or mall. Place did not matter; person did. The person has become the portal.

The development of person-to-person connectivity has been influenced more by innovations in communication than in transportation. When someone calls a telephone wired into the telephone network, the phone rings at the *place*, no matter which *person* is being called. Indeed, many place-to-place ties have connected households as much as individuals. By contrast, mobile phones afford a fundamental liberation from place, and they soon will be joined by wireless computers and personalised software. Their use shifts community ties from linking people-in-places to linking people wherever they are. Because the connection is to the person and not to the place, it shifts the dynamics of connectivity from places – typically households or work-sites – to individuals.[7]

The shift to a personalised, wireless world affords truly *personal communities* that supply support, sociability, information and a sense of belonging separately to each individual. It is the individual, and neither the household nor the group, that is the primary unit of connectivity. Just as 24×7 Internet computing means the high availability of people in specific places, the proliferation of mobile phones and wireless computing increasingly means the even higher availability of people without regard to place. From the point of view of people using mobile phones, their supportive convoys travel with them ethereally. They can link what they are doing at the moment to their far-flung network, just as I saw a young woman at a Rembrandt etching exhibition in Toronto describing her experience to her boyfriend across the continent in British Columbia (18 June 2000).

Although the switch from door-to-door to place-to-place has made possible communities of choice that were less constrained by distance, place-to-place community has preserved some sense of social context. The shift from place-to-place to person-to-person contact reduces this contextual sense: a caller contacts another by mobile phone or the Internet has uncertain knowledge about where that person is. Because mobile people frequently shift from one social network to the other at home or in the office, they contact each other in initial ignorance about their social contexts, unless like the Rembrandt-watcher they explicitly describe their surroundings. Rather than being embedded in one social network, person-to-person interactors are always switching between networks.

From inter-household networks to inter-personal networks

Even without door-to-door neighbourhood communities, the household and not the individual has been the key interacting unit in place-to-place communities. For example, in-laws are as supportive as own-kin, and wives frequently arrange visits with their husbands' friends and relatives (Wellman 1999a). The continuing shift in the western world to single-adult households – both adults working in married households, and serial marriage – has meant that married couples are no longer the demographic heartbeat of America.

Where high-speed place-to-place communication supports the dispersal and fragmentation of community, high speed person-to-person communication goes one step further and supports the dispersal and role-fragmentation of households. Does the switch to person-to-person connectivity mean that even stably married husbands and wives will be in separate communities? There may be a return to the separate marital lives that Elizabeth Bott documented over a generation ago in England (1957). 'The nuclear family may be on a comeback', a Rogers ATT mobile-phone advertisement says on Toronto radio (CFMX, 13 February 2000: 0813EST) with no sense of irony. Dad is bowling with the boys, Mom is on the road making presentations, son Dick is at his computer club, and daughter Jane is out of town visiting her biological Dad. Yet they all can stay connected at low cost through flat-rate national mobile-phone calling. Nor does the dispersion have to be far-flung: I know a couple in a wired Toronto mansion who communicate extensively by intercom.

Reading and responding to the Internet is more personally immersive than watching television or talking on the telephone. To net surf, someone must peer intently into a nearby screen as if praying to a shrine and finger keys as if they were prayer beads. This kinaesthetic focus on the computer, combined with the bulkiness of the screen, draws computer users away from simultaneously having face-to-face contact with proximate others. Family members have to compete for attention, for closer-to-the-eye computer screens afford less scope for joint interaction than television screens. Telephones allow much more body movement and glances at others than does personal computing. I doubt that many spouses tell their mates to leave the room whenever the telephone rings, just as I assume that most spouses refrain from opening each other's snail-mail. Yet some people are miffed when their spouses read their email. They regard their email address and alias as parts of their personal identity – not to be shared lightly and to be protected in divorce settlements (Cohen 2000).

Mobilisation

Until now, mobile phones have gone further than personal computers in affording person-to-person contact. At its most fully developed, mobilisation assumes that callers and receivers are always available, no matter where they may be. Hence mobile phoning suits and reinforces mobile lifestyles and physically dispersed relationships. It affords liberation from both place and group.

When mobile phones remain at home or in the office, they are just another form of place-to-place communication. When they travel in handbags, briefcases or belt-clips, they instantly afford person-to-person communication. My friend Janet has a single 'prime number' that first tries her wired telephone at home and then tries her mobile phone. Although I never know where I am reaching her when I call, I always know that I am reaching her and not anyone else in her house. I usually ask 'where are you?' when I call so that I can adjust the length, content, and intensity of my conversation. The context of place does matter, even in person-to-person communications. As Rebecca Adams commented: 'It is pretty hard for people to define someone's identity if they don't even know where they are in physical or social space when they talk to them on a cell phone' (personal email, 10 January 2000). Because mobile-phone costs are low in the United States and western Europe, they often take the place of traditional wired telephones.

As mobile phones proliferate, the norms of this inherently person-to-person system foster the intrusion of intensely involving private behaviour into public space (see also Lofland 1998). On Toronto's crowded Spadina streetcar in January 2000, Bev Wellman and I listened to a young woman carry on an intensely romantic mobile phone conversation with her lover. She seemed oblivious to my sitting next to her. Although we followed Erving Goffman's rules (1963) for behaviour in public places and gave her apparent civil inattention, her loud and personal talking transgressed the traditional place-based rules of public behaviour. Her intense involvement in her private conversation – and her loud voice intruding on our soft conversation – appropriated public space for her own needs. What if both parties had been seated side-by-side on the streetcar? It still would have been intrusive, but seeing both parties to the interaction would have provided a more appropriate sense of observational completeness. Observing this intense, one-sided conversation was more like observing masturbation than like observing a couple in love.

My sense is that such transgressions are increasing. Listening through earphones to music on tape and disc players is another example of the personalisation of public space. The listener is oblivious to passers-by, often walking into them, and unaware (and apparently uncaring) about the unwanted noise escaping from his or her earphones. People who withdraw inward in public space are unsettling, their behaviour signalling that their bodies, but not personas, are passing through. While enjoying the beauty atop the Milan Cathedral's roof in November 1999, Bev Wellman and I were startled when a young woman's mobile phone rang. 'Buon Giorno, Giuseppe,' she answered with a squeal of delight and proceeded to have an intimate conversation while standing next to us. Later, walking through La Scala square, we noticed a middle-aged woman dressed in a Gucci suit talking to herself. 'Even the mentally disturbed wear designer outfits in Milan,' I muttered. When she came closer, I saw that she was actually equipped with the latest in communication chic. With a tiny lapel mike pinned to her collar and a small 'ear bud', she was having a mobile conversation as she walked, the guts of her phone hidden in the Gucci. Watching her, I realised that wearable mobile phones can be a primitive version of multimedia, allowing one to talk simultaneously on the phone and with both hands. More seriously, they make it easier to use a mobile phone to net surf, as the phone no longer needs to be held up to one's ear for conversation.

Were the women on the Toronto streetcar or atop Milan Cathedral finding the community in wireless space that they would if they were talking face-to-face in a public space? Despite the women's manifest mobile-pleasure, it is likely that they and their lovers would be happier in person, using the senses of sight, sound, touch, smell and mutual cognition. I doubt that there will be androids or avatars up to the task in this century. But love is an extreme case. The more general question is: can people emotionally and cognitively experience relationships through computerised communication systems in the same ways that they experience face-to-face relationships?

Computerisation

My immigrant grandmother in the Bronx used to shout into the telephone for fear that she would not be heard 30 kilometres away in Brooklyn. A generation later, my Bronxite mother routinely conversed for hours on the telephone with her sister in Brooklyn. My generation thinks little of emailing: in our house the computer connection to the network remains live all day in case we have a bright idea we wish to share with our friends. (Such are the joys of flat-fee monthly rates.) Yet analysts still privilege email and wonder if it will be a good enough medium to sustain community.

If computer networks transmit information at the speed of light, just as radio or television broadcasts and telephone networks have done for generations, has computerisation enhanced community? Digital information in computer networks conveys more information per second than analogue telephone networks; computer networks combine the potentially wide reach of broadcast networks with the personalised communication of telephone networks. For example, I first floated an early version of this chapter on the email discussion list of the American Sociological Association's Community and Urban Sociology section: three hundred reasonably informed persons who know of me as I am currently the section's chair. Many responded to the group; some responded to me personally. I next tried a draft of this paper on my personal email list of '80 Best Friends': people socially close enough to give me a friendly critique.[8] The later version that you are currently reading is publicly available online, for computer networks support public address systems to strangers as well as personal communications and within-network broadcasts.

Because Internet accounts are personal and not place-based, they are already way stations on the move to person-to-person community. As high-bandwidth wireless computing becomes prevalent, communicating computers will break their tethers and become placeless. There are already leading-edge indicators of this trend. Internet cafés in malls or main streets allow travellers to keep connected, road warriors use global phone or Internet access networks to connect from hotels or businesses they are visiting, mobile phones are developing Internet capability, and a well-located few have higher-speed wireless modems on their laptop computers. I know a computer consultant in Silicon Valley who uses a wireless modem to check her email at 8.00 am while she watches her young daughter play in the schoolyard. As she sips her cappuccino, she is a multi-tasking harbinger of the convergent integration of a mobile phone's ubiquitous, portable connectivity with the multifunctional power of a personal computer. As satellite links develop and technical standards for wireless communications evolve globally, the same wireless phone-computer will be able to reach the Internet as easily in Bora Bora as in Silicon Valley.

As community moves out of the household and on to the mobile phone and the modem, there is scope for yet another re-negotiation of marital relations. Women had set the rules of the community game in place-to-place relationships and borne the burden of community keeping. If person-to-person community means that it is every person for himself or herself, then we might expect to see a gendered re-segregation of community (as in Elizabeth Bott's England, 1957) with the possibility that men's communities will be smaller than networking-savvy women (Wright 1989, Moore 1990, Wellman 1992a, Bruckner and Knaup 1993).

Is community viable online?

As computing power is increasingly used to prioritise and enhance interactions, the power of such person-to-person communication systems is poised to increase, for better or worse. Can true community be found online – in whole or in part – as well as in homes, on the phone, in the mall, or on street corners? When I circulated a draft of my argument online, political scientist Robert Putnam responded:

> I think you're a wild-eyed optimist to think that 'person-to-person' networks are 'just as good as, if not better than' old-fashioned door-to-door (or rather faces-to-faces) networks. But regardless of the differences between us in temperament, you surely cannot think that the two sorts of networks are 'essentially identical'.
>
> (personal email, 10 January 2000)

Several distinct issues should be addressed here:

First, *are community ties – and community networks – viable online?* Research shows that people interact happily and fruitfully online (for the most part) and in ways similar to face-to-face contact (Wellman and Gulia 1999).

Second, *the online–offline dichotomy may be overdone.* Many relationships do not exist only online but use online contact to fill the gaps between face-to-face meetings, not as substitutes for them. They supplement and amplify of face-to-face community ties, rather than replacing them.

Third, *are good online relationships as good as good face-to-face relationships where people can see, hear, smell and touch someone, usually in a social context?* Probably not, but the question may have an utopian assumption that if people were not online they would be engaged in stimulating community, household, or personal activities. Online relationships may be filling empty spots in people's lives now that they no longer can wander to the local pub or café to take up with their community members. Participating in online community probably replaces television-watching more than anything else (Nie and Erbring 2000). As the networked individual substitutes for the lonely crowd, online relationships may be increasing the frequency and intensity of community ties, although at the potential cost of strained household ties. Yet the studies that focus on this look principally at 'newbies' (Kraut *et al.* 1998, Nie and Erbring 2000): Our group's study of Unix users shows that these veteran Interneters flourish online (Chmielwski and Wellman 2000).

Fourth, *will the use of computer-mediated communication become more transparent as people get more experienced with it, and as such communication develops more verisimilitude through the use of video, and so on?* Or is the comparison with face-to-face relationships always a rigged game in which online relationships can never be quite equal, and we would be wiser to wonder if online interaction will develop its own strengths and create its own dynamics? These might be multimedia attachments of photos or developing new norms. We have already seen unique email dynamics in community-building: the folding-in of two disconnected friends into the same conversation, asking personal messages of posters to discussion groups and developing personal relationships, typographical conventions of embedding interleaved responses inside original messages, and responding to messages at the top of the message exchange rather than on the bottom. Most important, online communication seems to be extending the reach of networks: allowing more ties to be maintained and fostering specialised relationships in networks. People are increasingly known and related to only in terms of particular aspects of their persona: role-to-role instead of person-to-person.

Fifth, *even if not perfect, can online relationships be good enough?* Can people emotionally and cognitively respond to online relationships in the same way they respond to face-to-face relationships? The crucial difference between personal relationships and more specialised role relationships is the richness of their history (Banse 1999). To this, I would add the narrower bandwidth of online communication as compared with face-to-face and even phone-to-phone contact. Yet connecting online does have unique advantages. With respect to history, tracing memory in ageing online archives may be easier. I currently use an online personal directory that, besides supplying phone and fax numbers, primes my interactions with the names of people's spouses, children and mutual friends. In the future, it should be able to provide the titles, abstracts and text of the articles that people have written, as well as reveal their social ties with others in their networks (Contractor, Zink and Chan 1998).

Sixth, *in asking questions about the authenticity and usability of computer-mediated communication, we must differentiate between relationships based on online communication and those in which online communication is only one form of interacting.* Although many scholars and the mass media have been fascinated with online-only communities, our research group has documented what should be obvious to all community sociologists: people communicate with their friends, relatives, neighbours and workmates by any means available and necessary, online and offline.

Seventh, *as community increasingly becomes person-to-person (and not door-to-door or even place-to-place), people may continue to feel responsible for their strong relationships but not for the many acquaintances and strangers with whom they rub shoulders but are not connected.* Private contact with familiar friends and relatives is replacing public gregariousness so that people pass each other unsmiling on streets and highways. Such privatisation may be responsible for the lack of informal help given to strangers who are in trouble in public spaces (Latané and Darley 1976). It may also explain the paradox of well-connected people feeling lonely because of the lack of physically present community members.

Eighth, *to maintain anonymity and freedom of choice many do not want to be always – or often – connected.* Agency is a need as well as an analytic category. Just as computerised tools for finding others are developing, so are tools that block being found: spam-filters for unwanted email, cookie cutters to avoid being tracked on the web, multiple email accounts for different personas, and secretarial buffers – human and cyber. Science-fiction author William Gibson (the inventor of the term 'cyberspace') believes that in the near future 'people will pay money for something that will make them believe for a while that they are not connected' (quoted in Fulford 2000: B2).

Ninth, *does the shift to person-to-person networked connectivity mean that people can become more footloose, living almost anywhere as more communication becomes personal and not based on place?* For the developed world: yes, no and no. *Yes*, because many people for short periods can communicate effectively with the Internet, supplemented by the telephone (for nuanced, real-time conversations) and courier services (for the delivery of goods – documents now travel as attachments). *No*, because the narrower range of Internet communication makes face-to-face contact imperative for maintaining strong ties. *No*, because it is impossible to duplicate elsewhere the complex interplay of urban information, skills, goods, services and networks. Although Jane Jacobs (1967) pointed this out in antediluvian pre-Internet, pre-FedEx times, the joy and usefulness of face-to-face contact is still why Silicon Valley has such a high concentration of technology firms. Physical place matters, even for cyberspace firms. Travel time still matters for everyone, for, until the twenty-third century's invention of matter transmission, only bits – and not atoms – can flow through cyberspace.

Tenth, *will less-developed countries suffer a digital divide, and not experience the proliferation of computerised communication networks?* The less-developed world will add elements of person-to-person and role-to-role community to existing door-to-door, place-to-place communities. Transportation of people will generally be door-to-door, with intermittent place-to-place relationships. Communication beyond walking distance will become easier and cheaper as the lower infrastructure costs of mobile phones (and convergent wireless computing) facilitates contact of rural–urban and international migrants, specialised communities and information about global markets for products. Low levels of communication and electrical infrastructure, marked geographical variations in what infrastructure does exist and uneven distributions of wealth mean that any kind of telephone connection is rare in large areas of the impoverished 'fourth world'. Telephone density is less than two lines per thousand persons in Africa and forty-eight per thousand in Asia as compared with 520 per thousand in high-income countries (Marcelle 1998, Darkwa and Mazibuko 2000). These 'switched-off region[s] of the world' are in a state of 'technological apartheid at the dawn of the Information Age' (Castells 1998: 93–4). In areas with little wiring and low telephone density, communication will forgo wired systems and go straight to mobilisation. It is cheaper in such situations to erect wireless towers (and perhaps satellite ground stations) than it is to string a wired network. In outlying areas, mobile phones will often connect places, not persons: just as in rural America in the early twentieth century, the general store will be where people go to use the phone (Fischer 1992). Over time, personal mobile phones and wireless Internet devices should proliferate for the affluent and for travelling workers (see also Meier 1962, Castells 1998, Jhunjhunwala 2000).

Role to role

Specialised relationships

Many interpersonal ties are based only on the specialised roles that people play – not the whole persons. These relationships are between fragments of selves, rather than between whole selves. Such role-to-role relationships have already become abundant in place-to-place community. For example, our group's research has found that most community ties are specialised, with different community members supplying emotional support, information, material aid, social identity and a sense of belonging (Wellman and Wortley 1990; see also Fischer 1982). This means that people must maintain differentiated portfolios of ties to obtain a variety of needed and wanted resources. They cannot assume that all community members will provide all kinds of help. As noted above, person-to-person connectivity moves responsibility for well-being from the household and network to the two-person dyad. If role-to-role connectivity becomes increasingly specialised, who, besides spouses, will worry about the whole person? Specialisation means that the emotional supporters will not have to worry about material need, and perhaps will not even know about it. This will lead to lessened loads and pleasures of caring.

People often prefer some relationships to be specialised. For example, many collaborating scholars prefer the autonomy of emailing others at a distance to the more compelling, less specialised, face-to-face relationships. They attempt to balance a desire to function according to their own independent rhythms and a desire to obtain the intellectual, material and social rewards of membership in scholarly communities (Koku, Nazer and Wellman 2001). For example, among theoretical physicists, shifting from face-to-face contact to disembodied email contact is a possible means of obtaining autonomy: isolation is achieved without effort. These scholars can interact role-to-role without being constrained to deal with the whole person (Merz 1998).

What if computerised communication systems afforded greater personalisation and specialisation by role? Sophisticated telephone and computer response systems may have intelligent agents providing different sorts of responses to different sorts of callers: your spouse would hear a different message from your friends or tele-marketers. What if each person were reading a different version of this chapter, because I have used personal information to tailor the message that I most want you to receive?[9] Perhaps the emphases would be different; perhaps the content would change. I might leave out the anecdotes if high-status people logged on; I might use an appropriate personal example for close friends. If I knew you well enough, I might even use an appropriate personal example from *your* life. If I did not know you, my software might use heuristic rules to construct an appropriate version tailored to online information about your demographic profile, Internet-surfing tastes, or the friends we have in common. This would be computer-supported communication that was not only person-to-person but personalised role-to-role.

Specialised communities

Role-to-role community networks consist either of like-minded people – such as BMW 2002 fanciers – or of people with complementary roles – such as parents and friends, or violinists and cellists. While such communities are abundant now, they are flourishing on the Internet and will become even more abundant as the Internet's capabilities develop. People participate in many ways. They often subscribe to multiple discussion lists and newsgroups, letting others organise the membership and course of the communities. Discussion lists and newsgroups provide permeable, shifting sets of participants, with more intense relationships continued by private email. They can more actively send out messages to personal lists of their own making, perhaps keeping different lists for different kinds of conversations. Moreover, they can vary in their involvement in different communities, participating actively in some, occasionally in others, and being silent 'lurkers' in still others. The relaxation of constraints on the size and proximity of one's 'communication audience' on the Internet can increase the diversity of people encountered. At some undetermined size, an online community becomes an unstructured crowd.

The Internet affords the development of new connections and the acquisition of new information. Using email lists and newsgroups to ask distant acquaintances and strangers for information and advice is easy. Information may come unsolicited through distribution lists, chat groups, newsgroups, pointers by friends to interesting websites, and forwarded messages from friends who 'thought you might like to know about this'. Friends forward communications to third parties, and in so doing they provide indirect contact between previously disconnected people who can then make direct contact. When one's strong ties are unable to provide information, one is likely to find it from weak ties. Because people with strong ties are more likely to be socially similar and to know the same persons, they are more likely to possess the same information. By contrast, new information is more apt to come through weaker ties better connected with other, more diverse social circles.

The Internet's very lack of social richness can foster contact with more diverse others. The lack of social and physical cues online makes it difficult to find out whether another online community member has similar social characteristics or attractive physical characteristics. Thus the Net's lack of in-person involvement can give participants more control over the timing and content of their self-disclosures (Walther 1995). This allows role-to-role relationships to develop from shared interests rather than be stunted at the onset by differences in social status. For example, geographically and socially isolated Muslim women in North America find sociability, support and a sense of belonging in an online discussion group (Bastani 2000). This focus on shared interests rather than on similar characteristics can be empowering for members of lower-status and disenfranchised groups.

The proliferation of computer-supported specialised ties may also be providing the basis for intervening interest-based structures that provide support, partial solidarity and vehicles for aggregating and articulating interests. This would be an Internet *cum* Tocquevillean substitute for the decline of organised groups that Robert Putnam (1995, 2000) has identified as a key problem in America. Even in the pre-Internet France of the early 1990s, friendship and intimacy differentially linked occupational groups. Sales workers and executives were rarely connected, but clerks and blue-collar workers were (Ferrand, Mounier and Degenne 1999).

Such specialised communities, based on shared interests, can foster cognitive homogeneity. Despite the Internet's potential to connect diverse cultures and ideas, people are drawn to online communities that link them with others sharing common interests or concerns. They may be more diversified than 'real-life' community in their gender, ethnicity and socio-economic status, but they still communicate about only a limited set of topics and ideas.

Where person-to-person community is individualising, role-to-role community deconstructs a holistic individual identity. A person becomes only the sum of his or her roles, and there is the danger of alienation. The compartmentalisation of personal life – within the household and within the community – may create an insecure milieu where no one fully knows anyone (Detelina Radoeva, personal email, 12 January 2000).

Networks in cyberspace and physical space

The turn to cyberspace has affected the network basis of community in many ways.

- In the short term, it has made the household more important, as a base from which to operate one's computer-supported social network. This can lead to a rise in neighbouring, as home-based people take more interest in their immediate surroundings and use the Internet to neighbour without physical intrusion and to arrange visits (Hampton and Wellman 1999).
- Jointly with the mobile phone, it is emphasising the ascendancy of person-to-person community, thus contributing (along with other factors) to the de-emphasis of domestic relations.
- It has emphasised individual autonomy. Each person is the operator of his or her personal community network (see also Wellman 1999a).
- It has afforded greater involvement in communities of shared interest. Such communities have probably become more spatially dispersed.
- Online relationships and online communities have developed their own strength and dynamics. Participants in online groups have strong interpersonal feelings of belonging, being wanted, obtaining important resources, and having a shared identity. They are truly in cyberplaces, and not just cyberspaces (Rheingold 1993a, 2000, Wellman and Gulia 1999).
- Often, the comparison between cyberspace and physical space is a false dichotomy. Many ties operate in both cyberspace and physical space, using whatever means of communication is convenient and appropriate at the moment.
- It has increased the importance of network capital in the fund of desirable resources, along with financial capital, human capital and cultural capital. Such network capital is variegated. It consists of knowing how to maintain a networked computer, search for information on the Internet and use the knowledge gained, create and sustain online relationships, and use these relationships to obtain needed resources, including indirect links to friends of friends.

The good news is that the cost of computing is becoming so low that in the developed world, the digital social-class divide should get smaller just as the digital gender gap has. Even in the less-developed world, the growth of wireless computing has made affluent residents less dependent on the national communications infrastructure. The bad news is that our schools do not know how to teach such networking skills. Fortunately, poorer groups in society have always networked heavily for the want of other resources. The problem will be to move from local networking and migrant networking to cyber-networking (Lomnitz 1977, Roberts 1978, Espinoza 1999). It may be then that network capital may provide a partial way of coping with a lack of other forms of capital.

Acknowledgments

My thanks to Bev Wellman who identified 'place-to-place' and helped me think it through as we drove down the Sepulveda Pass on the 405, mobile phone clipped to my belt. I've also benefited from cyber- and meat-space conversations with Andrew Beveridge, Erin Bradner, Sarah Busse, Mark Chignell, Dimitrina Dimitrova, Keith Hampton, Caroline Haythornthwaite, Jerry Krase, Kristine Klement, Lyn Lofland, Michael Milton, Andrew Odlyzko, Bandana Purkayastha, Anabel Quan Haase, Detelina Radoeva, Karen Ramsay, Howard Rheingold, Charles Tilly, Chris Toulouse, Gerda Wekerle, Beverly Wellman, James Witte, Alesia Zuccala, Sharon Zukin, other correspondents at the American Sociological Association's Community and Urban section who commented on a preliminary mini-draft (http://www.urbsoc.org/communityweb/), and compatriots at the University of Toronto's Centre for Urban and Community Studies, Collaboration Laboratory, Knowledge Media Design Institute, Personalization Technology Laboratory (BCUL), and Virtually Social Research Network. The research that underlies this paper has been supported by the Bell Canada University Laboratories, the Social Science and Humanities Research Council of Canada, and the Tele-Learning Centre of Excellence.

This chapter was previously printed in *The International Journal of Urban and Regional Relations*, June 2001, Vol. 25.2. Permission for reprint and copyright holder is Blackwell Publishers and the editors of IJURR.

Notes

1 George Hillery showed a generation ago (1955) that sociology has and needs multiple definitions of community. Contemporary community sociologists have two main foci (Wellman 2000b): (1) the ecological juxtaposition of people in the same locale; (2) interpersonal relations (as defined above), no matter where they are located. Although my own work has focused on the interpersonal definition of community, I have always believed that community can be sought in neighbourhoods – and sometimes even found there (Wellman 1979, 1999a, Wellman and Leighton 1979). However, I object to confining our view of community to neighbourhood-based ones. Although not every network is a community – unless you think of NATO or interlocking corporate structures as communities – every interpersonal community is a network. Whether such communities are found in – or confined to – neighbourhoods is a secondary question. I am also encountering a third focus among Internet marketers: labelling as a 'community' disconnected aggregations of random visitors to websites (see also Henshall 2000). For example, 'Talk City', a commercial set of websites oriented to American women, has a

'Vice-President, Community', whose job it is to encourage women to chat, eyeball ads, and buy things (www.talkcity.com).

2 'Affordances' is a term widely used in the study of human computer interaction (Norman 1999). Erin Bradner (2000), writing for computer scientists, has coined the term 'social affordances' to emphasise the *social* as well as individual implications of the technological features of computer-supported communication networks and human–computer interfaces. See also Gaver (1996).

3 In theory, telegrams travelled at the speed of light, although limitations caused by human operators and mechanical failure inevitably made the actual user-to-user speed appreciably slower.

4 I assume at each end: 33 kilobit/second effective speed of telephone 'dial-up' modems: this will rapidly increase to 10 megabits/second in this decade.

5 Nozawa 1997 and Otani 1999 show that this non-localism is also prevalent in Japan, despite its many institutions to promote neighbourhood solidarity, support and social control.

6 Formally, groups are a special type of network: densely knit (most people are directly connected), tightly bounded (most ties stay within the densely knit cluster), and multi-stranded (most ties contain many role relationships). In practice, it is linguistically convenient to contrast groups and networks.

7 For a discussion of how this affects home-based teleworkers, see Salaff, Wellman and Dimitrova (1998).

8 The process gave me more, better and varied feedback than I had previously experienced when I had shown papers to a few face-to-face colleagues or circulated drafts by snail (postal) mail. I did notice that some online readers responded to me privately instead of to the group. Perhaps they were reticent about being critical in public. I also found that the comments kept on coming and coming, evoking revisions that stretched the forbearance of the *IJURR*'s editors. In some ways it would be nice if online articles could be left open-ended, to be revised when new thoughts and findings occur. However, scholars might never get closure and liberation to move on to the next thing.

9 www.doubleclick.com already does this for Web ads (Furger 2000).

Chapter 4

Creating community in conspiracy with the enemy

Erik Stolterman

Introduction

Shaping a networked society is an adventure in design. A public sphere in cyberspace will not emerge from technology itself. Rather, this public sphere must be designed. This chapter is about that design. I am working on the assumption that a public sphere has to be designed by the public. It cannot be defined by commercial or governmental actors trying to 'help' the public. In a democratic society, a public sphere in cyberspace must be defined and designed by the people who find such a sphere necessary for their own needs.

The idea that our traditional communities are challenged, and are even under attack, by new technologies has been circulating for some time. The telephone, radio and television have all been labelled as enemies of community values and community-building. Information technology is often portrayed as the latest and perhaps the most dangerous enemy attacking our traditional community structures and values.

Information technology is accused of promoting only the enjoyment and pleasure of the individual because it offers virtual social relations without sacrifices or obligations. This technology seems to be understood as an enemy of locality, commitment, solidarity, obligations, relations and pride – values connected with the traditional community.

At the same time, we can see an enormous variety of approaches and attempts all around the world to make that same technology a means for creating and developing communities. Given this fact, it seems relevant to ask whether it is at all possible to *create community in 'conspiracy with the enemy'*.[1] In this chapter I will argue that there is a solution to this seeming impasse. I will suggest that a solution may be approached by critically examining the assumption that information technology is an 'enemy' of community. A solution may also be brought about by contrasting fears of this 'enemy' with empirical results from studies discussing the development of a widespread social life on the Net. In the course of my discussion, I will introduce such concepts as *architectonic* and *tectonic systems*, *designability*, *intended functionality* and *unintended use*.

I will be drawing the conclusion that technology can be deliberately and consciously designed, and that it is, in fact, so designed every day. To find ways to foster new designs, we need to show respect for the enormous richness and variety of the way people already have chosen to work with technology to provide for their everyday need for community. An examination of this phenomenon demands more close attention to the community life already on the Net. Community research should focus on people already designing their lives 'in conspiracy with the enemy'.

The overall message of this chapter is that technology cannot be regarded as a ready-made tool that can be used to create community. There exist no fixed tools and no predefined functionality. There is, however, a 'soul' of this new technology.

The soul of the technology

Information technology is not just another type of technology with known matter, structure, appearance and functionality. It is an entirely new kind of technology that is extremely diverse in the kinds of activities it manifests. That is why there is a need for closer studies of the technology, with the goal of understanding its 'soul', or in other words its basic core. There are several possible ways to understand technology and how it influences society. Today almost everyone agrees that technology does not in itself determine how it can or will be used and what consequences it may lead to. In the writings of Bruno Latour, particularly in his book *Pandora's Hope* (Latour 1999), we can find thorough and eloquent argumentation for the idea that neither technology nor the social environment alone are sole determining factors. Latour argues that there is no 'divide' between them. To him, the idea of a divide is a modern attempt to rationalise our world. The divide is one example of how people have attempted to describe and understand the idea of modernity, but Latour argues instead, 'We've never been modern.'

Latour's perspective draws attention to the real world – to the reality where people live and in which technology is part of an everyday network of social and technological actors. According to this idea, it is, for instance, not possible to analyse the impact of technology by studying technology as a distinct entity in itself. At the same time, it is not possible to understand technological development solely by analysing the social sphere. Latour uses instead the concept of 'double aspect'. There is no reference that begins at one or the other of the ends, i.e. either at the technology (world) end or the social (world) end. Rather, as Latour writes, 'Instead of growing from two fixed extremities toward a stable meeting point in the middle, the unstable reference grows from the middle toward the ends, which are continually pushed further away' (Latour 1999).

This means that, if we want to discover the true meaning of technology in relation to society, we cannot find it at one of the two extremities. We will never be able to understand how technology influences or changes our society by assuming technology to be 'given' in any sense. Nor can we understand technology based on how people behave. One conclusion that can be drawn from Latour's observations is that we have to start at the 'middle' moving towards the ends. This raises the question: what is the middle when it comes to information technology?

The designability of the technology

Technologies can be described and categorised in many ways. One way is to talk about open and closed technologies. A *closed technology* is one that does not allow the user to change anything after it has been designed and manufactured. The structure, functionality and appearance of the artefact are permanent. When dealing with a closed technology, we might find general characteristics in the way the technology appears to influence the people around it. We might find that the technology seems to foster the emergence of certain situations and behaviours. The technology is a relatively stable variable in social settings. And when the technology is moved to another setting, we know it will remain the same as far as matter, functionality and appearance are concerned.[2]

With an *open technology* it is much more difficult to find such stable patterns. An open technology is always, in a more radical sense, in a dialectical relation to its user and the situation. At the same time, as someone is using the technology, he or she can also change its basic design and manifestation. An open technology allows the user to continue changing the technology's specific characteristics, and to adjust, add or change its functionality. When it comes to an open technology, changes in functionality pose a question not only of change in the way the existing functionality is used or understood but also of a real change in the artefact's internal manifestation.

Information technology artefacts are often examples of an open technology. They can be changed, and if they cannot be changed it is usually possible to add, embed, contain or surround the artefact with other technology in a way that radically changes it. When a technology is open in this way, we can recognise it as *designable*. A designable technology is by definition difficult to describe and define in a comprehensive way, since at any moment it might change. It is not uncommon for even a designable artefact to contain some kind of 'closed' aspect hidden deeply in its innermost core. One fundamental property of an open technology is that it is sensitive to how much it is used. With a closed technology, it does not matter if there is one user or thousands. But the more people use a designable technology, the more it changes. Functions are added or taken away. The structure is redesigned and its appearance might be changed continuously. This property of designable technology radically influences the notion of what it means to be either a designer or a user of the technology. The user is at the same time a designer, and the designer can be understood as a user. This blend of the two roles probably reflects a core aspect of truly open and designable technology.

Cyberspace as a tectonic system

Most designs can be described as systems; they consist of many parts interacting in ways that appear to be a single entity. We usually define a system by addressing its different aspects, such as structure, function, aesthetics and ethics. Sometimes we find these aspects implemented in a way that gives the system a sense of wholeness, or even a sense of being intentionally designed as a whole. This sense of wholeness might, if it is well worked out, serve users by giving them an overall understanding of the system, an understanding in which all details seem to relate and connect throughout the system, and each detail seems to have a relation to the whole. The system can be understood as a unit. We can label a system such as this *architectonic*.

Working in an architectonic way can be understood as a process in which the relation between details and the whole is at all times attended to by the designer, and every detail is considered as important as the whole. This way of working can very easily lead to a crisis of complexity, that is, a situation emphasising the importance of *organising principles* guiding the architectonic design work. Organising principles helps the designer to make judgements throughout the design process.

A system can, of course, be designed without an organising principle, or with only locally (or regionally) organising principles. We can label such a system *tectonic*. A tectonic approach is possible when we have a system based on a technology that allows new parts and new functionalities to be added without necessarily changing the basic structure and dynamics of the system. With information technology, we do not have to be architectonic, that is we do not have to design the whole first. A tectonic system can work without a 'super' designer, since the technology allows continuous adding and linking of new parts to the overall system.

Information technology has characteristics suitable for both architectonic and tectonic designs. One basic reason for this is that information technology is extremely open to design. The technology can be designed to be a system with an overarching structure, predefined functionality, and strict purpose and goal. But the technology also makes possible designs that are open to changes and redesign.

The ATM machine is an example of an architectonic IT-artefact. It has a clear purpose and a closed structure and functionality. As a user you cannot change the artefact. You are defined by the architectonic design of the system to be nothing but a user. A modern word processor sometimes has a built-in capacity to be customised by the user.[3] This means that the system can look and behave differently to different users. Usually these differences will remain within the architectonic design implemented in the artefact. This means there is still a distinct difference between being a designer and being a user.

An architectonic design often has a clearly defined purpose and goal, one that is usually well known and built into the structure of the system itself. A tectonic design does not have an overall agreed-upon purpose or goal. The system can evolve in many directions and is therefore more difficult both to predict and to understand.

Most information technology artefacts are results of architectonic design principles. But, as the technology changes, so do the preconditions for new forms of artefacts and designs. With the Internet and cyberspace, we are moving into a situation where non-architectonic systems emerge and evolve.[4] Cyberspace is a good example of a tectonic system that in itself both invites and reinforces new tectonic designs.

Intended functionality and unintended use

When it comes to cyberspace, the inventiveness of people has been fascinating. Underlying cyberspace is, of course, a core technological system with limitations and a basic functionality. But cyberspace is an open system with a strong tectonic character. This tectonic character lends people to be creative and to find ways to continuously redesign and add new designs to the overall system. This is one reason why it has been difficult to predict the way people will make cyberspace usable. Interacting with a technology in this way can be labelled *bricolage*. Bricolage happens when users do not take a system for granted. A bricoleur is a person who tinkers with the technology by combining and adding functions and parts, and by exploring hidden possibilities in the technology that makes new use possible (Lévi-Strauss 1962).

In a study on identity and deception in virtual communities, Donath shows the very delicate relation between behaviour and technology (Donath 1999). Donath describes how the designed functionality of transferring and communicating identity on the Internet breaks down when people find ways to 'fool' the system and to take advantage of possible but not intended capacities of the basic technological structure. What the study shows is that the realm for possible innovation is much larger than was probably intended by the designers, and that people are very good at finding new ways to act, i.e. new possible actions, in that realm.

One interpretation of this study is that people are good at finding new ways to overcome the limitations of the technology. They invent new ways of making use of the technology's present structure and functionality. But this is too narrow an interpretation, since it is based on the assumption that technology should be judged by its *intended functionality*. Judgement of technology must instead be based on an understanding of the total space of possible actions it creates. Technology is polypotent and cannot be judged based on how this potency is brought to existence in one specific context (Sclove 1995).

The study by Donath shows how difficult it is to distinguish clearly between use and design. This is definitely the case with tectonic systems. Since an architectonic system has a clearly defined purpose and stable functionality, and is usually a closed system, the idea is not to let users be part of an ongoing design process. The reason for this is that allowing unmonitored user contributions to design may open up the design for unanticipated and possibly dangerous use. It might even threaten the stability of the design itself. A tectonic system is, as a result of its fundamental structure, less threatened by 'bad' or unintended use. Instead, it usually invites new creative uses and constant redesign.

Some principles of tectonic design

If we assume that tectonic designs are always under 'attack' from user creativity, and if we want to design sustainable systems, we have to build these systems based on design systems other than those common in architectonic design. Since architectonic design has been the model for almost all systems design, it is very difficult to escape the basic principles guiding this type of design. Examples of architectonic principles are the idea of a well-defined purpose, the idea of pre-defined functionality and the idea of a consistent interface throughout the system.

These principles serve in many cases well as design recommendations. But design principles must be intentionally chosen in relation to the intended purpose of the final design. If we are looking for a stable, purpose-based system with pre-defined functionality, architectonic principles are suitable. But when we are designing for large numbers of users, users we do not know, and especially when we do not know how and to what ends they may want to use the system, other principles are necessary.

One of my intentions in this chapter is to argue that it is possible to establish design principles based on tectonic-design ideas that better fit the idea of a public sphere in cyberspace, and of community building in particular. These principles, as they are presented here, are still very abstract and not operationalised into practical tools for design. I will present and discuss them only briefly and without any priority. The basic idea is to understand cyberspace as a tectonic system and to create a tectonic system that we have to design in accordance with the following ideas:

- *Diverse functionality*. This principle focuses on the idea that a system should be designed to be open to changing functionality. A rich and diverse repertoire of functions should be intentionally implemented. Functionality should also be understood as something changing over time, and as something amenable to change by the users themselves.
- *Bricolage*. Every user should be seen as a prospective bricoleur. Thus, the basic assumption should be that any attempt by users to change and

redesign the system is part of the process of establishing user-needed functionality and appearance.

- *Character*. In tectonic design – design that invites modification and redesign – there is also a basic system demand with certain specific characteristics. A tectonic system needs to be *robust* to withstand 'attacks' from users. It also should be *forgiving*, which means that it has some ability to accept changes without demanding complete safety.
- *Richness*. In a tectonic system, *richness* is more important than user-friendliness. A system whose purpose is to evoke creative and radical use must present a sufficiently rich and complex foundation. Creative and unexpected use is not produced in simplistic and easy-to-understand contexts. Tinkering and bricolage happens when things can be done in many different ways and with many different tools.

This first attempt to conceptualise some principles of tectonic design is based partly on empirical studies. But it is still only conceptual speculation that must be further empirically tested and studied.

Implications for the shaping of a public cyberspace

In what way does the idea of tectonic design and its principles have implications for the shaping of a public cyberspace? It has relevance in at least two ways.

First, it has implications for the practical design work aimed at creating a public cyberspace. If we take these design principles seriously, they can work as *conceptual guidelines*. They will not work as practical guidelines in the particular design situation, but they can provide intellectual support in the overall design process.

Second, the idea of tectonic design might have implications for some of the ideas currently circulating in the debate about how to create a public cyberspace. For instance, these design principles to some extent challenge the quite common ideas of 'best practice', participatory design and user-friendliness.

The idea of 'best practice' is that we can learn from the specifics in a particular situation. Usually this is done by 'copying' behaviour and actions from one situation and applying them in other situations. The idea is that we can use others' experience without having to make the same mistakes. This might be a good strategy, especially if we are working with systems of an architectonic character, since these systems are based on the idea that users have common needs. With a tectonic system, the idea of 'best practice' is not as valuable, since it is designed to be changed and redesigned. The notion of generally applicable design solutions has a different meaning when it comes to tectonic designs.

Participatory design is another approach that might not be as suitable for tectonic design as for architectonic. In the redesign of a tectonic system, it is the everyday user who changes the system. The user is not participating with the 'real' designers. There is usually no designated designer with a close relation to the user as in a truly participatory design approach.

User-friendliness has been a key concept in systems design over the last decades. The idea is to create a system that shows itself to the user in such a simple and friendly way that the user will be able to use the system as it was intended. A tectonic system does not necessarily have these attributes, since it will be changed all the time. Instead, richness and complexity seem to be basic preconditions for bricolage to appear in a constructive way.

There are some indications in previous research that the principles of architectonic design do not fully apply to systems in which the public is the user, and in which there is no natural and given functionality. The shaping of a public cyberspace is more about designing a foundation that allows for a rich and diverse functionality, and for the appearance of bricolage. Maybe public systems should be designed with a very strong emphasis on tectonic elements, and with a strong intention of providing a design that opens up a large space for possible actions.

In cyberspace, it is possible today to identify a huge variety of 'uses'. In many cases these innovative uses could be labelled 'designs'. This is, of course, still a very general speculation that needs to be examined and tested in real design projects, and also analysed in relation to successful examples of public spaces in cyberspace.

Is information technology the enemy?

Maybe we have put ourselves in an impossible position by asking how we should *use* the technology to create and support communities. Perhaps you cannot answer this kind of question with this technology. Maybe this is a question suitable for technologies of a more closed and architectonic character. A designable and tectonic technology cannot 'be' anything. People change it all the time. It constantly evolves and develops. We will never be able to reach a full understanding of it. We can trace technology use back in time, but not, in any detailed way, foresee its future use.

So where does this take us if we want to find ways to use this technology to support communities and a public sphere in cyberspace? There are at least two possible ways to do research in this field that can generate general knowledge applicable in a prescriptive way. The basic premise of these two approaches is that people all around the world actually seem to succeed in creating and supporting a wide variety of communities with the help of this technology. We have to study these attempts.

But we have to study how they deal with and approach the technology, rather than focusing on what they actually do when they use it. The specific 'use' is and will always be context- and situation-specific, and it will probably not be possible to produce abstractions in a way that can subsequently be used to produce general knowledge. The important thing, rather, is to try to find out *how people understand and approach the technology*. Since this technology is designable, it can never be moved from one community to another without being changed. This means that a tool or a specific use that is copied will not work the same way in two different places. The tool can and will be redesigned. The most important question is, therefore, what kind of knowledge and understanding of the technology is needed to create a good foundation for that kind of context specific redesigns?

This is also in line with Latour. We have to start at the middle working our understanding in an outward direction. There are no fixed ends. When we study technology, we have to study both it and the people who deal with it simultaneously. We have to create chains of *circulating reference* as Latour calls it (Latour 1999). These chains of circulating reference can create a strong and viable understanding of how people relate to and deal with technology.

Information technology is no enemy. It is a technology that can be consciously and deliberately designed. We have only to learn how to deal with a designable technology. We have to learn how to begin our studies in the middle ground. We don't have to find the 'best practices' by describing how people use a specific technology.[5] We have to study how the people behind a 'best practice' understand and deal with that technology. It is more a question of method than of tools or use. We have to accept that we cannot find answers to questions about *how* the technology should be used.

This means that we *can* work in collaboration with the technology. Working with a designable technology makes it possible to design and redesign that technology to fit its specific and unique context and purpose. But we need to find new ways to extract and formulate the generality involved in the existing examples of successful use.

One last word of warning: even if a designable technology seems to be open for an almost endless variety of designs, it still has a core. Maybe the core in information technology hides something that we cannot see today. In the core, there might be an 'enemy' just waiting to change the world slowly in ways we can't even imagine today.

Notes

1 'Conspiracy' is here used in its traditional meaning of 'breathing together', i.e. working together for the same purpose in a close relationship
2 This is not as simple as I have presented it here. What can be seen as functionality in one setting can, of course, be understood as something else in another setting. I am trying not to delve too deeply into the difficult subject of determinism versus constructivism, since that is not my main issue in this chapter.
3 In some technological fields, we can find similar concepts that deal with the 'openness' of technology, concepts such as customization and tailorability. These

concepts differ from the notion of designable technology and the idea of tectonic systems according to the degree to which they are truly open to change. Usually these concepts are used in the sense of superficial changes, i.e. changes that are made possible by the original designer. True designable technologies are, of course, not restricted to information technology. Customizing cars, remodelling houses, and redesigning gardens are all examples of 'users' changing technologies. There are many more complicated aspects of the difference between degrees of designability that I will leave out of this discussion for the moment.

4 Most tectonic systems based on a specific technology rest on a foundation of the technological infrastructure of a 'host' system. Usually this infrastructure is an example of an architectonic design. This is the case with the Internet. The tectonic character of the Internet is a result of an intentionally very stable and architectonic basic design.

5 Examples and 'best practices' do still have a purpose. They can be extremely important in showing that it is possible to do things and that it is possible to succeed. They can function as forms of inspiration.

Chapter 5

The technological story of a women's centre

A feminist model of user-centred design

Eileen Green and Leigh Keeble

Introduction

This chapter focuses on the experience of introducing information and communication technologies (ICTs) into two women's centres in the north-east of England.

With new forms of ICTs being announced almost daily, promising access to super highways of information, leisure and pleasure, the pressure on individuals to get connected to the Internet is intense. The impact of ICTs is apparent in many aspects of our everyday lives, at home and at work, in schools, shops, banks and universities. But many of us are still wondering how best to use them. How do we make sense of the increasingly bewildering array of IT goods and services on offer? Which do we actually need and will they really enhance the quality of our lives? These are just a few of the key questions facing us in the twenty-first century as we struggle with tasks like finding the best Internet provider, and ponder whether we can afford or need interactive television, or a mobile phone with access to the Internet. What is clear is that traditional forms of communication are being transformed by ICT access, with the majority of workplaces, many households and increasing numbers of community centres getting connected to the Internet to maximise communication networks. As Scott *et al.* (1999) argue, ICTs sit amid 'a set of highly complex technosocial networks, from which social, economic and cultural change seem to spread with increasing speed'.

Set against these developments is the potential that the ICT revolution is reproducing traditional lines of social inequality. Although the majority of the UK population has used a personal computer at some time and over half now own a mobile phone, fewer than a third of the population have accessed the Internet. There is evidence to show that Internet take-up in deprived neighbourhoods and amongst socially excluded groups is lower than the national average (PAT 15 2000). In the case of women, whilst they use the Internet in Britain in growing numbers and by summer 2001 were set to overtake men as the prime users (Ramrayka 2000), only one in three of Internet firms founded each month across Britain has a woman behind it

(Hyland 2000). In common with other businesses and industries, the proportion of women at board level of Internet companies is negligible. At the same time, types of use of the Internet vary between women and men, with more men using the Internet to find out about financial products or services. Online brokering is also an area dominated by men (Moss 2000). Research has found that women spend less time surfing the Net and prefer simpler websites with easy navigation facilities (*ibid.*). Our own research found that the women interviewed were looking for community- and family-focused information or support and were discouraged from accessing the Internet because of the difficulties they found in obtaining this type of information.

The lack of access to the Internet in deprived areas and the marginalising of women's interests and issues to commercial sites such as handbag.com are central to the issues which are discussed in this chapter. The case studies which form the empirical data are gathered from two women's centres which are based in high levels of social and economic deprivation in the north-east of England (DETR 2000). This chapter argues that these two characteristics – being a woman and living in a deprived area, limit opportunities. We argue that maintaining the women's centres in these areas is central to ensuring women's continued involvement in the Internet and its growing business and economic implications.

Feminists, among others, are concerned to ensure that women's interests are represented within the changing structures and have argued that the gender–technology relation is a crucial area of study. Because ICTs are transforming 'the everyday', its impact upon gender relations is critical; but we need to ask questions about technology as a social, as well as a technical, process and whether or how new technologies can meet women's needs. The reluctance of many women to readily embrace contemporary technologies, or their apparent 'self-exclusion' from computer-related activity, is often interpreted as 'technophobia'. However, an alternative interpretation suggests it to be a rational response to the highly gendered cultures of masculinity which surround such activities. It has been argued that technology consists of more than the artefacts (hardware) and software and should also include the physical space or the 'bodily inhabiting' of the former and the social relations surrounding its use (Vehviläinen 2001). Numerous studies have shown that women tend to be more interested in the uses to which technology can be put than in the technology itself (Suchman 1991, de Cindio and Simone, 1993), which could be related to what Mortberg (2000) refers to as negotiations about the 'borders and content' of technology.

This chapter addresses the issue of the everyday design of technological systems, asking questions about the potential for members of the community, and in this case women, to become involved in a user-centred process of community-based design. The first section briefly introduces the case studies and summarises theoretical perspectives which have embraced the issue of involving users in the design process. This draws upon both the interdisciplinary work of those involved in IT systems-development methodologies which emerged in the 1980s and the more recently established field of community informatics. We argue that, although they are committed to user-centred approaches and recognise that technologies emerge out of processes of choice and negotiation between relevant social groups of users, what these two theoretical perspectives share is a failure to analyse the specific nature and position of those user groups.

The second section of the chapter draws on evidence from our empirical case studies. We assess the potential of feminist approaches to provide a 'lens' through which to explore the ways in which community-based design of ICTs might empower women users and place them at the centre of the design circle. Examining the issues of geographies of access, women's skills and training, confidence and self-esteem, we conclude by demonstrating the importance of establishing and retaining women-only spaces as places where women can be empowered as creative designers and users of ICTs and not just trained for work.

Case studies

The decision to base our research in women-only centres, rather than more general community settings where access to ICTs is available for a wide range of individuals, reflects the aim of our study which was to listen to the voices of the women in a physical and social context. This empirical approach builds upon the work of Green et al. (1993), which documented the importance of women-only technology-design circles in enabling women workers to participate in the process of human-centred design of an office information system for a major public library. This approach acknowledges the early work of Vehviläinen (1986) on study circles and also complements her more recent work around the evaluation of NiceNet, an EC-funded, women-only IT group based in a community centre in eastern Finland, between 1996 and 1998 (Vehviläinen 2000). Geographers and social scientists have long argued the importance of space to social interaction (Rose 1993). It is argued that human agents through everyday routine tasks and across space reproduce social structure. Accordingly, 'space' and 'the everyday' is the arena through which gendered social relations are '(re)created' (ibid.: 17). Taking gender as a set of relational processes which organise social practices, we are interested in establishing what women use the technology for, and whether and how they considered that ICTs could enhance their lives. To achieve these aims we decided to base our study in places where women are and where traditional 'masculine' cultures of technology are less likely to be reproduced or created.

The two women's centres which form the basis of this research are located in towns with high economic and social disadvantage. Both centres have been established for a considerable period of time.

Case study A

The first centre in our study was created by local women for local women, to provide a space for women. The centre provides a range of activities, not least of which is its role as a drop-in centre for women, and is seen as a place where women can socialise with other women and, if needed, seek advice from professional workers.

The town in which the centre is based was created in the 1850s[1] and was formed around iron mining and steel production industries. It was built on hundreds of acres of reclaimed marshland to become one of the most prosperous towns in the north of England. The town grew from nothing to a thriving industrial and commercial centre in the space of only forty years and continued to prosper for over a hundred years.

However, the decline of the town was as dramatic and as rapid as its creation. After the Second World War, the iron and steel industry began to flounder. By the late 1970s and early 1980s, many of the industries based around the area were in major decline.

The town in the year 2001 is a very different community from that of the 1860s to 1960s. By 1991 the population had declined from over twenty thousand to only eight thousand. Statistics from the population census of 1991 indicate that 68 per cent of the households in the town had no car and 76.1 per cent of residents were classified as coming from socio-economic groups 3, 4 or 5. There is little evidence to suggest that these figures have changed much in the ensuing ten years. The high levels of deprivation were reflected in the index of Multi-Deprivation Score (DETR 2000) with the town ranking only 64 out of 8414 British towns. The town is characterised by high unemployment, poor housing, low educational achievement, rising crime and high levels of child poverty (DETR 2000).

The picture so far presented of the town indicates an area of hardship and potentially a deterioration of community and family life. However, the reality is that, despite all its hardships, the town is a place of great community spirit and the local people have a strong sense of belonging and commitment to the area. Over forty voluntary and community groups have grown in the town, providing a huge range of services and activities in the area, and major injections of regeneration funding have had an impact. Not surprisingly, the women of the town are very actively involved in the regeneration of their area, and such an involvement led to the creation of the Women's Centre.

Moving to new premises in 1997, the Women's Centre now has nine staff and eight sessional workers and is directed by a management committee of twelve women. The centre also has a large number of volunteers who are passionate and committed to their work and endeavour to make a difference to all the children, girls and women who access their facilities. The facilities in the centre include a crèche, three training rooms, a main hall, IT suite, kitchen, smokers' corner and two officers. Whilst providing training facilities and a crèche, the centre provides a range of other activities, including participating in local and national campaigning and lobbying.

The centre has quite a long history of providing computer facilities and courses. A local college started delivering courses via laptops in 1996. Since 1997, the centre has had fifteen PCs. The computing courses offered at the centre have traditionally been in great demand from the women, and women using the centre have had access to basic word-processing and spreadsheet courses. The computer suite is also available on a free-access basis when the PCs are used for correspondence and for homework purposes.

In 1999 the Women's Centre went online because the centre manager realised that many of the women using the centre had never experienced using the Internet or explored different types of software beyond traditional word-processing packages. Once the line was introduced, a series of awareness-raising sessions were held. Approximately forty women attended the sessions and for many that was indeed their first experience of using the Internet. Most importantly, the women who attended the awareness sessions already accessed the centre for different activities and were very quickly making links as to how the Internet might help with other activities and courses they were involved in. The cost of buying a computer for home was noted by many women as being a barrier to their use. The costs of being online were also an issue. Evidence also suggests that, even when families do have a computer in the home, the male and children in the family are more likely to get priority of use (Morahan-Martin 1998).

Owing to enthusiastic demand, the centre is now running additional IT courses in basic Internet use and web-page design. The centre anticipates extending its courses to desk-top publishing and other multimedia-type activities.

Case study B

The second Women's Centre in our study was also created to provide support and training to women. The centre offers a variety of courses and activities, including basic literacy and numeracy skills, interest groups and GCSEs. The principal aim of the Women's Centre is to provide educational opportunities in the form of short or part-time courses within family-friendly hours. The centre takes a holistic approach to the general well-being of individual women and children, promoting a positive attitude to lifelong learning and assisting independent living. Offering guidance, support, confidence-building and awareness-raising, it aims to identify and remove barriers and encourage women who have felt excluded to participate in courses and activities.

The socio-economic history of the city in which this centre is based is similar to that of the town in case study A. The city grew around the ship-building and coal industries. The demise of these industries has resulted in high levels of deprivation in some parts of the city. This deprivation is reflected in the Average of Ward Ranks produced by the DETR, the city ranking only 15 out of 354.

The Women's Centre is located in the city centre and provides services for women from all over the city. On average, 450 women use the centre for a range of courses and services every term (approximately every three to four months). Recently the women's centre has started providing courses for asylum-seekers who have been entering the city. It employs seven women and has a management committee of fourteen women from the local community.

The centre has been running basic IT skills and word-processing courses for a number of years, and some women have attended more advanced courses in spreadsheets, power point etc., which have been held at the local university. The centre does have three computers, one of which is now online. At the present time, the centre does not run any formal courses in relation to the Internet or web-page design. However, women have indicated their desire to participate in NVQ Level II in Telematics in the future.

Both the centres have similar broad aims, that is, providing a space for women to explore self-identified activities, including those that are IT-related. They also provide professional support and counselling for women wishing to access their services. However, perhaps most importantly, the centres provide a social place for women to meet other women, a place where they can escape the isolation of their homes. Like NiceNet, the Finnish women's group described in Vehviläinen's study (2000), who enthusiastically began with concrete tasks like making canning labels and Christmas cards with the help of a PC, and the Sheffield library workers who struggled to understand how prioritising their existing work-based practices in the new computerised system was a radical way forward, it is the contextualised use of technology which is important here. Building on the concept of technology design as a socio-cultural process which embraces local activities and practices, bottom-up design which enables individuals to inscribe their own identities or what Bourdieu (1986) refers to as cultural dispositions or 'habitus', into the technology process, is the key to making it a meaningful part of the everyday experience, and thus sustaining its use.

In the following section we examine the ways in which information systems and user-centred design have impacted upon women's lived experiences of IT.

Information systems and user-centred design

Tracing the roots of user-centred design involves a brief summary of the interdisciplinary work which informed innovative IT systems-development methodologies which emerged during the 1980s. This summary draws the links between radical computer-systems design, social shaping of technology approaches and human-centred systems design. The practical applications of radical computer-system developers working within the Scandinavian tradition (Suchman 1991, 1994) was complemented by 'social shaping' of technology and social constructivist (Bijker *et al.* 1987, Murray and Woolgar 1990 etc.) perspectives from within the social sciences; approaches which moved away from traditional, determinist models of technology. Critical of the latter, theorists who focused upon the social-shaping model explored the boundaries between the social and the technical (artefacts and processes), arguing that they were negotiated, not fixed or given. This type of perspective was an important element of the work of sociologists influenced by the work of Braverman (1974) in the UK, which became known as the Human Centred Systems approach (HCS). This perspective emerged alongside radical Scandinavian interventions such as the UTOPIA project (Bodker and Gronbek 1991, Bodker and Greenbaum 1993). It is also work which engaged with and responded to growing evidence from the 1970s that large-scale office-computer systems design and implementation was failing. Not only were the systems themselves proving to be inefficient but they rarely met the needs of the users involved (Hirscheim 1985). What were needed, it was argued, were perspectives which developed the social or user-relations aspects of the systems-development process (Friedman and Cornforth 1989). In the UK, although the HCS tradition represented a radical strand in research on the design and use of computers, it was *gender-blind*, arising as it did out of initiatives to create 'socially useful production' (Cooley 1987) and computer systems which enhanced human skill in manufacturing contexts (Rosenbrock 1989, Gill 1990). Such initiatives formed the priorities of trade-union-inspired work, which challenged large-scale redundancies within the manufacturing industry and were based upon a commitment to maintain and enhance human skill within the manufacturing process. Social-class inequalities were at the forefront of such politically inspired work, however: although women workers were included in the equation of critiquing restricted opportunities for training and skilled work within emerging IT-related work, gender was ignored (Green *et al.* 1993). HCS perspectives took 'human' as read: human was male and typically a skilled craftsman in printing or engineering.

The gender–technology relation

It was within this shifting theoretical and design application context that an emphasis upon the gender of the users, and in particular office workers, emerged, stemming from a feminist interrogation of what counts as technical (Webster 1990, Cockburn, 1992, Wajcman 1991) or technological. At a theoretical level such a focus brings together literature from a variety of sources, including the sociology of technology and the coming together of feminist-inspired debates on the family, households and the organisation of everyday life. This builds upon a now substantial body of literature emanating from what is often referred to as the 'gender and technology' debate (Henwood 1993), a debate based upon research in the 1980s into the effects of 'new' technologies on women's jobs. Over the last decade, this has evolved into a series of linked debates about what is commonly referred to as the gender–technology relation (Wajcman 1991, Grint and Gill 1995).

Pertinent questions within these debates include: is technology inherently masculine? Are technologies implicated in women's oppression, or might they provide the means for their liberation? And can we separate theoretical understandings of the gender–technology relation from the empirical contexts within which they are studied? In the 1980s the quest seemed to be to extrapolate the components of a feminist theory of technology from empirically grounded analyses which constituted gender relations as a key focus. Two decades later, such 'grand' theorisation continues to elude us; but it may be that the only gender–technology relations worth studying are those which are inextricably bound up with everyday practices. Diverting our attention from 'the everyday' in pursuit of 'grand theory' may be misplaced in contexts where those everyday practices are becoming transformed by newly available and increasingly 'domesticated' ICTs.

Perhaps the most well-known and often-cited work on the gender–technology relation is that provided by Cynthia Cockburn (1983, 1985), whose early work focused on the relationship between technological change, deskilling and gender inequalities. Cockburn's later work on the technology relation (1992) argues that feminists and social shaping theorists (particularly actor network theorists) are asking different questions. Feminists are concerned with the continuities of gendered social relations which manifest themselves through each successive wave of technological innovation, whereas more traditional sociologies of technology assume the key question to be the relationship between technological innovation and social change. In the context of the design of community based technological systems, feminists (Scott *et al.* 1999, Page and Scott 1999) are questioning whether women in the community may become excluded from 'everyday practices' of technology which ensure their access to communication networks.

What feminists working in the area come together on is the premise that, rather than perceiving technology as having 'social aspects', we need instead to work from a base which represents technology (in this case ICTs) as social. Rather than focusing upon the possibilities of new ICTs to achieve the extraordinary, we need to be guided by perspectives grounded in everyday life and remember instead that it is the capacity of ICTs to become a routine part of the mundane, which is important. Gender is clearly about social relations, and to understand the multiplicity of ways in which gender and technology interact with and shape each other we also need to perceive ICTs as social relations (Cockburn and Fürst-Dilic 1994).

Community informatics perspectives

Some more recent attempts to link the technological and the social are grouped around the concept of the community, and represented in the work of community informatics theorists (see for example Schuler 1996, Loader 1998, Gurstein 2000b). Like the user-centred design approaches of the 1980s, community informatics is radical in its focus upon empowering the community to connect cyberspace with community place, but the concept of community involved needs critical examination.

Loader *et al.* argue that community informatics is an approach which recognises the transforming qualities of ICTs together with the continuing importance of community as an 'intermediate level of social life between the personal (individual/family) and the impersonal (institutional/global)' (Loader, Hague and Eagle 2000). The emergence in recent years of a range of community-based projects which attempt to extend access to new information and communication technologies as a tool for supporting local and global communication suggests the need for such a community-informatics approach.

> Community Informatics is an approach which offers the opportunity to connect cyberspace to community place: to investigate how ICTs can be geographically embedded and developed by community groups them-selves to support networks of people who already know and care about each other.
>
> (Loader, Hague and Eagle 2000)

However, the community-informatics model is not without its problems: like the majority of the user-centred design perspectives discussed above, it neglects to analyse critically the gendered social relations which characterise community contexts. Whilst it may have the primary focus of empowering individuals within social networks by means of the adoption and exploitation of ICTs, we would argue that its fundamental assumption that technologies should be embedded within existing cultural and social relations is gender-blind. It remains unclear as to what extent electronic spaces are influenced, amongst other factors, by real-life spaces which are often gendered and exclusionary. That is to say, to be a member of a community network can often involve accepting a specific set of symbols, values and language in order to be accepted (Castells 1997). Thus it could be said that it is those who define those symbols, values etc. who 'shape' such communities and, therefore, people's abilities to join or to be excluded. It is important to remember that community networks can reinforce existing inequalities and create new constraints as well as provide liberating opportunities.

Community informatics and access

We would contend that there remains an underlying assumption that, simply by putting technology into a local community setting, access by women and men will be equal. Evidence suggests that this is not the case (Spender 1995, Shade 1998). We have already noted that women's access to new technologies such as the Internet has increased and continues to rise (Moss 2000). However, the goal of equal access enshrined in the HCS approaches of the 1980s and contemporary community informatics assumes individuals to be active citizens with an interest in using ICTs as soon as they are available. Advocates of community informatics question these findings. Walker (2000) acknowledges that community projects involving ICTs have led to significant increases in access, but notes that the majority of those who explore the technology to any great extent either in community settings or in their own homes, are 'still white, male and middle-class'. Perhaps therefore, the assumption underpinning current community access does not take account of the gendered relations that already exist in these social networks. Advocating equal access as the goal represents technology as a neutral (technical) force, rather than the site of different sets of competing cultures and discourses, which are shaped by different definitions of and meanings attached to the technology. We would suggest that improving access for women is dependent upon the type of community group through which access is being sought. By placing technology into existing male-dominated community spaces we are potentially in danger of replicating the exclusion of women from such spaces. Our research suggests that many groups, however they are formed, reproduce gender inequalities which impact on how individuals explore the potential of new technologies, that is, women and men take on preconceived gendered roles which potentially limit access for women.

Loader *et al.* (2000) identify the complexities and ambiguities associated with the term 'community'. Literature has suggested that the 'community' can be a place both for women's emancipation and for their imprisonment (Williams 1993, Mayo 1994). It also suggests that, for many women, some parts of the community have traditionally been their place and their space. In contrast, the view of cyberspace enthusiasts has suggested that the Internet does potentially offer a 'new public space' and 'virtual communities' which are non-gender-specific, supportive and empowering (Barlow 1996, Rheingold 1994). Although women are increasingly using the Internet, the communities being formed in cyberspace appear to be, at least in part, excluding women, thus rendering their voice inaudible and marginal (Spender 1995). If women are not exploring cyberspace in a similar manner to men, their impact on the formation of the new communities that the cyberspace enthusiasts and Spender (1995) allude to is limited. This exclusion could be further exacerbated in view of the current apparent demise of existing communities based on collective memory, history, culture and identity and the new post-modernist version whereby moral and emotional commitments are perceived to be personal rather than collective. Mullard and Spicker (1998) suggest that in postmodern society 'community is not assumed to exist but has to be constructed around redefined values' (*ibid.*: 133); the exclusion of women from cyberspace and the demise of traditional communities suggests that, unless they develop alternative means of making space for their own definitions of technology and technologically defined communities (Vehviläinen 2000) there will be little space left for women.

The community-informatics model, by introducing and developing ICTs in community groups can potentially act to ensure that women remain 'locked into locality' (Scott *et al.* 1999) instead of providing a space for emancipation. The roles that women take in these groups are generally ones that are viewed as traditionally belonging to females, that is, secretary and helper (Loader and Keeble 2000). This tendency to reproduce existing gendered roles in community settings means that women will remain underrepresented and relatively powerless in this virtual space. As such, women are potentially being 'trapped' within the shrinking sphere of their own local communities and not fully participating in the emerging global informational community that the new technologies herald.

Design for getting on with 'the everyday'

In order to examine the ways in which developing community-based ICTs can empower women, we need to begin with an analysis of their situated experience within the context of their everyday lives. This means developing models which prioritise the 'ordinary', 'unexceptional' aspects of those lives, lives which are traditionally bounded by social networks of kinship, caring and obligation (Finch 1989, Morgan 1996). We need to include the local and listen to women's narratives about the spaces and places in which the everyday occurs. As feminist geographers note: 'For feminists, the everyday routines traced by women are never unimportant, because the seemingly banal and trivial events of the everyday are bound into the power structures which limit and confine women' (Rose 1993: 17). For geographers the assignment of place within a 'socio-spatial' structure assigns particular roles which in turn indicate capacities for action and access to power and resources. If we link this discussion with the geographical communities or communities of interest referred to above, it becomes clear that, if women remain confined to the traditional 'spaces' often defined by men, their capacity for empowerment through linked ICTs will remain limited. This is not to say that women's sense of local space cannot be embedded within the technology itself, indeed Vehviläinen's work has shown how metaphors of feminine domesticity, such as 'bottling preserves' (Vehviläinen 2000), can be inscribed within technology via the creation of labels through mail-merge. This evokes the ease and comfort of the domestic kitchen, which offsets the unfamiliarity of the computer artefacts and exclusionary 'techie' language which surrounds their use.

Women-only spaces and geographies of access

Whilst we have argued that community informatics, as both a theoretical perspective and a practical application, is potentially gender-blind, we also note that there are examples where such an approach may be positively beneficial to women. We accept Scott *et al.*'s (1999) concern about the potential of individual access to 'result in holes being punched in communities of physical locality', but would argue from our initial research that women-only centres are places where ICTs are being integrated into the everyday lives of users. We would argue that such centres which prioritise adhering to established strong aims and objectives potentially reinforce the notion of a strong community of physical locality which the technology can enhance rather than fragment. Women-centred networks reproduce and strengthen bonds of affection and support and they also function to produce, share and exchange resources (Balbo 1987) and perhaps more important, act as important sites of resistance to prevailing cultures of masculinity which have become embedded in technology. Many men also resist such traditionally masculine identities, as the following quotation from a male library worker in the Sheffield study commenting upon the shared understandings which developed between men who regularly played with the technology out of office hours, suggests: 'It's a bit more complex . . . I think that those men do [that], do it because they have no inhibition about being that sort of man . . . and the way you learn is to spend hours in front of a screen, and they've got hours to spend in front of screens!' (Green *et al.* 1993: 144).

ICTs can help to expand and strengthen a broader range of community networks (Page and Scott 1999). However, we are not suggesting that simply placing ICTs into women-only centres will ensure a sudden equalising of use of new technologies. The situation is far more complex than that. The women's centres which form the basis of our research do, as we have discussed, create space for women to explore their own interests and provide opportunities for women to meet other women and share their experiences, including their experience of ICTs. Another potential benefit to the actual space in the centres is that they are designed by the women themselves and may encourage ICT design. As such, they are not necessarily subject to the same codes and pressures that male-designed space can impose on women. The centres in our study provide a huge range of services which are often unique and vital; the diversity of services and facilities on offer in the women's centre was also found in other similar facilities (Page and Scott 1999).

The physical location of the centres are important in as much as they are accessible by local women but, perhaps more significantly, they offer a relaxed environment in which women can just 'be'. As one woman in a focus group described it, 'well it's the place as well, it's safe, relaxed – you feel relaxed'. This sense of safety and relaxation and being able just to be yourself was continually discussed by the women. Whilst they may not always able to identify why, the women were extremely conscious of a different atmosphere in the centres, and it would seem that this led them to explore activities which they had not previously considered. We would argue that this informal, relaxed environment that the women discussed represented an everyday environment and, as argued by Rose (1993: 22) 'examining the lives of women requires attention to the ordinary, to the unexceptional, because most women are excluded from arenas of power and prestige'.

This feature or aspect of the women's centres is equally important in relation to the women exploring new technologies. First, the 'placing' of the technology into this everyday environment suggests everyday use. Second, the relaxed atmosphere boosts the women's confidence and self-esteem and allows them to overcome their 'fear' of, or resistance to, the technology, and potentially enables them to strengthen existing, everyday practices which they value. Using the technology to enhance their ability to maintain links with family and friends creates a social space for women to act out active citizenship, and reminds us of the fluidity of the boundaries between what is considered to be the 'technical' and the 'social'. It is important, as Ormrod argues, 'to specify technology and gender as social processes where their boundaries and content are negotiated rather than pre-existing' (Ormrod 1995: 39): boundaries which are as much constituted by the placing of artefacts, as they are by the social relations of their use.

Locating the technology

In case study A, the computers are located in a separate room. However, the room is not set out in a similar manner to a classroom – the machines are placed around the edge of the room. The computers in this room are the only ones in the centre which are linked to the Internet. The remaining computers in the administration office have only office software on them. The issue of where the computers were placed in the centre was extremely important to the project manager. She was keen that they were not too separate from the other activities of the centre: they were to be an integrated part of the centre's work, not an 'add-on'.

The computers in case study B are situated in the main room near the entrance to the centre; located in front of a window which overlooks the street. Again, the project manager felt that the computers needed to be an integral part of the centre, so the room in which they are located is at the hub of the project's activities. In both, the aim has been to integrate the new technologies into the everyday organisation and activities of the centre.

Several UK governmental policies have been developed to try to achieve increased use of ICTs. Within those policies, is an implicit assumption that future jobs and employment opportunities are linked to computing skills. The apparent lack of computing skills by women suggests that women are making the wrong choices in education or in the job market (Bergman and van Zoonen 1999). For women to participate fully in the emerging information society both as employees and as what Scott *et al.* (1999) identify as 'full citizens and key agents', the issue of access to the technology needs examining. In particular, we believe that consideration needs to be given to examining how access needs vary between women and men (potentially also between individuals from different ethnic groups, different age groups etc.). However, we would argue that introducing ICTs in the women-identified types of spaces such as those in our case studies offers potential for women to explore and develop a range of self-identified skills and interests, which are not necessarily relevant to the gendered world of work. Such centres have the potential to empower women thorough increased networking opportunities. They might also offer opportunities for different types of employment for women, either from home or in community groups (Dyson 2000). Perhaps most crucially, the centres offer women the opportunities to explore the new technologies in a safe environment which is created around their own needs and values.

Women's confidence and self-esteem

The evidence from the pilot project supports earlier research (Dyson 2000) suggesting that for many women, particularly women returners, low levels of confidence and the lack of self-esteem is a major barrier to them accessing more traditional forms of education, especially in relation to information technology. Many of the women in our study acknowledged their lack of confidence and discussed their 'fear' of the new technologies. They also reiterated the importance of the centres in helping them overcome some of these fears.

> I think it's very difficult you know to sort of get started when you've been out of education for a while and you know your lifestyle, your housework you get out of the way you know of learning, your confidence is quite low, its difficult you know, it can be quite threatening when you go into a college.
> I think it is also to do with confidence though and your own self-esteem.

The women's centres offer the women a place in which they feel able to experiment: 'they don't patronise you, don't make you feel as if you are being stupid'. The environment and the support which the women receive both from the workers and from other women accessing the centres appears to give them confidence.

> it's just relaxing isn't it you're not frightened to say oh look I've done this or I've done that what do I do now, or can you tell us which way . . . You're not made to feel stupid. I mean in here they understand . . . It is absolutely brilliant, they are very understanding.

If P is busy there's somebody already to come up and show you what to do – it's great. It's that relaxed that you feel more confident with yourself I think. And we laugh about each other when you do something stupid so you just laugh about it and you don't feel stupid . . . it's great.

As discussed earlier, Balbo (1987) demonstrated how women-centred networks tend to be extremely supportive and encouraging: evidence of such support was clearly evident in our work. Dyson, in her evaluation of the Manchester Women's Electronic Village Hall (EVH), also demonstrates how women-only facilities can improve women's self-confidence, arguing that 'only another woman can restore another woman's confidence' (2000: 36). However, Dyson also notes that women-only provision should not be available merely for issues related to self-confidence. She suggests that such provision allows women to see themselves in new ways and to envision training, technology and society in general in new ways.

Women's skills and training

Whilst we consider that the introduction of new technologies in the women's centres should not simply be about improving women's skills, the high levels of economic and social deprivation in the areas surrounding both centres are characteristic of socially excluded communities. These levels of social exclusion are underlined for many of the women by their lack of computing skills and their need to be wage-earners. Some of the women are seeking employment after long periods of domestic and childcare responsibilities. McGivney (1994) argues that employment prospects are directly related to a person's previous employment. A lack of up-to-date skills restricts employment opportunities; this is particularly pertinent in the field of information and communications technology, which is developing and progressing at a rapid rate. Women who lack such skills can therefore incur considerable financial and career penalties (McGivney 1999). These concerns were aptly expressed by one woman who noted: 'I think as well when you don't work there's this awful fear that your skills are just not that current any more and you are lagging further and further behind and it is worrying. The whole new technology has just passed me straight by.'

Low expectations, career breaks and employment histories of unskilled or low-skilled, low-paid work, result in many women lacking the necessary qualifications and experience to access more 'traditional' education provision. In addition, cultural and institutional barriers can act to exclude women from more traditional classroom environments. This point was addressed by one of the women now studying at a women-only facility after attending a more formal course run by a local provider:

> it's very intimidating there because you get all these computer types, you know, people who are obviously very computer-literate and just switch it on and I'm thinking, oh my god, how do I log on and what do I do . . . obviously the teacher can't be with you all the time, you know.

What was apparent was that many of the women were acutely aware of their lack of knowledge of ICTs. They were conscious of 'missing out' on something and were aware that the introduction of new technologies such as the Internet represented part of a 'technology-led' future which could easily find them left behind. The following are just two examples of the ways in which the women expressed their concerns about not keeping up to date, especially in relation to the skills which their children are learning.

> they have got a computer and the Internet at the nursery, that's like 3-year-olds, they can go to the toddler group from 18 months, so from 18 months they can be using the computer. There was a girl, she was just gone 3, in the toddler group and she was sitting playing with the mouse. Clicking things and moving them around. She was not even watching the mouse when she was doing it, she was just watching the screen.
>
> It's so important to get used to computers these days. You're almost terrified that if you fail then that is going to be it. It's like not learning to read, my god, I'm not going to be able to function in this society . . . Especially with the children being so good – I mean, I don't know anything.

Directly linked to the issue of skills and training is the type of teaching and training methods undertaken by the women's centres. A key finding emerging from our research relates to the teaching methods, both formal and informal, used at the women's centres.

Bostock and Seifert (1987) state the case for women tutors in women-only environments. First, the tutor acts as a role model, and second, women tutors' attitudes towards their students are different from their male counterparts'. The importance of getting the 'right' tutors for formal training at the women's centres was clearly expressed by one of the project managers:

> it's not just getting on with the women but it's knowing what the women's centre is about which is really important to us and if we haven't got women who are sensitive to that then I don't even want them . . . for a tutor, enthusiasm, a sense of respect for the women, somebody who speaks very simply and doesn't try to complicate things, someone who doesn't speak down to them that has a good relationship with them, somebody with a sense of humour and somebody that's quite sensitive to all the issues like ageism, you know, sexism.

Equally, the women themselves expressed the importance of the right sorts of tutors, in particular in relation to the informal support they receive from the women's centres: 'she explains things in words you can understand, she doesn't use the jargon'. The evidence emerging suggests that the gender and attitude of teachers is extremely important to the women at the centres. Where the centres have had bad experiences with tutors, the numbers of courses have declined dramatically. Accordingly, the staff at the centres continuously strive to identify women who will work with women in a facilitating and empowering way.

Conclusion

The evidence emerging from our research suggests that the women's centres in our study provide women with opportunities to explore new ICT experiences in a safe environment in which they are not judged or criticised. One woman encapsulated these feelings when she discussed her experiences in a more formal training environment:

> The tutor said to me, he said, what do you do and I said, I'm a housewife, and he said, well what do you do all day, I mean what do you do all day . . . I remember once I hadn't logged on properly, I'd got into the hard disk instead of the A disk or whatever and the tutor announced, 'she hadn't logged on properly'. I felt he was saying this stupid woman who doesn't look quite sure what she does all day, but she does not know how to log on.

Williams contends that it is important that we should 'understand . . . the "networks and communities of value" which we inhabit, through which some of our needs for "due recognition" might be met' (1999: 675). It has been argued that the prospects for ICT-facilitated empowerment of citizens are dependent upon embedding electronic networks within existing social, economic and political community networks (whether geographic communities or communities of interest) (Hague and Loader 1999). Community networks, which Williams identifies as 'networks and communities of value' (1999), establish ownership of the technology and control over the uses to which it is put at the community level. However, ICTs are subject to social shaping and, as such, are embedded within a variety of often conflicting discourses and might be harnessed in pursuit of a variety of competing objectives. We believe that it is vital to identify those 'values' that are central to the pursuit of an empowerment agenda and to locate those values within contextualised environments. For some women, women-only spaces offer 'safe', comfortable environments which can place women in the centre of the design circle. Spaces such as women-defined and women-owned centres provide a unique setting within which women can participate in the design of technologies which enhance and extend their own aims and objectives. It is essential for women to retain and improve upon access to their own gendered cyberspace; women-only spaces are but one part of such a strategy.

Much of the work of the Community Informatics Research & Applications Unit (CIRA)[2] is focused on small, locally based voluntary and community organisations that are characterised by an ethos of self-help or mutual aid. We would argue that the latest ICTs potentially lend themselves to increased bureaucracy and the entrenchment of existing gendered power relations, just as much as they do to user-empowerment and the promotion of more democratic outcomes. The direction which is taken is highly dependent upon the social values that shape their design and implementation.

Whilst the culture of smaller and locally focused organisations renders them potentially well placed to utilise ICTs in pursuit of community empowerment, alternative agendas in relation to ICTs are pursued within these organisations which can also marginalise groups such as women. Ultimately, exploiting the full potential of ICTs for all citizens may be dependent upon how successfully the underpinning values of the groups can be promoted and defended.

Notes

1 The historical information about the town was produced by Sian Basker, CIRA, University of Teesside, and Linda Taggart, Women's Centre. The information was presented at the ESRC Seminar 'Community-based initiatives for women: Democratising ICTs', which is part of the seminar series 'Equal opportunities online: the impact of gender relations on the design and use of information and communication technologies.' The paper was entitled 'Embedding ICTs in Grass Roots Women's Organisations.'

2 The Community Informatics Research & Applications Unit (CIRA) was established by the University of Teesside to investigate and analyse critically the social and economic factors shaping the development and application of new information and communication technologies (ICTs), such as the Internet, and their consequences for community-development, economic restructuring and social exclusion. It is a multidisciplinary unit where social scientists, computer scientists, software engineers, project managers and designers are encouraged to combine their respective talents on particular research projects.

Chapter 6

The safety Net?

Some reflections on the emergence of computer-mediated self-help and social support

Nicholas Pleace, Roger Burrows, Brian D. Loader, Sarah Nettleton and Steve Muncer

Introduction

By the mid-1990s commentators such as Rheingold saw in computer-mediated communication (CMC) the chance for a new form of social interaction, in which relationships were not limited only to those people one physically met. Like-minded people in cyberspace could form 'communities of shared interest' and relationships that were unconstrained by time and space (Rheingold 1993a, 1996). Some also thought that the virtual environments within which CMC took place could be seen as small 'societies' in which new behaviours were emerging (Dibbell 1996, Reid 1994, 1996). For the Electronic Freedom Foundation (www.eff.org), CMC offered, and still offers, the potential for an effectively ungoverned hyper-individualistic liberal 'e-society'.

Yet in the late 1990s, when the Internet became accessible to others besides the North American upper-middle class and academics that had been using it and talking about social, political and cultural revolution, the predicted social changes failed to emerge. The rise of CMC was not insignificant, but it was having mixed effects rather than causing the absolute change that had been predicted. At the time of writing, in the reality of mass access to the Internet, the talk of one form of revolution has been largely replaced by talk of another, that of e-commerce. In turn, as the reality of e-commerce settles down and is understood, some of the wilder claims of the end of all shops being just around the corner (Leebaert 1999) will be replaced with more reasoned discussion of what will again emerge as mixed and sometimes limited effects.

Before mass access to the Internet arrived, there were those who thought they foresaw a social problem rather than the positive revolution seen by commentators such as Rheingold. Varying degrees of decline in social interaction were predicted as a result of the emergence of cyberspace, with the 'postmodern turn' in the social sciences arguing that simulations and representations of reality may increasingly be preferred to 'real' social interaction. Just like television before it, the Internet was seen as keeping people inside their homes following 'inauthentic' synthetic image-centred relationships, when they should have been outside forming 'real' relationships and interacting with one another in the flesh (Kraut et al. 1998).

Again, this breakdown in normal social interaction through living a 'virtual life' seems to have failed to arrive with mass access to the Internet. Of course, it's relatively early days yet, but it may be the case that, rather than blurring the lines between the real and virtual and undermining our relationship with the 'real', the Internet has instead become another channel, perhaps even just another, albeit more elaborate, shopping channel. Again, this does not mean that the effects of the Internet on social interaction are unimportant, but simply that they seem set to be less extreme and more mixed than the whole-sale change in social interaction that some predicted at a time before mass access to the Internet was in place.

In summary, the Internet is unlikely to cause either a massive social revolution or a massive social problem. Rather, as Wellman and Gulia (1999) and Parks and Floyd (1996) argue, the impact is likely to be more varied and less extreme than the early commentators expected. What seems to be occurring is a much more complex and subtle interaction between individuals and technology as CMC is absorbed into daily life (Nettleton et al. 2001).

So the revolution is not coming, or rather it has arrived and it is not what we expected it to be. Yet at the same time, the convergence of ever-cheaper digital technologies means that the Internet will become ubiquitous, making the potential impacts of CMC difficult to ignore. These impacts will be varied, perhaps sometimes subtle, and perhaps even sometimes rather mundane.

One area in which CMC may have quite significant impacts is that of social policy. The use of newsgroups and other forums for CMC for virtual self-help or social support is a potentially significant development. The potential of computer networks to function as mutual support networks was recognised early on by medical researchers in North America, and there were early experiments with people with HIV (Boberg et al. 1996) and cancer (Weinberg et al. 1995). However, as Denzin (1998) observes, the combination of a positive attitude towards technology and an orientation towards 'self-help' in the US soon led individuals to begin setting up their own online self-help groups. Studies have been conducted in the US examining self-help groups for people recovering from child abuse (Mousand 1997), disabled people (Finn 1999) and recovering alcoholics (King 1994). The development of online self-help groups with a UK focus soon followed (Burrows and Nettleton, 2000). This self-help is part of the widespread health-related activity on the Internet. By some estimates, the second most common use of the Internet, after sex-related activity, is in seeking health and health related information (*Guardian* 1999, Eysenbach et al. 1999).

To understand the impact of the use of CMC for self-help and social support, which can be broadly described as computer mediated social support

(CMSS), it is of central importance to understand the context within which these technologies have arisen. CMSS arrived in a context in which its capacity to allow for increased self-reliance is in tune with a general movement towards increased self-reliance in society. To use the sociological argot, it could be argued that there is a powerful *elective affinity* between the techno-logical facilitation of new modes of being and social connection on the one hand and broader social processes of individualisation on the other. Family and other social networks are less robust than they perhaps once were, governments have taken a decision to reduce the size and scope of the welfare states, politicians seem unable to manage economies in a globalised world effectively, science seems less and less capable of dealing with disease and other problems, and consequently we feel increasingly on our own. It could be argued that CMSS gives us something new to turn to. The benefits of CMSS for those using it can be extensive. Help, advice, support and information are all available via CMSS and sometimes in forms that were not available before. Centrally, CMSS can potentially offer individuals access to a supportive peer group with *shared needs and experiences* on an almost constant basis (Burrows *et al.* 2000).

However, like the other changes that are arriving with mass access to the Internet, CMSS seems unlikely to be a revolution. People remain physically distant from each other and this limits the extent to which they can provide each other with some forms of social support, particularly practical support (Muncer *et al.* 2000). In addition, CMSS often takes place in unregulated environments, in which various risks are attendant (Burrows *et al.* 2000). Most fundamentally, many of those individuals with health and social care needs who are in a situation of socio-economic disadvantage seem unlikely to get Internet access or the right sort of Internet access to use CMSS, which may have set a limit on any effects it might have.

Computer mediated social support and the new insecurities

Globalisation, which is a shorthand term for the speed with which capital can now move between locations and sectors of the economy, is widely regarded as creating a new type of social insecurity. These movements of capital, aided by developments in information and communication technologies in what Castells calls the *informational economy* (1996), create unemployment and insecurity of employment as capital moves rapidly from one economic sector to another, and one area to another, chasing profits. In an attempt to retain and encourage investment, developed economies have generally aimed to reduce taxation levels and employment costs. This has created a situation in which most developed economies have reduced the extent of their welfare states at the same time at which increased unemployment and insecurity have arisen as a result of globalisation (Jordan 1996).

For Giddens (1994), the crucial point is that this economic uncertainty has been accompanied by general uncertainty. Science is now viewed with suspicion as environmental and other damage caused by what were regarded as 'advances' has become apparent and this mistrust has spread towards 'professionals' and traditional authority more generally. Religion, ideology and tradition have become harder and harder to relate to the instability of daily life, and national politicians seemingly have little power to reverse the change from economic certainty to uncertainty. Giddens argues that citizens in this situation have had to become increasingly reflexive. They must find their own path to economic and ontological security, becoming as self-reliant and as adaptable as possible to find their way through an uncertain world.

It can be argued that, when CMSS was introduced into this situation, it provided individuals with access via a tool with which to live an increasingly reflexive life (Burrows and Nettleton 2000). If one is worried about whether one's doctor knows what they are doing, or whether one's health authority is actually providing the best treatment for one's health problem, it is simply a matter of looking it up on the Internet. It has been reported that GPs already have patients who arrive at the surgery with printouts about their condition and the treatments available (Hardey 1999). Computer-mediated social support provides access to another form of data, the experience of others in the same position as oneself. In a context in which orthodoxy and tradition have become increasingly questioned, those with uncertainty about conventional approaches can instead draw on *shared experience*.

The forms of computer-mediated social support

Computer-mediated social support is a form of self-help conducted via a number of different forms of CMC using the Internet, Usenet and the World Wide Web. Fora for CMSS function by *sharing experiences* and by providing *emotional support*.

It is important to draw a distinction between CMSS which has its origins in self-help (Denzin 1998) and the provision of scientific information and services by professional bodies on the Internet. NHS Direct (www.nhsdirect.nhs.uk), for example, is the provision of health information by professionals. Similarly, online medical databases such Medline and other publicly accessible records of professionally endorsed peer-reviewed information do not constitute CMSS. Internet-based service provision by the voluntary sector, such as the use of the Internet by the Samaritans (www.samaritans.org.uk/), is professional and organised care service delivery, not the virtual self-help that can be described as CMSS.

Although health and health-related concerns remain the predominant focus of CMSS, it is not restricted to these areas. Two examples of this in the UK are the use of Usenet for sharing and providing information on parenting (uk.people.parents) and the use of the Internet to provide self-help to people who are having their homes repossessed (www.home-repo.org/).

The main means by which CMSS is provided and accessed are probably the newsgroups that are accessible via Usenet (www.usenet.org/) and which in recent years have also become accessible via the Web through sites such as deja.com (www.deja.com/usenet/). A newsgroup is an asynchronous form of CMC that is in effect an electronic notice board that allows individuals to 'post' messages to which other individuals can then respond. A series of messages on the same topic, grouped by their subject, become a 'thread' and an active newsgroup may contain many threads at once (M. Smith 1999). The newsgroups on Usenet that exist for CMSS range from the long-established and highly active US groups such as alt.support.depression or misc.health. diabetes or alt.parenting.solutions through to the more recent British additions on the UK Usenet (www.usenet.org.uk/) such as uk.people. disability, uk.people.parenting, uk.people.support.cfs-me or uk.people. support.depression. Some use is also made of email mailing lists, which are also sometimes known as mailbases or discussion lists. The Listz search engine at www.listz.com/ lists almost a hundred thousand mailing lists, a significant number of which deal with a variety of health and social care topics.

Interactive websites are also used for CMSS. Sometimes individuals organise groups of resources for other people with a shared problem, which might also be combined with newsgroup or similar facilities and other forms of CMC accessible via the website. Two examples would be the AAMolly website set up by a recovering British alcoholic to help others with alcohol problems (members.aol.com/aamolly/aamolly.html) and, again, the UK Home Repossessions page. These sites offer email interaction and may have web-based newsgroups and chat facilities. In some instances, individuals use the Web also to convey their own experiences of dealing with a health problem in a way that is not really interactive, using a website to tell their own story. It is difficult to classify such sites as self-help or social support because they are not interactive, but they nevertheless perhaps fall into what could be broadly described as CMSS (Hardey 2000).

Those technologies allowing synchronous communication, perhaps best understood as typed conversations, such as Internet Relay Chat (IRC), the text-based virtual realities such as Multi-User Domains (MUDs) are less widely used. However, Mousand (1997) has examined the use of a MUD by adult survivors of child abuse, and research carried out by the current authors has looked at the use of an IRC room by people recovering from an alcohol dependency; more recently there has been work looking at an IRC room for problem drinkers (Pleace et al. 2000).

The nature of CMSS varies between different virtual environments. Some groups have a much clearer focus on information, in Usenet terms being 'on-topic', while others are characterised by often being 'off-topic' and by containing exchanges that are more about play, social companionship and friendship than the exchange of information (Danet *et al.* 1998, Muncer *et al.* 2000; Pleace *et al.* 2000). The types of exchanges that take place in fora providing CMSS can perhaps best be categorised into two main types – *informational* and *emotional*. Informational messages are those concerned with the sharing of personal experiences and other information, but not intended to provide emotional support to any single individual. Emotional messages on the other hand are designed to provide emotional support or reinforce relationships between individuals. In broad terms, this also includes the playful exchanges that are such a strong feature of much CMC (Danet *et al.* 1998).

Although these two types of exchange can obviously co-exist within the same newsgroup, Muncer *et al.* 2000 found that a newsgroup for people with depression was largely, although by no means exclusively, characterised by emotional exchanges while another, for people with diabetes, was almost entirely devoted to informational exchanges. Both groups had a high volume of traffic, but, while the depression group had a core of regular users, the diabetes group was characterised by a greater number of individuals visiting on a more infrequent basis.

In the following informational exchange, an individual has posted on one of the many newsgroups on Usenet dealing with depression a request for information on the side-effects of a drug they have been prescribed.

First Post
Well I finally got the courage up to ask my doctor to prescribe me something for my constant anxiety and worrying. He has started me on 10 mg of [name of anti-depressant] once a day for a month. He wants me to come back in about 3 weeks and see him. What kind of experiences have people had on this medication? Good – Bad or what? Is there a better time of day to take the medication? Morning or Evening?

I have only been on it for 24 hours and I don't seem to have any of the side-effects that he told me about – do they show up later? (I just had a little trouble getting to sleep last night.)

Today, I did feel much happier than I usually do, I don't know if that is just a matter of finally feeling like I am doing something to get better or is the [name of anti-depressant] working that fast?

Second post (in response)
I've been taking [name of anti-depressant] since '93 and, at first, I had trouble falling and staying asleep all night; I would fall asleep then wake up 4 hours later and not be able to fall asleep again, so I started taking [name of anti-depressant] in the morning and, after a while, I had no problems with falling asleep and staying asleep all night. Maybe you should try to take [name of anti-depressant] in the morning to see if your sleep patterns change.

The original poster who was asking about the effects of an anti-depressant received nine posts in response, all of which were based on the experience of other people who had been prescribed it. The exchanges were informal and quite friendly, but they were concerned with exchanging information based on personal experience for social support and not with providing emotional support.

The following post, also from a newsgroup concerned with depression, is emotional. In this instance, someone has detected tension building up to a possible argument between two of the participants and is trying to defuse the situation.

> I like you two. Do you think it would be best if you didn't carry on this thread – it's just I recall comments between you stating you rubbed one another up the wrong way. I know how Scarf gets upset sometimes in relation to Fluffy as she is caring, and, speaking personally, I feel Fluffy is a nice person, yet sometimes people want to reach out to Fluffy, and she cannot accept it, as she gets into a very negative state about herself. Now I'm not criticising Fluffy, or telling her what to do or how to behave. I'm just trying a bit of conciliation for you two, as its a shame to see two people becoming upset, especially when I view it as the depression and not the person inside causing the hostility.
>
> I wish you both the best
>
> ((((Scarf)))) (((((Fluffy)))))
>
> Raven

Neither information nor experience is being exchanged. Instead, someone is trying to mediate in a dispute between two of their (virtual?) friends. The individual with the nickname 'Raven' also 'hugs' the other two individuals involved, called Scarf and Fluffy, which is denoted by the use of multiple parentheses on either side of their names at the bottom of the post.

The way in which individuals use CMSS varies according to their experience and attitudes and the type of fora that they visit. We suggest that participation in CMSS can be classified as falling into one of two broad types: *passive* and *active*. *Passive participants* are individuals who simply read the posts in newsgroups that provide CMSS or visit websites with a CMSS function but never send messages or provide information themselves. In Usenet terms, this group is referred to as 'Lurkers' (M. Smith 1999). *Active participants* on the other hand are individuals who provide information or who comment upon the information provided by others.

Each individual using CMSS might stay consistently within one pattern of behaviour or might change over time or behave differently in various virtual contexts. An active participant in one newsgroup may be a passive participant in another newsgroup. A topic of concern to an individual, or a crisis point in their or someone else's life, might also lead a generally passive participant into a period of active participation. Just as individuals could move from passive to active forms of participation in CMSS, they could also become involved in both informational and emotional exchanges.

Mixed effects? Experiencing CMSS

In order to understand how people are beginning to experience CMSS we interviewed (face to face, by telephone and via CMC) a total of fifty-one people with a range of experiences to relate. They were recruited in a number of different ways. Some agreed to participate after being approached by us via email following our observations of their postings on a number of the newsgroups and discussion lists. Others were recruited by 'opting in' to the study following postings made by ourselves to a number of different newsgroups. The sample is thus unlikely to be representative of all UK-based users of CMSS but it is certainly diverse enough to explore in a meaningful way a range of different analytic issues (for a more detailed discussion see Nettleton *et al.* 2001). The sample contained twenty-one men and thirty women based throughout the UK with a diverse range of ages, incomes, household circumstances and many different health and social support needs. All had in common some experience of using the Internet for CMSS of some kind. The greater number of women than men in the sample may simply reflect the nature of our sampling strategy and the form and content of the virtual fora from which the sample was recruited. However, and perhaps not surprisingly given what we know about the highly gendered nature of informal health and social care work, health is the one category of online information that is accessed more commonly by women than by men (Eysenbach *et al.* 1999) and, consequently we may also expect more women than men to be using CMSS.

There is now a broad consensus that social support can have a beneficial effect on health and well-being. According to the 'buffer' theory, social support is held to protect people from the stresses of life, while according to the 'main effect' model, social support acts constantly on self-esteem and one's sense of well-being. In essence, the argument is very simple: people with good friendships, family relationships and sexual relationships are both less likely to become ill and more likely to recover from illness than people who lack such relationships, other factors being equal (Cohen and Willis 1985, Callaghan and Morrissey 1993). Clearly, if CMSS can augment or replace otherwise inadequate social supports, it is reasonable to suggest that it can have a beneficial effect on those using it. Referring to the US, Finn (1999) has argued that the sheer proliferation of self-help groups both off and on the Internet illustrates that they are providing the people using them with benefits. For many of the active participants taking part in the research, the social supports offered by CMSS were a major attraction and benefit. For example, one woman in her twenties said:

It's hard to explain, I used to get very depressed but being with other people on the Net has helped a lot. People are very supportive and club together. If I see something that I know someone else on the groups I use would like, I either post it or email them privately depending on what it is, and others do the same. We provide emotional support for each other too and some groups meet in real life every now and then.

Shared experiences, in terms of life events, such as recently having had a child, or having shared health problems, was one of the major attractions for the individuals using CMSS. The shared understanding that is a central feature of CMSS was in itself supportive according to some of the people who participated in the research. When this shared understanding was coupled with the ability to communicate anonymously and at a physical distance, it could make some online support groups very helpful to those who participated in them. As another female respondent put it:

It's, instead of getting you know twelve people in a room who've all had the same experience and you sit there and talk about it . . . you become more intimate more quickly this way because people will post things that perhaps they wouldn't say on the first night. I mean I'm sure you've been to meetings and you walk in and nobody says anything for ages and everybody's a little bit frightened to say something, whereas a keyboard in front of you it's very easy to write, type in, exactly what you're feeling and without, honestly without that board I would have gone crackers in that first week especially, I wasn't sleeping till sort of two, three o'clock in the morning.

For some passive participants, CMSS was more about the gathering of information than emotional support or friendship, but they nevertheless generally felt that they drew benefits from the data they collected. Crucially, too, CMSS provided sources of information other than from the doctor or another professional and this did seem to be an attraction to some of the participants. As another women explained:

Well, you get lots of information. I think that what you get is you get a different viewpoint from what you get at the doctor's. I think you know in this world, you go in and out of the doctor's really fast. You don't get the information you want and they don't really know any more than what they've been told. You know that certain conditions are treated in certain ways and that's that. And so you get much, much more information on different alternatives.

Since CMC first started, many academics and other commentators have discussed the extent to which it 'conceals' gender, ethnicity, income and other characteristics and visual clues that would otherwise influence or perhaps even prohibit conversation (Reid 1996). With the apparently increasing use of audio and video communication through the Internet, it is uncertain how long existing forms of CMC will continue to predominate. However, during the course of the research, some individuals reported that CMC in itself was beneficial in terms of social interaction and social supports because it could overcome prejudices and attitudes that might otherwise have been a problem. As a man in his twenties explained:

> I suppose it's almost, being blind, it's easier than meeting real people. You're not always addressing, you know, if you go out, I don't know say you go to a pub or whatever there's always somebody coming over and patting your guide dog and wants to talk about the dog or wants to talk about you being blind or wants to talk about how you got there and how you find the buses and this sort of thing. On the Internet you don't get that, people don't know about you so you can talk about what you want to talk about. You're not constantly trying turn the conversation round your way or whatever.

While the individuals using CMSS generally found it helpful and were able to talk about its benefits, some questions remain about the role of social support in health and well being. For some researchers, there are issues related to how well any effects that social support might have can be measured, as for example, higher levels of social support are associated with higher socio-economic status, which is in itself associated with better health (Cohen *et al.* 1999). For others, the absence of an easily measurable definition of social support is seen as a problem in assessing the impacts that it has on health (Callaghan and Morrissey 1993).

A related issue regards the nature of the social support that CMSS is able to provide. Social support can be classified in several ways, such as social companionship, informational support, esteem support and instrumental support (Cohen and Willis 1985). While CMSS can arguably provide the first three forms, as communication can provide companionship, provide information and reinforce self-esteem, it cannot provide the practical assistance or other tangible support that can be classified as instrumental support (Muncer *et al.* 2000). In summary, people may feel that they benefit from the social support that CMSS can offer them, but actually defining and measuring the effect of this support is problematic. It is also the case that CMSS cannot offer the full range of support available from social contacts in 'real life'.

While some individuals had formed relationships in 'real life' with the people that they had met online, for example travelling to the US to stay with friends from newsgroups, a few of the participants were a lot less willing to treat their CMSS relationships in the same way as they treated 'real' relationships. Several people differentiated between online friends and 'real' friends to the extent that they would not telephone or meet the former. For example, in one computer-mediated 'interview', when asked 'Would you say that you've ever formed friendships or any other kind of relationship using Newsgroups, email or any of the other services?' one respondent answered: 'Definitely, but they remain "Internet" friends – with no "offline" relationships by telephone or visit happening or planned.'

There was also sometimes the problem of hate messages from 'trolls', individuals who move between newsgroups offending people and starting fights for fun. For most of the research respondents, trolls were just unpleasant individuals such as one might meet occasionally in real life, and the usual tactic appeared to be simply to wait for them to go away, which they would generally do if they could not get a reaction. As a man in his thirties related:

> I mean everybody, I mean I'm pretty recently diagnosed with this, but there's, if you think that there are people that, that have had it ten, twenty, twenty years on there . . . and then, and then some guy comes on and he says, 'Oh I think the, the power of the mind can overcome all this', you know, and 'I think it's just willpower and all you lot haven't got any willpower', and all this lot, you know. And I mean he attracted a phenomenal amount of people going back to him and telling him what they think but to be fair the majority of them were quite civilised about it. But then others deliberated on whether or not he was actually like a troll and he was just, you know, you get people come every now and again and say, 'Oh right, I'll try this newsgroup, I'll put something down and see how many people I can wind up.'

Sometimes the activities of some of these individuals were disturbing, such as a lengthy post placed on a self-help newsgroup for people with depression which detailed various methods for committing suicide. The extent to which danger exists for vulnerable people using the Internet is uncertain, but the perception of risk among some participants was enough to ensure that they did not release any personal details over the Internet, and some used remailers (computers that disguise an original email address) to avoid even their real email address becoming known.

Another potential problem with CMSS, according to some of the participants, was what Americans call 'snakeoil'. Snakeoil refers to the perhaps mythical 'miracle cure' sold off the back of a wagon by an untrustworthy salesperson. The Internet equivalents were posts in self-help newsgroups advertising a website that offered the 'forgiveness of Jesus' as a cure for only $99.99. None of the participants who took part in the research seemed to have been taken in for a moment, but the mere fact that these posts were made and these sites existed suggested there was money to be made from sometimes highly vulnerable individuals.

In addition to confidence tricksters, there was also the concern that individuals might give each other incorrect and possibly even harmful advice. In a context in which scientific and professional information is viewed with increasing uncertainty, access to information based on personal experience did provide an alternative to medical or other professional opinions, but this alternative was potentially something of a doubled-edged sword. Concern among medical professionals about the quality of the information on the Internet has been growing for some time (Abbot 2000).

Some commentators have also suggested that CMSS forums might be used by some individuals not for social support but for entertainment. Just as American television programmes such as *Oprah* and its clones, unfortunately now including British versions, sell individuals' negative life experiences as entertainment and spectacle, so the use of CMSS by one individual might inadvertently provide entertainment for another. Individual experience or health problems might become commodified and consumed in the same way as soap opera (humdog 1996).

The safety Net?

While CMSS may provide Giddens's reflexive individuals with resources based on shared experience that may enable them to counteract the problems they encounter more effectively, it remains an often *inaccessible* resource. This inaccessibility flows first and foremost from individual and family financial resources and, while one no longer needs to have a high income to afford Internet access in the UK, CMSS is not something readily available to a family or individual living on a low income (Burrows *et al.* 2000: 97–8). As Holderness (1998: 37) views it: 'it remains the case that the sharpest, most clearly enumerable divides in Cyberspace are those based on where one lives and how much money one has'.

In addition, while the Internet is an increasingly open system it is still a largely North American, rather than a truly global, network. People from minority ethnic groups, individuals who do not speak and read American English and, depending on the environments one visits, women can still encounter problems using systems largely designed by and for young white American males. The attitudes of the 'nerds' who first used the network, which can be racist, misogynist and generally contemptuous of those who do not feel the need to understand the intricacies of TCP/IP, are also still firmly in the mainstream across the Internet (Spender 1995).

The danger that the Internet could exacerbate existing inequalities has long been recognised and policies are being put in place in the UK to attempt to counteract such an eventuality (IBM 1997, PAT 15 2000). In terms of CMSS, the potential problem is that it will reinforce the capacity of an increasingly self-sufficient and reflexive middle class to place themselves in an advantageous position. Rather than counteracting the undermining of social insurance and the welfare state resulting from successive governments' expenditure cuts, CMSS could be part of the Internet acting as a *catalyst* towards greater social division and inequality alongside other aspects of the Internet such as e-commerce (Castells 1996).

An Internet guru might address these concerns by pointing to the convergence of digital technologies and the arrival of Internet access through the television, mobile phones and a host of other devices. While lower-cost access to the Internet will arrive, the extent to which it will be really universal remains uncertain because the means of access seem set to change so radically. Attention also needs to be paid to the main engine behind encouragement of widespread access to the Internet, which is capital seeking new markets through e-commerce. The motivations behind the current UK government's attempts to secure mass access to the Internet, while not wholly economic, are nevertheless greatly influenced by such economic considerations.

The Internet that might arise from these motivations might not be much more than a computer-mediated shopping centre. Satellite digital television in the UK, for example, offers at the time of writing not actual Internet access but a limited facility for e-commerce and email. Other Internet service providers (ISPs) operating in the UK also emphasise home shopping and email above anything else that the Internet might have to offer. For most people, the Internet may not be about CMSS, or even information in general, but about broadcast and narrowcast advertising and shopping, with any CMC restricted to the same sorts of use that are currently made of the telephone.

Computer-mediated social support is also inherently limited by participants not being in the same room as one another: it cannot offer the practical, instrumental support of a real self-help group or a real friendship or relationship. There are also a range of potential problems, though the most tangible and perhaps the only real one of these is the concern about the quality of information people are getting from one another when participating in CMSS. The popular media love scare stories about dangerous people stalking anyone who dares to venture on to the Internet and about Internet con-artists because they pander to the anxieties that this technology creates in much of the population, but like the trolls in the newsgroups the actual impact of these risks, while tangible, is also perhaps negligible. There are also the fears about the commodification of misery by CMSS, which seems quite plausible, but when this takes place it will be the extension of an existing trend in society that already permeates the popular media into a new means of broadcasting and narrowcasting offered by the Internet.

Yet while there may be significant problems with the extent and nature of access to CMSS, there do seem to be some important benefits attached to the use of the Internet for social support. Otherwise socially isolated individuals had contact with other people, which sometimes moved into relationships being established in real life. Information, advice and help were provided that could be beneficial, and individuals were given an alternative source of information to professionals who might either withhold the full picture or be unaware of new developments or alternative treatments or approaches.

Although it would certainly be an exaggeration to describe some of the self-help newsgroups our research has examined as approaching the communities of shared interest that Rheingold (1993a) and others envisaged, individuals with shared needs and experiences are nevertheless able to meet in a way that would not have been possible before. The importance of being able to find someone or a group of people with shared experiences should not be underestimated.

In essence, CMSS is something that can have beneficial effects, but those effects are limited by its very nature. It cannot replicate the benefits of real social interaction in a real self-help group, nor can it offer the multi-dimensional social support of real relationships (Muncer et al. 2000, Pleace et al. 2000). Arguably, although it cannot compensate for a lack of social interaction and social support, CMSS can however provide at least some elements of social support, acting as a perhaps poor substitute, but as a substitute nevertheless, where other social supports are not available. It could also augment existing social supports where these are not always available or not as extensive as an individual needs.

At this point however, just as we have to acknowledge something of a link between CMSS fora and Rheingold's communities of shared interest, we also have to acknowledge some of the worries of those who were concerned that the Internet might undermine 'real' social interaction. While CMSS may be beneficial, it is no substitute for the real thing, and anything approaching reliance on CMSS in any individual is perhaps something of a concern. While it might mean a real increase in the quality of life for housebound individuals who are excluded from most social interaction, it should be seen as something that might help their situation rather than as an answer to the problem. Isolated individuals with CMSS at their fingertips may be less isolated than someone without access to these resources, but, equally, they could well still be very isolated.

In the end, CMSS is a mixed blessing. There would be risks in pretending it can offer more than it can, as it is no substitute for being in a real social network, and there are risks that it might provide people with information that is incorrect or dangerous. At the same time, it can improve individual quality of life, augment existing social supports and provide useful, empowering information that can really help an individual with a health-care problem or social-support need. This mixed blessing for the moment exists in a context in which most of the population cannot use it, and questions remain as to whether, when they get access, they will use these resources. Like the Internet as a whole, it is with us, but we cannot be quite sure how things are going to turn out.

Acknowledgment

The work reported here was funded by the ESRC (award number L132251029) under the auspices of its 'Virtual Society?' programme.

Part II

The experience of community informatics

Chapter 7

Community networks and access for all in the era of the free Internet

'Discovering the Treasure' of community

G. Casapulla, F. de Cindio and L. Ripamonti

Introduction

This chapter first discusses the issue of access in this era of so-called 'free Internet' use[1] and shows that a major role still exists for community networks if we are to take the 'access for everybody' goal seriously. It then presents the idea of facilitating access through 'cyberhunts', and describes how they have been designed and implemented within the Milan Community Network. 'Cyberhunts' have been successful because they integrate the well-known pedagogical principle that you will retain longer and understand better what you have learned through play. This approach underpins how the basic principles of *community* network have been explored.

Community networks and the access issue

In North America, as in Europe, one of the major goals for community networks (CNs) since their inception has been to provide people with access to the Internet. This is no longer relevant as free Internet connections are largely provided by private-sector organisations to attract more and more visitors to their sites (now called 'portals').[2] However, free connectivity does not guarantee real access for everybody. Many people need support, help and motivation to understand why and how making the effort to learn the Internet is worthwhile. They need to discover what opportunities it offers and what threats it holds. People need to be supported in exploring how the Internet can be used to communicate, to share knowledge, to support and spread ideas and to create a virtual environment which mirrors the dynamics of their local community. Last but not least, people need help in identifying what the most innovative technologies are and how to use them.

As Clement and Shade (2000) observe, mere connectivity – what ISPs and a variety of commercial sites offer free or at very low cost in a growing number of countries – is at the bottom of a hierarchy of needs that must be taken into account in moving towards universal access. Meeting their original main goal – to involve more people in the networked society, thus reducing the risk of a 'digital divide' – obliges CNs to deal with issues such as:

- making the use of information and communication technology (ICT) affordable for everybody
- motivating the different categories of citizens by making them aware of the online services and opportunities that are available to them
- avoiding frustrating experiences by monitoring the quality of the services offered online by public and private organisations
- making everybody aware that the possibilities the Internet offers are always open to further extensions since 'citizens are free to invent their own uses'.[3]

The above points may seem trivial, but they are not. They contrast the ways in which commercial companies are exploiting and colonising the Internet today, attempting to shape 'the global market' in the way they find most profitable. Let us compare the above points to what people in general experience and read or hear from traditional media (radio, television and newspapers) about the Internet.

First, *affordable use*. To fight the 'hits battle', webmasters try to make their sites more and more attractive by using the latest technology. Sometimes this provides real benefit (such as offering a more secure protocol for online transactions); sometimes the newest version of a technology solves problems present in earlier versions. But often this is not the case, and people are requested to download new versions or plug-ins, wasting time – and sometimes money as well – without getting any real improvement. People feel out of date, unable to keep pace with the racing virtual world, and give up.

Second, *motivations*. According to popular advertising, people are encouraged to approach the Internet for motivations such as:

- being informed on the financial markets and becoming millionaires or billionaires – but most people don't have the money or skill to become investors
- interacting in new ways with their municipality – but then people realise that this means reading the proceedings of the city council, paying taxes and fines, or sending emails to the mayor, which, at best, will be answered by a member of his staff
- chatting – which is probably not so intriguing for the large majority of working people, charged with work and family duties as they are
- visiting hot sites – no comment.

Very little attention is given to motivating people by recognising diversities: the best we see in a few sites is the chance to personalise a homepage. But this is good only for those who are already able to identify services useful to them. On the contrary, a technology as rich as ICTs are today, with the large investments being made in the field, should and could allow us to differentiate the offerings by taking into account factors such as age, disability, language and possibly income and gender.

Third, *the quality and user-friendliness of services*. At least in Italy, the current quality of online services is low, and therefore only people fully familiar with ICTs can use them. Let us take as an example the documentation that one of the biggest Italian banks gives to those who ask and pay for its home-banking service. It does not include the URL of the site to which one should connect. The User ID, password, and 'secret codes' to be used at the various levels (to enter, to order 'cheap' transactions, to place larger orders) are differently named in the written documentation and the online interface. Completing a transaction requires people to use their own knowledge and ability to overcome the faults of the online service. If you do not or cannot, you feel lost. Again, the result is that people feel unable to keep pace with the virtual world, and give up.

Fourth, *new domains of possibilities*. The 'openness' of the Internet has been its main engine of development. 'Open' means that everybody can set up her or his site, add her or his own content, develop her or his project, and use the Internet itself to find partners and resources or to make the project feasible. So 'openness' also implies that one can be an active player rather than a passive reader, contrasting with the attitude promoted by the broadcasting media. These characteristics are very well known to those familiar with the Internet's origin and development, but are less evident to those who enter now. In many cases, websites offer a predefined set of possibilities. Sometimes, these include an opportunity for people to make comments and offer suggestions, for example a new service that one would like. However, this is usually in the form of an email to the webmaster or to the web staff, that is the input is private or closed or reserved. There are several commercial sites that allow people to develop their own pages as a way to build customer loyalty, but this differs from and is something less than suggesting that people should develop their own project on the Internet. Claiming access for everybody should mean transmitting awareness, showing and teaching ideas, and bringing them into everyone's reach.

Even though, at first glance, the role for CNs seems to have diminished, and might even vanish because of the rapid development of the so-called free Internet, the above discussion shows that if we take the 'access for everybody' goal seriously, the kind of opportunity offered by the private sector is insufficient and deepens the digital divide. The engagement of CNs in pursuit of their original goal must therefore be renewed. CNs need to find ways to attract people who are not now interested in the Internet, to re-involve those discouraged by an unsatisfactory approach and to show both of these groups the new domain of possibilities that the Internet offers to each of us, according to our own condition, interests and role in society. Only if we succeed in this will we manage both to preserve the original Internet spirit and to avoid deepening the 'digital divide', the gap between people who 'have' and 'have not' access to the information society. Otherwise, the Internet will never benefit from the creativity, compassion, intelligence and dedication people can express which could be harnessed to help address the multitude of major problems humanity is asked to face in the globalised world.[4]

The value of the community: 'You are the network'

To realise that in the era of free Internet access CNs still have a relevant role to play, is less trivial than one might think. Without this awareness, and considering that the sustainability of these not for profit initiatives is always a major problem, CNs might either increasingly become mere providers of city hall's online services (in the case of CNs promoted and managed directly by the city hall), or attempt to become commercial enterprises, as was the case of the Amsterdam Digitale Stad. However the awareness of this role is just the first step, the more difficult ones being: finding effective ways to satisfy the needs expressed in the four points above; and in parallel, developing a model for sustainability, which has to be consistent with the goals the CNs are pursuing.

A deep discussion of this second issue is out of the scope of this chapter. However, it must be borne in mind because it defines the context of CN activity especially when considering that addressing the first issue cannot be on the basis of huge resources. While, for instance, commercial portals have money for advertising campaigns, CNs cannot do the same. Money for contacting people through the traditional media and presenting them with the CNs' vision of the Internet is scarce. Historically, CNs have relied on volunteer work, that is, on the community itself to carry on the activities needed to survive. We did this in managing Rete Civica di Milano (RCM), the Milan Community Network (see, for example, Casapulla *et al.* 1995), but were careful to allow volunteers to develop their own projects. A very small, paid staff handles its core activities. Since RCM maintains its original roots – its operational headquarters – in the university (at the Information and Computer Science Department of Milano State University), the staff is, from time to time, supplemented by students during a stage of their university curriculum in the RCM Laboratory. Such (extended) staff members carry on activities needed to keep the network running, both at the technological level and at the 'social' level. This includes managing and updating the computers and the network and guaranteeing adherence to specific netiquette rules, which we call 'Galateo'.[5] They also manage relations with local government institutions, launching initiatives that show potential (new) uses of the Internet, opening new areas of particular importance and, last but not least, supporting projects proposed by individual or group members. In this way, the volunteers are not simply dedicated to pursuing activities conceived by someone else but are also supported in pursuing their own projects.

From a learning environment to a learning community

Let us reconsider points one, two, and four above and show how they can be better fulfilled in a community framework.

First, people may need support to get connected. Modem set-up and proper web-browser configuration may still represent a barrier that individuals are not able to solve alone. After the connection has been set up, new problems may arise such as identifying the cookies that one is forced to download while visiting a site, or the configuration of the proxies of some ISPs.

A *community of helpers* (sometimes they are called *computer angels*), such as the ones that exist in RCM and in many CNs, offers this kind of support. They are volunteers, often students, although there are also retired people doing this. These individuals either offer support by telephone or make house calls to solve the most critical problems. Compared to the ISPs' call centres, the difference is that the latter conceive of people merely as customers, while the former give people the feeling and awareness of being part of a community that does not leave you to fend for yourself.

Second, people need support to understand which software is necessary or useful. There is such a large number of applications around the Internet that it is increasingly difficult to identify which software *must* be installed on a PC to access the majority of sites and services properly. There is software that *may* be useful to have, and this may depend on your specific interests (video, music etc.). Finally, there is software that is strongly promoted by some sites simply for marketing purposes. Not everybody can be informed as new standards emerge, not everybody wants to spend time reading technical magazines (for instance, women often do not have the time or enjoy doing so).

Third, once these problems are solved, people may still need a guide to navigate the Internet. Everything seems easy, but when one looks for a specific site, for some specific information or for a particular functionality, problems arise. The search engines are still far from being easy to use, and the initial efforts, such as trying to find a specific photo to be included in one's child's homework, can be very frustrating. Many sites consist of databases; computer professionals are designing interfaces for users who are assumed to have specific training.

A *community of users and experts* is an appropriate environment for addressing the second and third points. Sharing experiences and knowledge has been, and still is, the major reason for Internet newsgroups and mailing lists, when they are appropriately managed. People who are not familiar with such communication facilities must be introduced to the kind of co-operation these make possible: everybody should learn to 'waste time' answering questions when they can. They should also learn to read (at least, to scroll through) the FAQ file before asking a question: the point is to avoid wasting other people's time and attention, the kind of careful behaviour a community requires. Moreover, each RCM forum has one or more 'moderators': staff members who take care of the forum, promote discussions, erase obsolete messages and store important threads. They must accept or reject messages according to two major criteria: first, whether the message is consistent with the RCM Galateo; second, whether it is pertinent to the forum's interests and goals. Sometimes the forum is proposed and handled by a professional, who makes their expertise available to the community. They do this as volunteers, though it may also be a way to acquire clients. RCM hosts several of these online consultancy forums from experts in different fields, including technology.

In this context, we need to educate citizens to consider the forums in such a rich way.[6] In particular, they need to realise that the 'moderator' (the name, due to the software platform RCM uses,[7] is probably not as appropriate as one might wish) is more the forum's housekeeper, who keeps it clean and in good order, rather than a censor. But moderators also must be educated to manage the communication properly: for example, when they reject a message because it is not pertinent, they are strongly encouraged to suggest a different forum where it can be accepted. They need to treat forum participants on a peer-to-peer basis. It has been known for some moderators to become small 'bosses' of the forum. Communities of users are to some extent *communities of experts*. In any field, others' experience is of invaluable importance.

Cyberhunts

How can we teach all these abilities? How do we encourage people to 'discover the treasure' to be found on the Internet and in its community, bypassing and forgetting the trivial advertising? How can this be done cheaply and attractively? During the first year of RCM, we organised once-a-week meetings for citizens interested in being informed about our initiatives and the Internet. But there were only three staff members. As RCM and the general interest in the Internet grew, we were no longer able to sustain such load. We began to realise the need to teach the Internet through the Internet. But this could not be done as a kind of computer-aided education, with online courses and the like. As a result, we conceived the idea of 'cyberhunts'.

In 1996 RCM proposed its first cyberhunts, that is, a 'treasure hunt' to be played partly in the virtual dimension and partly in the real one. The clues to carry on with the hunt could, in some cases, be found online (in a newsgroup or on a website) and in others, at a physical place in the real town (such as a shop or a city-hall office). This mix of virtual and real is one of the major design principles of RCM cyberhunts. Another principle is that, unlike traditional role games (even in their online versions), people play with their real names and identities.

The design principles of RCM cyberhunt corresponds to the design principles of RCM itself. The virtual town and the real one are not disjointed; rather there is mutual interplay between them. People get to know each other in the real world and then communicate, co-operate, meet, play and so forth through the Internet. But the reverse also applies: people first meet each other via the Internet, through, for example, an interest in the same forum (for example 'movies' or 'HTML'). As the CN is locally rooted, this can then lead to a meeting in the real world to play (for example going together to the cinema) or work (for example becoming partners in developing websites).

Activities in one dimension have effects in the other dimension too. RCM members are identified by their 'real' first and last names; moreover each presents herself or himself to the online community through a personal self-portrait (which also resolves ambiguities for those with the same names). Different or multiple identities are not allowed and only in specific cases can messages be anonymous.

By applying and playing the cyberhunt, people implicitly acquire these principles. Also, the registration procedure becomes natural. To play, you have to register and read the rules of the game, which is subscribing to the 'Galateo' (the behavioural code that RCM members commit to following).

These hunts have always been aimed at conveying knowledge and making people more confident with ICTs, with the structure and the possible uses of the CN itself, and with the Internet. For example, hunters were asked to find a specific message[8] and to reply in a specific way ('to the sender', 'to all but not to the BCC'), to solve problems or to uncover clues that either required using certain specific features of some relevant software or required discovering a given forum (such as the 'helper' or the 'expert online' forums, so that people then learn that there are places where one can get help). To win the game, people spontaneously assume a proactive approach. In that way they learn the fundamental principles of the appropriate use of network technologies while enjoying themselves, according to the well-known pedagogical principle that you will retain longer and understand better what you have learned while playing. Moreover, in a treasure hunt, you are also spurred both to co-operate (with the members of your team) and to compete (among teams) thus learning to use the Net as a platform for co-operation and competition.

The first edition of the treasure hunt dates back to 1996, and was aimed at the whole RCM 'virtual population', to familiarise people with the features of FirstClass (our BBS software) and to strengthen the 'sense of community' among RCM members. It did not have a specific graphic interface, but heavily relied on text and emails. Step by step, this interface has evolved, and in the 1999 edition a specifically developed website and several multimedia applications were included. In that way, we met the need to keep people up to date with the evolving technology. The 1999 edition, for the first time, was also published in CD-ROM form and promoted outside RCM by selling the CD with a magazine. In 1999, RCM was also asked to design and manage a cyberhunt to launch the Varese Community Network, hosted by the local university.

These hunts were designed by a team that consists of one member of the RCM staff (let's call him 'the community enlivener') and two volunteer collaborators: one for the graphics and the other for the scenario (that is, the writer of the story that provides the background for the game); the former did the work to demonstrate his graphics abilities, while the latter did it simply because writing stories is his favourite hobby.

In terms of access, we registered constant growth in the participation from one edition of the hunt to the next. Growth was linear over the first three hunts (doubling each year and reaching four hundred participants in 1998), while the last edition attracted about five thousand participants who began the game (thanks to the 'boom' of free Internet access). However, with such a large number of players, it is difficult to evaluate the real success of the hunt with respect to its educational goals. We realised that we needed specific tools to track players' behaviour, as well as more sophisticated parameters and corresponding automatic tools to monitor the liveliness of the community. As a result, we began to develop such tools (Longhi 2000) before designing a new cyberhunt.

Scopri il Tesoro (Discover the Treasure)

The truly outstanding result that RCM has obtained with the cyberhunts is 'Scopri il Tesoro' ('Discover the Treasure'), an online educational game for children.

The first attempt dates back to 1998. The idea was to reproduce the cyberhunts with the specific goal of attracting children (under 16) to both the real and the virtual museums in the town. Unfortunately, this project did not 'take off'.

The idea was then adopted by a group of teachers at several elementary schools in Milan. They were already managing the 'Città della Scuola' ('City of School') forum in RCM, dedicated to a sub-community of people involved in teaching and studying and, more generally, were concerned with school and its problems. They set up an association, CODINF (for COordinating committee of teachers interested to INFormatics). RCM and CODINF are the promoters of 'Scopri il Tesoro'.

The first edition of 'Scopri il Tesoro' started in the spring of the 1998–9 school year. Despite an inauspicious start, within a couple of months (April–May 1999), four hundred students had got involved, organised in 'crews'. It was impressive to meet these four hundred 'pirates' at the awards day, which took place on a hot, midsummer Saturday morning, after schools had already closed. This success, which took us by surprise, demonstrated beyond any doubt the validity of the hypothesis about the use of games, namely treasure hunts, as a means to convey education in ICT. Therefore, partly under the pressure of several teachers, CODINF and RCM decided to organise a new edition the following year: 'Scopri il Tesoro 2000' [Tesoro00]. Launched at the beginning of the 1999–2000 school year, 'Scopri il Tesoro 2000' involved more than four thousand children. Starting from the Milan schools, the news of the game spread all over the country leading to approximately three hundred crews from every corner of Italy and from Switzerland taking part.

The participants are grouped in 'crews,' each with a 'captain'. They are asked to use the means best suited to their age to obtain the clues they need to carry on with the game (for example very small children mainly draw and then scan their art works to put them online, while older ones use more sophisticated techniques). The clear aim of the game is to discover a mysterious treasure, while the 'hidden' goal is learning to use computers and to interact with other crews through the Net.

The whole game is integrated into the educational programme of the schools. A key factor for its success is that the volunteer teachers who design and co-ordinate the game (called 'spiriti guida', or 'guiding spirits') develop the game's steps in 'real time', adapting it to the achievements and needs that arise while playing. In more general terms, 'Scopri il Tesoro' is built on the methodical application of the participatory design principle, which inspires the RCM's overall design and implementation (Casapulla *et al.* 1998). This, of course, requires a big effort (in terms of time) on the part of the co-ordinators. Therefore, the number of 'guiding spirits' has had to be expanded from the original two to nine. RCM staff support them by maintaining the 'Scopri il Tesoro' website, providing graphics according to their specific requests and paying special attention in registering the people involved in the game. Increasingly this means not only teachers and students but also parents, brothers, sisters and sometimes even grandparents. In addition to school crews, we admit home crews as well, so spreading out the educational benefits. The schools and the university (as noted, RCM is hosted by the Computer Science Department) actually fulfil their task of being a point of reference for the overall community, which directly fits with RCM's mission of facilitating access to the Net. 'Scopri il Tesoro' can in fact be seen as a kind of learning community, which incrementally introduces ICTs to people of all ages, making them active citizens of the information society.

In March 2000, a thousand children gathered in one of Milan's major theatres for one of the stages of the game, again mixing the real world with the virtual one. It was an unforgettable day. The enthusiasm of the pirates and their awareness that they were part of an educational game helped convince the somewhat sceptical authorities – the Provveditorato agli Studi (Board of Education), the University Dean of Sciences and the City Superintendents – of the major role RCM can play in introducing people of all ages to the information society (as evidenced in interviews conducted that day and video-taped).

Thanks to the success of 'Scopri il Tesoro', the local office of the Ministry of Education, which had not initially paid any attention to the co-operation between RCM and the schools, has now discovered how fruitful such co-operation is. People who were very cold towards RCM are now anxious to co-operate with us. It seems that 'they' have finally 'discovered the treasure': the value of the community.

We are now at the beginning of the third edition of the game (Tesoro01), and the number of requests from teachers definitely confirms its success. The first edition was about learning the elementary functions of the net (email and newsgroup and attachments of different formats for dealing with images and sounds) mainly in the framework of a community network. The second edition introduced the Internet, maintaining the community network as the project's intranet. The demand for the third edition is leading schools to develop their own websites. The game increasingly becomes an educational environment (and community), which, step by step, leads people (the 'crews') to reach an educational goal.

Conclusions and future developments

We believe that cyberhunts are successful because they integrate the well-known pedagogical principle that you will retain longer and understand better what you have learned by playing with the basic principles of a *community* network. Cyberhunts are designed with these principles in mind.

In the case of 'Scopri il Tesoro', two further factors are relevant. First, the existence of a network of relationships between teachers, which developed and strengthened thanks to the early use of RCM and, thus, of the Internet. It is on the drumbeat of these networks, both real and virtual, that 'Scopri il Tesoro' has spread, first in Milan and then throughout the country and abroad. Second, thanks to the existence of a specific netiquette (the 'RCM Galateo'), teachers felt secure in involving children in online playing, unlike what happens at private companies' sites (which also try to attract students and teachers). We are now getting requests to produce new cyberhunts, aimed at simplifying network access for people experiencing different kinds of barriers (economical, cultural etc.), including employees of the most conservatively bureaucratic organisational environments (such as trade unions and public institutions).

Moreover, RCM cyberhunts, with their interplay between the 'real' and the 'virtual' worlds, can be very attractive for marketing purposes. For commercial enterprises, a cyberhunt is a way to stimulate people to navigate their site. For a local institution, it is a way to make citizens discover their home town, their home region and so forth, in both its real and its virtual aspects.

Finally, we believe that cyberhunts may be effective in helping small and medium enterprises (SMEs) explore the opportunities that ICTs offer the economy. Field studies (for example Formaper 2000) indeed show that educational ICT available for SMEs do not take into account their special needs and constraints. For SMEs, especially the very small ones with fewer than ten employees, which are a fundamental part of the Italian and Lombard economies, it is often not feasible to send employees away even for a one-day course. They often ask their employees to use their own time to learn new tools. And, overall, there are a lot of people who need to keep themselves up to date with the evolving technology. Community networks in general and cyberhunts in particular can be exploited for this purpose and can evolve towards a specialised distance-learning platform for SMEs, for networking applications, groupware and ICTs in general (see also De Cindio 1999).

RCM has had a range of requests from different kinds of organisations, including trade unions, local public institutions, and private companies in various fields. Moreover, the group of 'Scopri il Tesoro guiding spirits' and RCM itself have had requests for co-operation from a leading group in distance learning. Therefore, we believe that exploiting this idea, and preserving its original educational purpose, can indeed fulfil the goal of involving more and more citizens in cyberspace in a – let us say – 'correct way', while also contributing to the sustainability of the community network.

Acknowledgments

Special thanks to Marco Godi (for computer graphics) and Andrea Spalla (scenarist), who, along with Giovanni Casapulla, designed, implemented and managed the several editions of the cyberhunt. Laura Fiorini, Loredana Gatta and Cesare Riva are the 'guiding spirits' who have conceived, organised, co-ordinated and managed 'Scopri il Tesoro', again with the support of Marco and Andrea, respectively for the graphics and the story. All the RCM staff supported the cyberhunts and 'Scopri il Tesoro' teams with very special attention. Without their voluntary and passionate work all our games would not have been possible. We also are grateful to Philip Grew for critically reviewing our English grammar.

Notes

1 'Free Internet' in this context means access to free or low-cost email accounts, web space and other services (e.g. personal calendars) that in Italy are given without charge by several Internet providers. It does not mean 'free' access to the Internet; there are still telephone and connection charges involved.
2 This is what M. Gurstein observes in the introduction to the book on 'Community Informatics' that he recently edited: 'Initially a number of CNs were established as a means to provide Internet access and particularly email accounts to those unable to acquire them in other ways. However, with the very rapid proliferation of low-cost email and even free email accounts by companies such as HotMail, this role for CNs has diminished very significantly.'

3 Quoted from Clement and Shade (2000); but this is also the ultimate meaning of the slogan 'La Rete siete Voi' ('You are the Network') which has appeared – since its inception – on the desktop and homepage (RCM) of the Milan Community Network (see below) to inspire everyone who logs on to be an active member and promoter, while the staff act as a sort of 'enabler' to the community.

4 Rephrased from the 'Seattle Statement,' www.scn.org/cpsr/diac-00/seattle-statement.html.

5 Each subscriber must accept the 'Galateo' in order to become a member of RCM.

6 To some extent, this is more difficult and more important now that many commercial sites and portals host similar forums, without any specific attention to their appropriate management.

7 The software RCM uses as 'community server' is the FirstClass Intranet Server by Centrinity Inc. (previously SoftArc Inc.). RCM architecture also includes a web server which enriches the FirstClass Intranet Server with programmable facilities, e.g., for handling statistics, for developing specific applications etc

8 A simple but not trivial example is this: Find a message that should not have been approved because it is outside the scope of the forum, and find a forum where it might have been sent instead.

Chapter 8

On crafting a study of digital community networks

Theoretical and methodological considerations

Nicholas W. Jankowski, Martine van Selm and Ed Hollander

Introduction

All too often, initial activities undertaken in designing and preparing a research project are left unmentioned in subsequent reports and publications. This tendency can camouflage much important preliminary work that may, in fact, determine the subsequent direction of the research conducted. In this chapter we describe some of our considerations in developing a research project around two digital community networks in the Netherlands. The first section provides a theoretical backdrop, situating this project within the tradition of community media studies at the University of Nijmegen. The second section of the chapter sketches two community-network sites being considered as foci for a longitudinal study: *Residentie.net* and *Purmerend Punt En El*. A preliminary study was conducted of *Residentie.net*, situated in The Hague, and the results are reported in this section of the chapter. In the third and last section some of the tasks involved in developing a formal proposal for a long-term investigation of these two community networks are reviewed. Concerns regarding the theoretical perspective and methodological approach are also addressed and the overall theoretical framework for the study is presented. We conclude by indicating issues of continuing importance in developing this and other investigations of digital community networks.

Theoretical backdrop

Staff members of the Department of Communication at the University of Nijmegen in the Netherlands have been involved in the study of community and locally oriented media for the past quarter of a century. Since the introduction of local radio and television services on cable television systems in the mid-1970s, Nijmegen has been following these and other small-scale media developments in the country. The most extensive research project from this period was a panel survey examining the introduction of community television in four Dutch municipalities (Stappers, Hollander and Manders 1978). This work was complemented by an action-oriented field study of the introduction of community television in a new housing estate on the outskirts of Amsterdam (Jankowski 1988). Both projects were concerned with identifying transformations in media use whereby residents could become producers of media messages, and both were concerned with the possible contributions of these media to the sense and development of community among residents in the respective communities.

Several other projects followed these early studies: an overview of the historical development of small-scale electronic media in Europe (Hollander 1982) an edited volume of European initiatives with local radio and television (Jankowski, Prehn and Stappers 1992), an examination of the relation between local media and local governments (De Goede, Hollander and Van der Linden 1996) and – most recently – a collection of theoretically oriented studies of traditional electronic and more recent network-based community media (Jankowski and Prehn 2001). These contributions to the literature have helped establish Nijmegen as one of the main European centres for community media studies.

One of the core concepts emerging from this work is appropriately called 'community communication'. The primary focus of this research tradition is the communication behaviour of individuals in a specific context, that is, the local community, rather than as an element of a mass audience (Hollander and Stappers 1992). 'Community' in this concept refers to either a geographically delineated region or a bonding based on common interest. In the case of geographically based communities, people are addressed by community media as residents of a specific region – a neighbourhood, district, town or city. Because of this position they are able to appreciate the relevance of the topics presented in community media – not politics in general, but local politics; not national sports, but local sports; not crime somewhere else, but crime in the community. The same applies to membership in communities based primarily on interest, cultural or ethnic bondings. Community communication involves, in other words, mediated and non-mediated communication behaviour of individuals in specific contexts, be the contexts geographically situated or topics of interest not bound by location in space.

This notion of communication-in-context has inspired scholars to develop concepts that 'capture' the relationship between a social system and its corresponding communication system. The German concepts *Kommunikationsraum* (communication space) and *lokale Öffentlichkeit* (local public sphere) are illustrations of this effort (Hollander 1988, Hollander and Stappers 1992). One of the aspects these concepts have in common is the conceptualisation of communication as a form of 'sharing' rather than merely the 'transmission of messages' (Carey 1989, Chaney 1978). These concepts have also contributed to the influence of community characteristics in the study of communication processes and content, and to the examination of the differences between communities and their respective communication activities.

This approach of German origin has not, however, been related to a more empirically oriented research tradition in the American-oriented field of community media, a tradition going back to the work of Janowitz (1952) and Merton (1949) on the community press. This tradition concentrates on factors operating at the individual level, which partially determine the use of community media. This research tradition, spanning a period of more than forty years, has been systematically evaluated by Stamm (1985). Stamm considers the results of empirical studies on the use of community newspapers and presents an overview of 'community ties' as antecedents to or consequences of community newspaper use. Stamm further distinguishes between 'ties to place' (such as length of residence), 'ties to structure' (such as membership of local organisations) and 'ties to process' (such as participation in local activities), and proposes these as the main factors operating at the individual level which are associated with the use of community media. Although Stamm restricts his investigation to community newspapers, other local media could also be considered regarding potential contributions to community ties. And the interactions between such local media and other forms of community communication – individual exchanges, group communication and various forms of mediated communication – can also be considered in the analysis of community ties.

On viewing the tradition of research on community and communication overall, two central issues related to the use of community media become apparent: the matter of causality and the choice between a static and a dynamic theoretical model. The issue of causality dates back to the difference between the theoretical approaches of Merton (1949) and Janowitz (1952). Janowitz envisioned community newspaper readership as a contributing factor to the integration of people in the community; Merton, in contrast, postulated readership of the local newspaper as a result of integration in the local community and of local orientation.

Researchers since then have generally taken a pragmatic view on this issue, depending on the aim of their investigations. Stamm (1985: 8) suggests a solution to this dilemma by presenting a cyclical model regarding use of community newspapers; see Figure 8.1, which reflects one point in a time sequence. With this dynamic view on the process of becoming and remaining a reader of a community newspaper, Stamm assumes that at different points in time community newspaper readership helps in establishing community ties and vice versa. The main innovation in this perspective is the departure from the older, static conception regarding the relation between community newspaper use and community ties. The static perspective assumes that the relationship between community newspaper use and community ties is linear. The dynamic view assumes that the relationship between community media use and becoming involved in a community is a two-directional and circular relationship. The processes involved are different, but nevertheless related: the process whereby people establish relationships across time with the

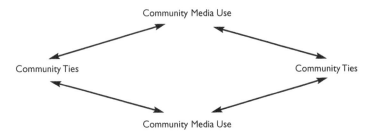

Figure 8.1 Community ties and community media use
Source: Stamm (1985: 8)

community in which they live is distinct from but related to the process whereby people attend to different community media at different points in time for various purposes.

Apart from causality and the time factor, a third theoretical issue has emerged in the debate on the use of community media: the change in perspective from a sender-oriented approach to an active audience or social-action theory approach (Bauer 1984, Renckstorf, McQuail and Jankowski 1996). This change in theoretical perspective is not specific for the study of community media, but has affected mass communication theory generally (see McQuail 2000, Baran and Davis 2000). It explains, for instance, why Janowitz (1952) maintained that community integration is a result of community newspaper use. Today, expanding on Stamm's (1985) work, community integration is seen as both a consequence and/or an antecedent of community media use.

The rich tradition of research on communication and community has produced numerous studies. Theoretical work has focused on the level of the social system and empirical investigations have been directed at the use of community media by individuals (for example Halloran 1977, Beaud 1980, Van der Linden, Hollander and Vergeer 1994). Researchers working within the conceptual domain of community communication, however, have not been very successful at accumulating and integrating this intellectual labour. Although Stamm's general concept of 'community ties' covers a range of concepts and variables, they differ widely in theoretical scope and operation-alisation. In other words, a general theory of community communication is still needed which elaborates how these processes are related across time.

One of the aspects of this yet-to-be-developed general theory involves attention to two levels of analysis: first, the individual level involving personal actions, motives, expectations and aspirations, and, second, the level of the social system, that is, the specific context or community: city, neighbourhood, women's group, ethnic or cultural group, special interest group etc. At the individual level, it is assumed that people differ in their actions, attitudes and their attention to community media. Accordingly, it is assumed that at the level of the social system communities differ with regard to characteristics such as homogeneity, history and population size. In addition, these differences affect both the members of the community and the attention of these members to community media.

Much of the theorising on community communication and community ties seems relevant to the study of a wide variety of community media, including digital community networks. The issues and characteristics of these networks, or digital cities as they are sometimes called in the European context, seem to resemble many of the issues and concerns evident during the early period of the introduction of electronic community media. The expectation that community networks can contribute to the development and improvement of the localities in which they are based is similar to the intention of community radio and television initiatives launched two-and-a-half decades earlier (see, e.g., Jankowski 1988). It is not surprising then that those of us in Nijmegen concerned with the study of community communication have became interested also in the digital community networks emerging across the country.

Preliminary study

We have been negotiating access to two possible sites for an extended study of digital community networks: *Purmerend Punt En El* in the city of Purmerend and *Residentie.net* in The Hague. The cities in which these two community networks are situated are briefly described below. This is followed by a description of a preliminary study conducted around *Residentie.net*.

Candidates for study: Purmerend Punt En El, Residentie.net

Purmerend, located some 25 km to the north of Amsterdam, has become in the course of the past two decades a modern and expansive satellite to Amsterdam. About half of the 68,000 residents of Purmerend are immigrants and look to Amsterdam for their economic, social and cultural well-being.[1] This relationship has been the source of long-time concern among community organisations and members of the city council in Purmerend; there is much interest in building more of a sense of community *within* Purmerend. One of the initiatives related to this concern is construction of a virtual reflection of the geographically situated municipality. An initiative to construct a site began in 1998 and emerged from a division of the city government concerned with the automation of government activities. Several city employees of this division witnessed at close quarters the development of another community network, *Digital City Amsterdam* that was launched in 1994. In addition, the major growth of websites initiated by other municipalities and regional governments across the country since then, providing informational and transaction services to their citizens, has been identified (see, e.g., Snijder and Flos 2000).

In 1998 the Purmerend city council established a task force to investigate the possibilities of a digital version of the city, and in January 2000 that task force commissioned a feasibility study. By the spring of 2000 a commission of interest groups was established to develop and give form to the site under construction, *Purmerend Punt En El*. A prototype was also developed for the site by technical staff of the city. Most recently, in August 2000, the city council approved a proposal to expand the initiative further with the intention of having an operational site by early 2001. At the time of the preliminary study, *Purmerend Punt En El* had not been launched and it was decided to postpone study of the initiative until a later date.

A second candidate for possible study was *Residentie.net*, located in The Hague. This city is the administrative capital of the country and, with a population of some 441,000 residents, it is one of the largest municipalities in the Netherlands. The population is diverse: both diplomatic staff and immigrant labourers reside in the city; at the same time, a large part of the working population lives in surrounding towns and villages. Many international organisations are located in The Hague; industries such as tourism and telecommunications play a major role in the city's economic climate. In sum, The Hague contains the cultural and recreational facilities associated with a large city as well as the problems regarding social and economic inequalities, crime and urban blight.[2]

We approached the director of *Residentie.net* for permission to conduct a limited course-based research project during the early phase of development of the community network shortly after the site was officially launched in April 2000. He agreed to provide basic documentation on the initiative and to assist in arranging interviews with staff and other involved persons. Students in the seminar followed up on this arrangement and secured interviews with an editorial board member and with a volunteer responsible for one of the 'virtual neighbourhoods' on the site.[3]

The community network *Residentie.net* is the result of an alliance between the local government of The Hague, the Dutch telecommunication company KPN and the local cable company Casema. The site is one of the initiatives developed when the community council in the late 1990s began to expand a so-called 'I-vision'. This vision involved, first, the creation of Internet access for all residents of the city, second, the provision of a wide diversity of local news information, and, third, the development of stronger projection of the city's image as an international centre of administration, justice, industry, culture and tourism. In 1998 a decision was made to develop a digital community network, and local government, companies and organisations were earmarked as potential providers of content for the site. The site became operational in April 2000 and can be accessed via the Internet and Teletext.

The site is organised with familiar city features in mind – city squares, traffic intersections and boulevards – and contains a conventional three-frame site structure. The left and right frames consist of hyperlinks intended primarily for consumers and commercially oriented visitors (links for creating websites, advertising, sponsoring, shopping) and for visitors interested in local activities and information (boulevards, traffic intersections, city squares). The centre frame is reserved for news and information items. Registered members are offered special services, such as chat, email and home page construction.[4]

Social capital

The main theoretical concept chosen for this preliminary examination, *social capital*, was popularised by Putnam (1993) during a study of governmental units in different regions of Italy. In that study he observed:

> Although all these regional governments [in Italy] seemed identical on paper, their levels of effectiveness varied dramatically. Systematic inquiry showed that the quality of governance was determined by long standing traditions of civic engagement (or its absence). Voter turnout, newspaper readership, membership in choral societies and football clubs – these were the hallmarks of a successful region.
>
> (Putnam 1993: 66)

He proposed the term 'social capital' in order to describe societies or communities in which norms such as trust, reciprocity and social networks make collective action possible (see also Foley and Edwards 1999: 142). Foley and Edwards (1999) note that Putnam's study inspired much scholarly work, both theoretical and empirical, by political scientists, sociologists, economists and scholars from other disciplines. Foley and Edwards reviewed forty-five publications reporting research in which social capital played a central role. The authors conclude that in the majority of studies social capital is treated as an independent variable affecting a variety of societal characteristics (such as economic growth, school attendance, and neighbourhood stability). In other studies 'social capital is treated as a dependent or intervening variable, with particular emphasis on the sorts of voluntary organisations said to produce it' (Foley and Edwards 1999: 147). Foley and Edwards criticise both types of studies of social capital because they mainly refer to attitudes, as measured by survey questions, without attention to the context in which social capital is believed to be present. To solve this problem, Foley and Edwards proposed a model that explicitly accounts for the context-dependency of social capital and allows for differentiation along the unequal distribution of access to and possession of resources (1999: 168).

In another study, Riedel *et al.* (1998) treat social capital as a dependent variable of a community network in a rural town in Minnesota. The authors consider electronic democracy initiatives as a means to enhance equality of political participation. Such equality involves, broadly speaking, access to information technologies and to the skills necessary for using the technologies. They suggest that fostering such equality online can be achieved by accentuating social or group-based forms of participation. They consider social capital a useful tool in examining this inasmuch as 'the theory of social capital deals directly with equality by predicting the conditions under which those lacking resources can co-operate to accomplish collective ends' (Riedel *et al.* 1998: 375). In the empirical section of their study, they examine the effects computers and network use may have on what they consider the three essential components of social capital: interpersonal trust, social norms and association membership.

We adapted the work of Riedel *et al.* (1998) to our preliminary study of *Residentie.net* inasmuch as the components of social capital discerned therein – interpersonal trust, social norms and association membership – are applicable to characteristics of computer-mediated communication (CMC). Electronic environments have, for example, their own set of social norms, known as 'netiquette'. Anonymity, moreover, is a typical characteristic of CMC and is a widely discussed topic in the literature (e.g., Lee 1996). Anonymity can be related to the component interpersonal trust. And the third component, association membership, can be understood in terms of virtual communities. For these reasons, the components of social capital formulated by Riedel *et al.* were adapted to this preliminary study of *Residentie.net*.

The objective of this study was to look for indications of social capital in the intentions expressed by the initiating organisation of the community network, in the content made available on the site and in the assessment of the site by community residents. The following material summarises the findings along these three divisions.

Organisational objectives

A member of the editorial board of the community network was asked to reflect on the objectives of *Residentie.net*. His comments were analysed in terms of the three components of social capital proposed by Riedel *et al.* (1998). Indication of the first component, *interpersonal trust*, was found in the presence of the trust between users of the site and trust in the organisation responsible for the site. *Residentie.net* discerns between members of the network and visitors to the site, a practice common among other digital cities in the Netherlands. Registering as a member requires filling in a form requesting personal data such as surname, address and date of birth. By such registration it was believed that the authors of any inappropriate behaviour (such as racist expressions) could be identified and appropriate action taken by the editorial board of the network. However, very few visitors to the site took the trouble to register during the first weeks after its official opening. Moreover, both individuals and the national consumer union reacted negatively to the collection of such personal information on a public website. The main objection involved uncertainty as to what purpose collecting the information served. These reactions prompted the editorial board to modify this requirement. Now, only a nickname and a password are requested when registering on the network. The only regulation of behaviour on the site currently is through volunteer adherence to a list of rules posted on the site.

With respect to the second component of social capital, *social norms*, we asked the editorial board member whether site behaviour was monitored. He indicated that the board regularly reviewed exchanges on discussion-oriented locations such as the town squares in order to check for inappropriate behaviour. During the first months of operation, only one instance was detected, and the person responsible for the square was requested to modify contributions because of racist utterances. In extreme cases, the site administrator has the authority to withdraw site membership; the board member emphasised, however, that site visitors and members are expected to regulate minor disputes or infractions themselves.

An indication of the third component of social capital, *association membership*, was gained by asking the board member whether community-building, generally speaking, was an objective of the site. He indicated this to be the case, but at the time of the interview he did not sense much evidence of community-building on the site. More lively debate and more activity, he felt, is needed before the label 'community' can be assigned to the site.

Site content

Part of the content of the website was examined through an exploratory qualitative content analysis, guided by the three dimensions of social capital suggested by Riedel *et al.* (1998) – interpersonal trust, social norms and association membership. As indicators of interpersonal trust, we looked for the presence of anonymity (of visitors) and the accessibility of information on the site. For social norms we looked for references to rules of behaviour and netiquette. And for association membership, we checked for the presence of organised groups or communities and representation of local 'real-life' associations on the website.

Given the expansiveness of the site, only four regions were examined: the section containing a registration form, the town squares, traffic intersections, and boulevards. These areas all contained interactive tools through which involvement of citizens with the site might become apparent. Table 8.1 summarises the information found in these areas.

Table 8.1 Arenas of *Residentie.net* and components of social capital

Social capital	Residentie.net			
	Registration form	*Town squares*	*Traffic intersections*	*Boulevards*
Inter-personal trust	Expected	Expected	Real names and private telephone numbers made available	Real names and private telephone numbers made available
Social norms	Rules and conditions for participation	Rules for behaviour	Netiquette	Rules for behaviour
Association membership	Encouraged to become member	Open to (invited) members	Membership not required; few traditional associations	Membership not required; few traditional associations

Regarding the *registration form*, the objectives of the site are described at the top of the form. Visitors are encouraged to become members with the statement: '*Residentie.net* is for all of us. Register and become an active participant in this community!' We considered this an indication of *association membership*, as the importance of becoming a member is emphasised. In addition, visitors must indicate that they have read and agreed to a list of rules and conditions for participating on the site. This can be considered indicative of *social norms*, as members must actively 'promise' to live up to these rules and conditions. Initially, *interpersonal trust* was expected, as persons were accepted as members only when they completed a form requiring personal data (surname, home address and birth date). Anonymity of members, in other words, was not accepted. This requirement, however, was abandoned because visitors were reluctant to register. Hence, it seems that measures taken to increase interpersonal trust resulted in distrust of the initiators of the site.

Regarding the *town squares*, the site contains a number of squares related to specific topics. Squares are interactive locations where members meet, discuss and exchange news, computer files and photographs. There are two ways to participate in a square: as a guest or as an active member. Members can also initiate their own squares and set additional rules for membership and behaviour. *Interpersonal trust* is expected from founders of a square, as personal data (nickname and password) are required. These data will, in most cases, be open to all members and visitors of *Residentie.net*. Potential founders of a square are asked to live up to general behaviour considered acceptable on Internet services such as discussion lists, which suggests the presence of *social norms* on the squares. Some squares are open to all visitors; others are open only to (invited) members. In the first months of site activity, associations active within The Hague were not represented in the squares.

As for *traffic intersections*, there are six areas, some with general locally oriented information (such as city government information) and news about local activities, and others with human-interest stories and trading information. The traffic intersections have a policy of open access: no registration is required and visitors are free to participate (for example by sending email messages to the editors of traffic intersections or personal messages to acquaintances). Most of the messages sent to editors of the traffic intersections were signed, it appeared, with the real names of the persons; sometimes private telephone numbers were also added. This, together with the openness on the intersections, suggests a form of *interpersonal trust*. Similarly to the other areas of the site, *social norms* are present in the form of 'rules of the game' and netiquette. Traffic intersections are accessible without registration requirements. Few indications, however, could be found for *association membership*, and few traditional associations seemed represented on the traffic intersections.

The site *boulevards* are organised around specific groups of residents in The Hague, such as seniors, students, business representatives and women. Similarly to the traffic intersections, the boulevards are open to all visitors without registration. Participants are free to withhold personal information in their contributions, but home addresses and private telephone numbers are often given. Both the accessibility of the boulevards and the presence of personal data provided by the visitors can be considered indicators of *interpersonal trust*. The posting of rules for acceptable behaviour on the boulevards can also be seen as an indicator of *social norms*. Although visitors are encouraged to participate actively in the boulevards, registration is not required. However, several real-life associations were represented on the boulevards and served as indications of association membership.

User experiences

In this part of the preliminary study we examine how users of *Residentie.net* experienced the three dimensions of social capital formulated by Riedel *et al.* (1998). We decided to concentrate on the town squares, which were reflective of a real-life counterpart, that is, existing geographical neighbourhoods in The Hague. By proceeding in this fashion, we felt it would be possible to compare the social capital experienced in the physical neighbourhood with that on the website. After inspecting a number of town squares, it seemed as if few members of *Residentie.net* were actively participating in the squares. We eventually selected for further study a square with the most activity: the 'Zeeheldenkwartier'. An obstacle to finding potential respondents for this part of the study, however, was the absence of email addresses appended to postings on the square. We therefore decided to conduct an interview with the initiator of the square whose email address was available. During the interview we asked whether characteristics of social capital could be identified among residents living in the neighbourhood and among the participants in the community network square.

This person indicated that the neighbourhood has a socially and economically diverse population; both house-owners and persons living in low-rent housing estates reside in the area. She described the neighbourhood as generally relaxed with an open atmosphere. The neighbourhood also has a number of committees consisting of residents who organise various annual events. In some sections residents collectively work together in, for example, cleaning the pavements and other public areas. In the opinion of the square initiator, there is a sense of community or social capital in the neighbourhood inasmuch as people care for the area and collectively engage in periodic activities.

The town square for the neighbourhood on *Residentie.net*, however, does not have a lively discussion forum. The initiator of the square suggested a number of reasons for this situation. First, the community network is not yet very well known among residents of The Hague. Also, people may feel reluctant to register on the square for reasons of privacy. Most of all, however, there is another website for the neighbourhood containing much the same information as the one established on *Residentie.net*. This other site is very popular and visitors engage in considerable interaction. The town square on *Residentie.net*, in other words, must 'compete' with this website. Overall, the initiator of the town square on *Residentie.net* does not feel the vibrancy which exists in the real neighbourhood; in this respect, the social capital of the neighbourhood seems greater than on its virtual counterpart.

Research project

The preliminary study described above was admittedly limited; a much more extensive empirical base is necessary before any conclusions can be drawn. Still, the exercise was valuable in several respects. First, it provided an opportunity to reflect on the concept of social capital and consider applying it to an empirically oriented study. Second, it allowed us to consider various issues related to an analysis of community-network websites, such as comparing real-life environments with the characteristics of their virtual counterparts, and to examine citizen interactions on such sites.

The preliminary study also allowed us to reflect on some of the suggestions Harrison and Stephen (1999) make for the investigation of digital community networks. They advocate, first of all, that evaluation research should be conducted across time and be comparative in nature. They also suggest taking note of the organisation perspective in these studies and in soliciting input from a number of actors involved in the initiatives. Perhaps most importantly, they call on academic researchers to become engaged in the creation of community networks through critical and constructive study and consultation.

Regarding social capital, we feel the term strongly resembles features traditionally associated with previous academic and practitioner-oriented discussions of community, community ties and community-development programmes (see Bell and Newby 1974, Stamm 1985). In some ways, it seems as if usage of the term 'social capital' is a product of current academic fashion and the alluring siren of social change. Social capital may, in fact, be more limiting than what was previously understood under the older, more traditional, term 'community'. One of our first tasks during the development of this research project is to examine the relation and differences between these two terms.

Whatever result that exercise in comparison of concepts may provide, earlier investigations of community radio and television suggest that the potential contribution of media to community-development processes is limited (Hollander 1982, Stappers, Olderaan and De Wit 1992). The same may be true for contributions to the social capital of a community. As with community media, community networks may reinforce the social capital of an area when components of social capital are already present, but contribute little to improving the situation faced by localities lacking in social capital – a situation often faced by new housing estates and municipalities dependent on other social, cultural and economic centres. Put more bluntly, those geographic communities already rich in social capital may become richer thanks to community networks, and those communities poor in social capital may remain poor. This is a possibility we intend to explore in this research project.

As we elaborated in the first section of this chapter, theoretical and empirical research on community media has a long tradition. At the moment however, there seems to be a tendency to study the Internet and, more specifically, digital community networks as a theoretically new and distinct field (Van Den Besselaar, Melis and Beckers 2000, Gurstein 2000). The intention of this research project is to investigate digital community networks from within the conceptual domain and methodological framework already established for research on community media. In this manner it will be possible to draw on the experiences gained from earlier projects concerning community media and to study the functionality of digital community networks in relation to the functionality of other forms of community communication such as community newspapers, local radio and community television.

Speaking more generally, the emergence of the Internet has, like that of almost any new medium, given rise to hopes and fears about the impact of new media technology on the fabric of society as a whole and on urban communities in particular. This research project focuses on the potential of digital community networks to stimulate involvement of new groups – young people, immigrants, women – involved in the local community previously excluded from community media participation. The aim of this project is twofold: first, to conduct an in-depth comparative investigation of the participation of these groups in digital community networks and, second, to ascertain what conditions operating at the community level facilitate participation of these groups in the community networks and community activities. Digital community networks may be, in other words, valuable instruments for encouraging new groups to become involved in their local communities. This project will focus on these groups on their participation and input in digital community networks and on the consequences of that participation for other forms of community communication and involvement in the respective communities.

Community communication: point of departure

Digital community networks provide, much as traditional community media do, a shared location of identification for residents. At the same time, Internet facilities with possibilities for interactive communication provide opportunity to extend beyond the physical boundaries of a particular locality and to engage people on the basis of shared interests, independent of geographic location. The question, however, is whether community networks are merely an extension of already existing forms of community communication such as interpersonal communication and community newspapers, radio and television, or whether these networks constitute a radical break with these media.

The planned research project is to address the functionality of community networks for citizens in terms of media substitution, competition and extension (Lerg 1981). The basic hypothesis of this project is that community networks will not replace existing community media and other forms of community communication but will develop a functionality of their own, while at the same time community media will adapt to the new situation.

A second hypothesis is that groups, different from the groups involved in traditional community media, may become involved in community affairs via digital community networks. It is known from other studies (Hollander, Vergeer and Verschuren 1993, Westerik forthcoming) that community newspapers and local and regional forms of radio and television draw their audiences mainly from the older segment of the population. The rationale behind this phenomenon is that people first have to settle in a community in order to develop community ties and become involved in the community (Stamm 1985; Westerik forthcoming). On the other hand, the Internet has the potential to attract new groups of users, such as young people. Digital community networks may be a valuable instrument for encouraging new groups to become involved in local communities.

Community characteristics

· Population size and homogeneity
· History
· Urban/rural dimension
· Social, political and cultural issues
· Relation to surrounding region

Figure 8.2 Components of community communication and digital community
networks

Inasmuch as the communicative patterns of individuals are to be investigated in a specific geographic context, two levels of analysis are being considered: first, the individual level of personal actions, motives, expectations and aspirations of community members and, second, the social system level, that is the contextual aspects such as the city or neighbourhood, ethnic or cultural group. At the individual level it is assumed that people differ in their actions, attitudes and participation in community media and online community networks. At the social-system level it is assumed that communities differ in characteristics such as homogeneity, history and infrastructure and that these differences affect both the members of the community and the participation of these members in digital community networks. A diagram suggesting the relation of these features is shown in Figure 8.2; the characteristics noted are only illustrative of the features and should not be considered as complete. As with the dynamic model developed by Stamm (1985), described in the first section of this chapter, the relations posed in this model are also contingent on situations at specific points in time. The direction of the relations may change, in other words, for different time frames and for different community and individual characteristics.

The community characteristics in the figure are sometimes described as the social capital of a region (see Putnam 1993, 1995, Riedel *et al.* 1998). Further, Blanchard and Horan (1998) suggest that computer-mediated communication can help to generate social capital when virtual communities, such as digital community networks, overlap face-to-face networks and facilitate the density and flow of information within networks. Social capital can, in other words, serve as a condition and also as an outcome of community networks activities.

We plan to apply this framework in our investigation of community networks in the Netherlands. In order to include both levels of analysis a comparative study is proposed of two cases where existing geographically based communities (such as a city or a neighbourhood within it) are involved in various forms of community communication and a digital communication network. We have been in discussion with representatives from two community network initiatives: *Residentie.net* in The Hague and *Purmerend Punt En El* in the city of Purmerend. Both initiatives are in an early stage of development and offer the opportunity to perform extended case studies. Various distinctions in approach and setting between these initiatives (such as the role of city government, degree of social cohesion, variations in the social capital of the communities) may provide explanation for differences found between the two cases.

Methodological concerns

The case studies of both initiatives are to be conducted across time, drawing on field-research techniques developed in the community-study tradition within sociology (see Jankowski and Wester 1991), in the action-oriented tradition within community media investigations (Jankowski 1988, 1991) and in the interpretative approach to investigating online activity (Mann and Stewart 2000, Hine 2000). The researcher will perform participant observation in both the virtual and geographic manifestations of these communities in order to develop in-depth understanding of crucial phases of the two initiatives. These observations will be supplemented by electronic survey research among community-network participants, and standardised questionnaires for measuring media use will be adapted for this purpose. Content analysis, quantitative and qualitative, will also be conducted of the local media content and network sites in order to determine the nature of mediated communication within the communities. In the event that the log data for the community networks is made accessible, this content analysis will be supplemented with an examination of site traffic. This multiple method approach will facilitate the triangulation of findings and thereby provide a richer and fuller awareness of the communication processes within these communities.

We believe that a research design involving an integrated range of methods for data collection and analysis offers – in principle – the possibility of a richer understanding of the object of study. We realise the value in being able to verify what people say with what they do, particularly in a virtual world. At the same time, we are aware of the difficulties in 'triangulating' findings from one source of data with those from another when no base standard exists.

We are also concerned with how to incorporate an action component in the research design. We are aware of the difficulties such an approach may involve: having to choose sides during internal conflicts, having insufficient competence to consult actors properly during complex internal decision-making processes, lacking ability to meet the overall high expectations of the host organisation (see further: Greenwood and Levin 1998, Stringer 1999, Reason and Bradbury 2000). There are also potential rewards to such an approach, especially the possibility of contributing to a better communication structure for a community. Selection of an appropriate form of action research will be made in consultation with the digital community network organisations in the respective communities.

Finally, and perhaps most importantly, we will be asking much from the field researcher selected to conduct this study: willingness and ability to engage in intensive and extended interactions with persons at various strata in the localities and the digital community networks. The researcher must be familiar with a multitude of methods for data collection and analysis, and have the ability to integrate the findings into an overall theoretically grounded analysis. Such long-term, holistic projects are not common in the field of community media, but recent examples provide sources for inspiration (Hampton and Wellman 2000, Silver 2000). With such a field researcher, and with agreement on the above theoretical and methodological issues, the groundwork will be laid for contributing to a greater awareness of the value digital community networks may have for geographically based communities.

Notes

1 See further: http://www.purmerend.org.
2 See further: http://www.denhaag.org.
3 We wish to thank the following students for their contributions to this preliminary study during a graduate seminar: Sandra Goudswaard, Ivo Kersten, Ralf Knippenburg, Eef Oosters, Reneé van Os, Inge Verburg and Karin van de Wetering.
4 See further: http://www.residentie.net.

Chapter 9

Community networking in Russia
Identifying the research agenda

Sergei Stafeev

Introduction: community networking in Russia

This chapter explores the development of a 'digital divide' between not-for-profit, non-governmental organisations (NGOs) in Russia. It explores the particular problems faced by NGOs in Russia and suggests means of bridging the divide.

Russia has been experiencing a technological revolution. However, this revolution has resulted in a significant growth in a 'digital divide'. This divide is particularly apparent for those social institutions which do not seek to make commercial profit but which challenge a range of social problems in Russian society. Non-profit, non-governmental organisations (NGOs) in Russia are the front-line troops tackling problems in civil society along with a range of development issues. Social change is often a 'thankless' matter and NGOs have to work with no resources available for promoting their ideas or for attracting appropriate attention from sponsoring agencies, government and business. Historically, Russian NGOs have survived largely by owning their information and that of their users. This constituted their value and took the place of financial assets.

Usually NGOs have a vital role in the development of a democratic society. Russian society is in transformation from communism to an open democratic society. NGOs have blossomed throughout the region in response to the changes in society. Their health and fitness is crucial in the process of transformation. Analysts and experts attest that most of Russian NGOs remain in a primitive state.[1] However, most have developed in response to local community needs but do not have the capacity to play their full role in transforming Russia into an open democratic society.

The problem raised here is that, while we are witnessing a technological and information revolution and the rapid development of the Internet, a huge number of socially-oriented institutions in Russia are being placed in a strict information hierarchy. The information owner sets the criteria and price for its dissemination, which is not affordable for the vast majority of Russian NGOs. This makes them miss out on one of the most significant achievements in information and knowledge distribution systems. Potentially this will result in making it even harder for NGOs to continue implementing their missions.

The Internet has broken down the information hierarchy by eliminating obstacles to global information-sharing, thus potentially equalising the relationship between those who own information and those who want it. The Internet provides a lot of information. However, skills are needed to ensure that those needing the information can filter it and interpret it and turn it into useful knowledge. Whilst I acknowledge that the Internet is only a tool for NGO activities and much more is required to achieve their goals, the use of the Internet for information-sharing can encourage individuals to be socially active, which is the ultimate aim for further developments of NGOs.

Urban and rural FreeNets and community networks, especially in the United States, European countries, Canada and Australia, have created a radically different worldwide public sphere.[2] Emergence of this new public sphere presages a profound transformation where local information, for the first time, has begun to shape national and international networks.[3] Effects of this change on the policy environment will have a significant impact on the democratic rights of individuals and communities to pursue their visions for the future. This is especially important for post-communist countries, where administrative orientations and priorities regarding the significance and development of ICTs are fairly different from those in developed countries.

Significant differences exist between the levels of development of ICTs and the communication infrastructure in Newly Independent States (NIS), the United States and Europe. Besides the current differences in both hard and soft infrastructure there is a different historical background and tradition in NIS regarding ideas of self-governance and community-building on the local level. This background heavily influences the perspectives of Internet NGO resources and Public Information Technology (PIT) development. In fact, the worldwide trend of non-profit information resources is based on the already existing local community-access centres being united into broad regional and nationwide information networks (CTCnet in USA, CAP in Canada etc.).

The representative system of municipal governance created in Russia in the beginning of the 1990s is constantly changing. It now has inherited features of the former Soviet system of limited public participation in the political process and it lacks a number of significant and vital functions that are performed by communities in developed countries.

Nevertheless, today in post-Soviet countries we have identified a need for innovation, which will provide the basis for a wide range of changes within public administration. This development is often referred to as the transition from government to governance (see for example DETR 1998).

Developing ICTs in Russian NGOs

Our activity has to do with introducing new technological tools and knowledge into the Russian NGO sector. The main mission of this project is to address the challenge of making the NGOs in north-western Russia become aware that information once unique to them is now widely available over the Internet. Whilst recognising that the new ICTs are only a tool for NGO activities, this approach has to do with their being socially active as the ultimate ground for any further development. Some NGOs have excellent initiatives but are not ready or do not know how to partner with others to give their projects leverage. Others may seek project-funding but are not able to gain access to phone networks to communicate with external funding foundations or just do not know how to search the Internet for potential funding organisations. Bearing these issues in mind, the project aims to address the 'digital divide' in the non-profit sector in Russia by striving for equal information access and distribution through the creation of a community information network for all civilian and NGO initiatives in north-western Russia.

Successful community networks are driven by a broad set of social ideals and goals – the foremost being how modern information communications technology can be used for community-development purposes (Schuler 1996). Just as with modern public libraries, civic networks are worth supporting because of the greater public good resulting from their availability and use.

This programme aims to help communities develop community networks to provide services of genuine local relevance and benefit for the local community. An additional aim of this project is to demonstrate how these technologies can be used for fostering communications and information-sharing between Russian communities.

These same technologies offer benefits on a global scale as well. A community network will carry the full content of the larger Russian NGOs' projects locally and its content will be mirrored in other parts of the world through the Internet. In addition to the local content developed for local purposes (and, of course, published in the Russian language) each participating site will also publish some material in the English language that will be of interest to the global community. The goal is to help demonstrate how technologies can be used to effect partnerships with individuals and organisations in other parts of the world.

One of the primary objectives in establishing an information community network is to extend access and use of local, regional, national and international information and communication services to the local public who might not otherwise have the possibility of such access. Of equal importance is the ability of civic networks to offer the same individuals the ability to publish information. This can prove to be of vital importance as it can give 'voice' to such groups as NGOs, educators, government agencies, religious organisations, senior citizens etc. But the most important objective of civic networking is to establish a broad consortium of participants from various sectors of local community life who agree to work together to develop a shared information and communications resource of genuine benefit to the local community.

Through the programme we aim to help communities develop their own information services and provide the software for constructing interactive bulletin-board systems, email list servers, interactive chat sessions etc. The community networks will provide software, which will allow access to a basic Internet service such as email, the World Wide Web (WWW), telnet, FTP etc. However, it will also make possible the easy construction of a WWW-accessible version of the local information and communications network. The software must support local language content (initially handling Russian and English languages) and must provide facilities for handling the different Russian character set encodings.

Current activities on community networking in Russia

So far almost all of the projects connected with the development of non-profit access to information resources services (above all the Internet) and the Russian NGO sector have been implemented through educational institutions, particularly through universities. The Open Institute (G. Soros Foundation) supports the 'University Internet Centres' providing free public access to the Internet.

Another example of a successful project is the not-for-profit initiative 'Friends and Partners Civil Networks'. This is a joint Russian–United States planning and demonstration project, supported by the Ford Foundation, the Eurasia Foundation and other interested organisations. It aims to promote development and the widespread availability of advanced telecommunications technologies and civic networking to enhance the delivery of social services and generally serve public interests; to promote access to government information and increase civic participation; and to support the advancement of a nationwide civic networking infrastructure in Russia. The main strategy of this project is the building of a national Friends and Partners network through setting up a number of regional centres of free public access to informational resources (Internet) on the basis of existing active social groups.[4]

The third example is a Russian–British project, 'Gardarika', which will provide the experimental ground for our research. Together with its British partner, Community Education and Development Centre (CEDC) Studio of Computer Design, 'Gardarika' established the Centre for Support of Public Initiatives in St Petersburg at the Russian Christian Humanitarian Institute (RCHI). The remit of the project includes arranging an educational research centre into the problems of the non-commercial sector. In addition, at Vyborg, Leningrad Oblast, a municipal centre of support for NGOs was set up. The municipal centre provided an opportunity for a group of specialists from Great Britain, St Petersburg and Vyborg to review the principles of the co-operation between NGOs, municipal administration, business and the mass media. A working model of the regional informational net of NGO support was also created (St Petersburg–Vyborg). It allows users of the network (non-commercial organisations of the region) to take advantage of the Internet in their activities. This project laid down the foundations for the creation of a regional network of NGOs in the region of Leningrad.[5]

The general principles of the research

Our activity has to do with introducing new technological tools and knowledge into the Russian NGO sector. The first step of this introduction is the implementation of a research programme. The main mission of this research agenda is to make NGOs in the NIS aware of the fact that the information which was once unique to them is now widely available over the Internet. It was also intended to construct an information network that would act as a resource for NGOs, for federal and municipal bodies and for mutual business interaction. We remain aware that the new technologies are only a tool for their activities and the organisations involved still have to act alone to pursue their goals. However, this approach is intended to encourage the organisations to be socially active, our ultimate goal for any further development.

Another important direction of our research programme is the development of a nationwide informational infrastructure for NGOs in community networks. Generally, community networks are based on several principles and goals, including first, content provided by the members, second, bi-directional communication, and, third, focus on local affairs (Schuler 1996).

We realise that setting up a proper, autonomous, not-for-profit informational infrastructure in a small territory requires a great deal of organisational and financial resources. It is possible to draw on those resources which already exist (commercial, governmental etc.). The main aim of our project in this direction is to investigate and clear up the necessity of a telecommunications infrastructure.

We consider that a community information infrastructure (CII) is not simply about hardware – wires, modems, servers, routers etc. The term is not limited to how communities provide access, increase individual computer literacy or extend connectivity. Rather, CII refers to the nature of the information infrastructure, for example the content, structure and relationships among discrete information resources, providers and users, and the intended social function of the CII. To this degree these key aspects correspond and create a new 'public sphere'. Democratic decision-making and community-building are enhanced.

There is a lack of government funding for national programmes for Internet development in the NGO sector together with a lack of recognition of the value of the Internet in terms of it being a tool for sustainable economic development. A brief policy analysis reveals the underlying priorities of economic efficiency and competitiveness of governmental information social policy and highlights their inherent techno-economic determinism.[6]

Altogether these factors create serious obstacles for the successful integration of the countries of the former Soviet Union into the global information society, leading those countries into the so-called 'digital divide' zone. However, there is not much discussion about the 'digital divide' in the NIS and, in comparison with the US and Europe, the policy of restricted information access already has a negative impact on social and economic development in those countries.

Because of the factors identified above we consider it is vital to establish *an independent interdisciplinary and inter-professional research organisation* responsible for the implementation of:

1   *scholarly and critical research*: observations and analysis of social, cultural, economic and political situations; resource analysis; analysis of existing projects in the public interest technology (PIT) field and other happenings in this field. PIT concerns the development of a family of resources for community networking, recycling programmes, assistance to other non-profits and free access centres etc.
2   *joint national and international projects* regarding the analysis of existing successful experiences in this field in various countries, analysis of interpretation and the appliance of such experience to NIS. These projects will be conducted in partnership with a wide range of various research organisations, experts and specialists from all over the world
3   *independent recommendations for policy-makers and law-makers* in NIS. The research organisation would also co-operate with them suggesting alternative versions of governmental and municipal programmes in the community-networking and not-for-profit-ICTs realm. It would develop recommendations and guidelines for international organisations interested in supporting not-for-profit ICT projects in NIS
4   *the creation of working models* of not-for-profit Internet resources access networks on regional and local levels
5   *the analysis of public involvement* in the discussion of national policy in the field of ICTs usage
6   *the organisation of regular conferences* to provide a forum in order that those engaged in research and practical work in the field of PIT can meet and exchange information about their work
7   *the sponsorship and dissemination of information* about our research through the publication of a site on the WWW and through other

scholarly and popular publications. It would also act as a clearing-house for information about research resources in the field of PIT and encourage their development.

The principles of the research methodology

Much of the work would be focused on small, locally based voluntary and community organisations (NGOs) that are characterised by an ethos of self-help or mutual aid. Whilst the culture of smaller and locally based organisations renders them potentially well-placed to utilise ICTs in the pursuit of community empowerment, alternative agendas can potentially marginalise these groups. It would appear that exploiting the full potential of ICTs for all citizens in post-Soviet countries might be dependent upon how successfully the underpinning values of the groups can be promoted and defended.

Several main fields are valuable in the establishment of an encompassing research programme. These fields differ from each other because of the methodology involved in investigation of each.

ICT and social life in community-networking aspect

The prospects of ICT-facilitated empowerment of citizens depends upon embedding electronic networks within existing social, economic and political community networks (whether geographical communities or communities of interest) (Gurstein 2000b). In ICT experiments, the use of technology is the central theme. In experiments in the social field, the method for solving social problems is important. In community networks, establishing ownership of the technology and control over the uses to which it is put at the community level is crucial. However, ICTs are subject to social shaping and, as such, are embedded within a variety of often conflicting discourses and might be harnessed in pursuit of a variety of competing objectives. It is vital to identify those 'values' that are central to the pursuit of an empowerment agenda and to locate those values within the contextualised environments. Community projects must work to meet the needs of the under-served groups such as minorities, low-income, homeless, elderly, disabled, immigrant population in urban and rural areas. These community networks should be an integral part of the community groups they serve.

Comparative investigations and analysis

When looking at the technical and social aspects of already implemented projects it is important to distinguish between projects run at national, regional and local levels. Projects can also be categorised in terms of the kind of activities addressed, distinguishing those focusing on work activities from those focusing on everyday life and those focused in civil society as a whole. Three main types of trails serve to assist in this categorisation:

- *technology trails* – in which prototype components and systems are developed and tested in an operational environment
- *service trails* – in which advanced communication services are demonstrated and tested by network operators and service providers
- *usage trails* – in which end-users of advanced services experiment with and demonstrate innovative uses for their own business, public service or personal interest.

As a result, there is a need to develop a national methodological knowledge base of design, development and implementation strategies. From this base NGOs or communities can, after reflection, select methods appropriate to their specific needs, or be inspired to develop their own. Also such a knowledge base would highlight the potential for the social shaping of ICTs. In this field the main tool will be the analysis of 'best practice'.

Case studies in informational policies

In this area there is a need to analyse and examine existing international and national governmental policy documents and related texts and to examine the implications at the micro level to address social exclusion through not-for-profit ICTs initiatives.

There is also a need to provide a nationwide overview that can in turn be fed into the development and implementation of local plans and to establish a framework of methodological tools to inform policy of more inclusive and collaborative pathways to more equal society in post-Soviet countries.

Problematic areas

We shall consider nine problematic areas. First, *community informatics studies*. This encompasses the research of already established and formed community information infrastructures. This would cover the content, structure and relationships of discrete information resources, providers and users and the intended social function. It should be noted that communities are vital social entities where there is an active, inclusive information infrastructure involving mass media, gossip, community forums, friendly conversation on the street and messages emanating from various community organisations. It also comprises studies as to how ICTs can help achieve social, economic, political and cultural goals for a community.

Second, *NGOs and digital divide*. NGOs are the front-line troops tackling civil-society and community-developmental issues. Often, Russian NGOs have already developed the credibility, the network of contacts, the understanding and the trust of the community they serve. It is proposed that NIS should develop networks of non-profit access to informational resources and PIT (access centres, community web resources) by relying on the most active and prominent local non-profit organisations and initiatives. To demonstrate this methodology a special pilot project is to be launched in the Leningrad region to educate not-for-profit organisations in the use of newer information technologies to strengthen public participation in policy development. The 'Gardarika' project, in collaboration with CCNS, will start an online resource centre to share emerging not-for-profit case examples and research and technology resources for public policy activities.

Third, *communication policy and the new public sphere*. The advancement of communication technologies, along with the abundance of information in today's knowledge-based society, is creating a new, integrated global information society. Achieving a successful balance between the demands of the open market and the need to maintain and promote cultural sovereignty and national identity will be key to maximising gains from the global informational society. The centre's research studies should contribute to the information social-policy discourse by examining existing tensions between policy and attempts to address social exclusions through ICT initiatives in NIS. This research programme plans to build a nationwide base of local, regional and national groups interested in public access, developing tools to promote the public's right to know and making specific recommendations for improved public policies. There is a need to research and record the process, the impediments and the key components of success and to develop models which can be used in this particular cultural setting.

Fourth, *community networks and economic development*. Many successful examples exist in various countries showing how community networks can effectively address many important social issues, such as unemployment, business development, social cohesion, technology training and access to technology. It is necessary to analyse those examples to determine their potential for transfer and implementation in NIS. This is especially important in developing independent strategies applicable to NGOs in the NIS so that they maximise their ability to manage their activities and fundraising campaigns for ICT initiatives and programmes.

Fifth, *education, training, community learning networks*. A major and rapidly emerging area for non-profit ICT network activities is in education, training and life-long learning. A number of successful projects in distant education have been implemented in some academic centres and universities in the NIS.[7]

However, all of these projects focus only on a narrow group of the population, which realises the importance of education and can afford unrestricted access to the Internet. Unfortunately there are no successful non-commercial projects of ICT usage for community education, working with disabled groups or telemedicine at the local level. The objective in this area of research would be to examine proven experience in this field in order to develop and test practical recommendations and working models of free access.

Sixth, *ICT in rural communities*. It is important to determine the impediments to a more equitable distribution of PIT around the country – especially to small towns and rural areas. It is particularly important to research the feasibility of not-for-profit Internet access centres to be established with minimal financial and technical investment in remote areas. These areas do offer great potential for the employing of new communication technologies, for example satellite channels.

Seventh, *models of networking*. Experience demonstrates that all tools of public-interest technology – public access, low-cost hardware and dial-up access, training and technical assistance, online conferencing, non-commercially driven community publishing, web and listserv hosting – can be delivered more economically and efficiently when local resources are pooled. Consequently, existing models of networks in various countries need to be examined on local, regional or national levels. The principles of interaction between different social groups (NGO, governmental bodies, mass media, business etc.) for better co-operation need to be examined within these networks in pilot projects.

Eighth, *free or community access centres*. Possible organisational, financial and technical grounds for such centres need to be defined for application in the NIS. Research in this area will develop the documentation necessary for setting up a typical centre (guides, rule books, examples of best practice etc.).

Ninth, *using PIT for public involvement or public participation*. As pointed out above, we need to study ways of involving the public in decision-making using PIT (for example how ICTs can reinvigorate a young representative democracy in post-Soviet countries). This activity will investigate the possibilities of vertical communication between state institutions, government and self-government on federal or regional and local levels, and citizens, including:

- electronic publishing of information, from government to citizen
- electronic gathering of information, from citizen to government
- informal online discussions
- formal consultations using online debates etc.

Conclusion

The purpose of this chapter has been to raise issues pertinent to the community networking research agenda for the Russian Federation developed by the Centre of Community Networking and Information Policy Studies (CCNS).[8] Central to our vision is the idea that CBO (community-based organisations) and other NGOs, which are being encouraged to take over more and more responsibility for local regeneration and for service delivery worldwide, cannot only access but also produce and manipulate data in the public domain. Equally, public service planners and managers must have, and be able to value and use, data and other information produced at a community level.

One of the main activities of CCNS is to provide assistance to develop the information resources for the civil society of Russia. We are sure that at present it is very important to strengthen efforts aimed at the integration of Russian society (including low-income citizens who do not have the opportunity to use the Internet) into the world information space. This informational openness of society, the practical realisation of citizens' rights to have free access to information and citizens' participation in information exchange through up-to-date ICTs is, we consider, the most important prerequisite of democratic change in post-communist countries.

Notes

1 There are a number of Russian books which support this statement, for example, V. Kasho (2000) *NGO: Questions and Answers* (Krasnoyarsk), pp. 7–25.
2 A good collection of articles and links on this can be found on http://www.tachoon.net.
3 An example of this can be found at the very dynamic site Seattle Community Network, http://www.scn.org.
4 http://www.friends-partners.ru.
5 http://www.cspi.org.uk.
6 A good example is the White Paper on the National IT Policy, 2001 available online at http://www.soi.ru.
7 For example http://www.sitc.ru – a successful project on distant learning in Yakutsk, Siberia.
8 http://www.cspi.org.ru/ccns.

Chapter 10

Some lessons of social experiments with technology

Birgit Jæger

Introduction

Denmark was one of the first places where social experiments were used as a process for introducing information and communication technology (ICT) to ordinary people. In the middle of the 1980s the first wave of experiments was introduced into rural areas in Denmark. Since then several other experiments have been carried out. Many things have changed since the 1980s. The goals have changed, the technology is different, target groups have shifted and new groups of actors are involved. In this chapter the development of social experiments with ICT in Europe, and especially in Denmark, will be described, and the chapter will try to identify what the outcomes of all these social experiments were and what the lessons might be for future developments.

Background

For many years the study of technological development has focused on the research and innovation process – often in the laboratories of large companies. The development of technology was understood as a linear process in different stages, such as invention, innovation and diffusion. Thus technology was understood as a determinant of social structure (Smith and Marx 1994). This way of understanding technology and the development of technology has been questioned in recent decades by another theoretical approach, where technology is understood as shaped or constructed through complex social processes. From studies within this framework we have learned that it is not appropriate to describe the development of technology as a linear process in distinct stages. Studies have shown that there are still processes of innovation going on even in the stage of diffusion (Bijker 1995). This new approach has led to a need for studying technology in a broader context where social processes both in the lab and in the everyday use of technology are drawn into the analysis.

Within the framework of the social construction of technology, a recently completed European study, called the SLIM study,[1] emphasised the processes of social learning in the European uptake of multimedia and ICT. One way to analyse the learning processes was to study social experiments with ICT. Based on descriptions from the eight participating European countries, the SLIM study wanted to analyse social learning, which resulted from experiments. This chapter draws heavily on the work undertaken by SLIM but it also draws on work from earlier evaluations of different Danish social experiments. Mostly these experiments focused upon ICTs, but, where appropriate, experiments from other fields are also included.

In the first section of this chapter social experiments will be described in a broader political context. Social experiments will be discussed as a tool for innovation and development primarily within the public sector. In the next section the chapter discusses what a social experiment actually is. In working on the SLIM study it soon became clear that one could not take the concept of social experiments for granted. The concept had different meanings for the different participants in the study. The chapter will go on to present a theoretical understanding of social learning which arose out of the SLIM study. Finally, the chapter will describe different lessons learned from social experiments mainly in Denmark.

Social experiments as a tool for innovation and development

The 1980s saw a boom in both ICT experiments and other government-sponsored experimental programmes in Denmark. It seemed as if every minister with a little self-respect had his or her own programme. There are several reasons for this boom. One of the reasons is that after approximately thirty years in power the Social Democrats stepped down and four parties from the political right (led by the Conservative Party) took over. This new government saw it as a major task to reorganise public administration in Denmark.

Another reason for the introduction of social experiments could have been the influence of social movements. Especially within the field of social policy, social movements had been very active. Many social workers were not satisfied with the methods for tackling social problems. Attempts to restructure traditional public administration structures and procedures had been limited by the rigidity of the system, and new means of producing changes were being sought (Hegland 1990). Thus the social policy field was one of the first areas where experiments were introduced and in 1989 one of the biggest governmental programmes was introduced. It was the so-called SUM programme (SUM stands for The Ministry of Social Affair's fund for development), which supported approximately 1700 local experiments spread all over the country. A total of 350 million DKr was used in the next three and a half years to find new ways to solve all kinds of social problems

(Jensen 1992). (Sums in Danish Kroner should be divided by ten to give an approximate equivalent in sterling.)

A third reason for the boom can, to a certain extent, be found within the public administration's planning system. For a couple of decades the planning had been more or less automatically an extrapolation of the budget on the national, regional and local levels. In the 1980s it became clear that big changes in society (stemming from facts such as an increasingly overstretched economy, growing unemployment, the introduction of information technology and increasingly poor industrial relations) demanded other solutions than those previously used. In other words, there was a need for innovation and development in public administration as well as in private companies. The first social experiments with ICT in Denmark were also evaluated as a method of planning. The conclusion of this evaluation was that social experiments cannot replace traditional physical planning but they can supplement the planning because they are very useful to explore what is possible, the inexperienced, the alternative and the unexpected (Marling 1991: 205).

No matter which reason is the most important, a need for innovation was identified, which led to a wide range of changes within public administration. Today this development is often referred to as the transition from government to governance (Rhodes 1997). This transition consists of a lot of different elements (decentralisation of local administration, user boards, privatisation and so forth) which together have resulted in a breakdown of the traditional hierarchy of public organisations. Instead new networks have appeared where the borders of the organisations are not clear at all (Andersen *et al.* 1999a). The stream of publicly funded experimental or developmental programmes can also be understood as one element in this transition.

To give a picture of the prevalence of ICT experiments I have listed some of the experiments in Table 10.1. It is mainly a list of experiments which are anchored in local communities, funded by the Danish government and played out in public administration (I have excluded experiments taking place in private enterprises and funded by the enterprises themselves, the EC or other sources). A more detailed description of some of the ICT experiments is given in the SLIM review of multimedia experiments and trails in eight European countries. Table 10.1 is a rewriting of the Danish review (Jæger and Hansen 1999a: 111–19). I do not claim that it is a complete list, but they are the best-known public experiments.

All the experimental programmes, with ICT or within other fields, produced a lot of results within each cohort; for example the SUM programme resulted in a lot of new ways to solve social problems for disabled people, refugees, older people, the unemployed and so forth. But the most important result of all these governmental programmes was that experiments became accepted as a tool for innovation and developing new approaches to public administration. In the TMU programme (introduced below) it was presented as a major breakthrough that the people managing the programmes

Table 10.1 Danish ICT experiments

Name	Objectives	Date	Resources	No. of experiments	Evaluation
The telephone companies experiment with online service	Development of a Danish online service	1982–4	30 million DKr from the telephone companies	2	Yes, by independent researchers
TUP (Technological Developmental Programme)	Introduction of ICT in private companies	1984–9	1500 million DKr from the government	Unknown	Yes, by independent researchers
TMU programme	Regional development with ICT in rural areas	1986–9	30 million DKr from the government, 100 million DKr in total funding	16	Yes, singly and at an overall level. Carried out by independent researchers
Kommunedata's[2] experiment with online service	Development of a Danish online service for the local authorities	1989–91	Kommunedata and the two involved local communities have funded the experiment. The total amount of funding is unknown.	2	Yes, by independent researchers
Kommunedata's experiment with local election	Development of support for electronic local election	1997	Unknown	1	Yes, by independent researchers
Spearhead municipalities	Use of ICT in different parts of the local administration	1996–7	Only local. The amount of funding is unknown	10	Yes, followed by the National Association of Local Authorities in Denmark
The elderly's use of ICT	Development of applications to raise the quality of life of elderly	1999–2003	33 million DKr	6	Yes, by independent researchers

had learned the value of experimentation (Cronberg 1990 and 1991). They had learned how to apply for funding, how to organise the experiment and how to manage its implementation. This was new knowledge in Denmark at that time. It was also a theme in the social field. In 1991 a study of the experiments (Adamsen and Fisker 1991) concluded that there was a battle going on between two different kinds of organisational cultures: the system culture and the experimental culture. Today we can conclude that the experimental culture won the battle. Today experiments are widespread as a method of innovation in public administration. Even the smallest Danish local community knows how to establish an experiment and the larger and regional agencies know how to apply to the EU for funding. Thus we can conclude that this is one of the long-time results of all these experimental programmes.

This victory of the experimental method has led to them becoming an accepted approach to policy-making. Today one seldom hears anybody talk about social experiments. Nowadays, politicians and civil servants talk more about developmental projects or just activities. This shows that experiments have become mundane – a part of everyday life within public administration.

The large governmental funding programmes have however been replaced by smaller programmes focused on a specific sector. Some of these are described as *permanent pools* which are focused upon local developmental activities. These smaller programmes and pools can be found at every level of public administration. At the national level funding for a specific programme is often a part of a political negotiation around the objectives of the national budget. At the regional level and sometimes also at the local level the politicians often have a special account on the budget for experiments and policy development.

Because of these trends it is not possible to obtain an overview of all the experiments going on in Denmark today. Many activities are not defined as experiments: they are just seen as a way to develop public administration. In the 1980s the experiments were very easy to recognise, because they were matters of public debate. That is not the case today. What is at stake in the public debate today is rather a question of whether or not we have gone too far in the experimental direction. The Danish Finance Minister, for example, has recently raised the question of whether there are too many programmes and suggested that it may be dangerous not to have a coherent overview of these fragmented and diverse small pools and programmes.

To return to Table 10.1, the fact that experiments have become mundane means that there are a lot of activities which are not on the list, simply because to obtain a complete picture would require a survey of every local community. As an example I will mention the field of tele-work. Tele-work is mentioned in the national ICT policy for implementation of the information society,[3] but there has never been a central initiative to establish experiments in this field. Notwithstanding, the increasing interest in this issue has led to a lot of activities. The Danish trade union for office workers and trade has made a homepage about tele-work.[4] On this homepage eighty-four activities were registered in April 2000 (an increase from thirty-five activities in July 1998). Some of them are called experiments, others are labelled as projects of development. A few of these activities are just one single person who is tele-working, but in other projects more than a hundred people are involved. Some activities are taking place in public administration, others in private enterprises.

Another similar example is the emergence of public-agency homepages on the Internet. The national ICT policy encourages every public authority to make public services available on the Internet for citizen access. As a result of this there has been a boom in local authorities present on the web. In July 1998, eighty-seven out of 275 Danish municipalities and all fourteen counties had made a homepage (Jæger and Hansen 1999a: 110) and in April 2000, 217 municipalities had a website. There are of course big differences in the quality of these homepages. The simplest ones contain just a picture of the mayor and a few pieces of information from the town hall, while one of the most developed homepages (Copenhagen) can be characterised as a 'Digital City' (Jæger 1999).

What is a social experiment?

In the SLIM study our discussions of how to understand social experiments soon ran into questions such as: What is a social experiment? How social does it have to be? Does it always include the users? Who is learning? And what do they learn?

By analysing experiments from all eight countries it became clear that there were many features which could lead to different ways of categorising the experiments. In this study we ended up with a continuum of different experiments with technological feasibility studies at the one end, over commercial trials and pilots to classical social experiments at the other end (Jæger et al. 2000). This continuum describes whether the experiment takes its point of departure in technology, market or users' needs. But we also identified other features that could serve to make categories. There is a big difference between experiments that are privately funded and those that are publicly funded (not to mention the experiments which are a mixture of both). We could also distinguish between experiments run at a national, regional and local level, just as we could categorise experiments in terms of the kind of activities addressed, distinguishing those focusing on work activities from those focusing on everyday life and those focused on civil society as a whole.

The distinction between trails, pilots and experiments is also reflected in the European ACTS (Advanced Communications Technologies and Services) programme. This programme distinguishes three main types of trial:

- *technology trials*, in which prototype components and systems are developed and tested in an operational environment
- *service trials*, in which advanced communication services are demonstrated and tested by network operators and service providers, both to validate protocols and to stimulate demand and new applications
- *usage trials*, in which end-users of advanced services experiment with and demonstrate innovative uses for their own business, public service or personal interests (Jæger *et al.* 2000).

The SLIM study also showed that there were national differences in the understanding of what a social experiment is. The Danish and British cases illustrate these differences. In Denmark the classic social experiment has been dominant while in the UK the more commercial multimedia pilots have been the norm. At least some of these differences can be explained by different national policies in the field of technology. Whereas UK policy since the late 1970s has almost exclusively focused on the commercial factors, and in particular competitiveness, the Danish policy has been focused on citizen-involvement in the assessment of technology. In Denmark citizen-involvement became an essential element of the societal appropriation of technology (Andersen and Jæger 1999).

The SLIM study does not reach conclusions as to whether one kind of trial or experiment is better or more correct than another. Rather the conclusion is that experiments will always be very context-dependent, and what is the right experiment in one context can be the wrong in another and vice versa. However, we still have not defined what a classic social experiment is.

If we go back to the first wave of experiments with ICTs in Denmark we recognise that there was not a clear-cut definition of social experiments at that time either. This wave of experiments was actually a by-product of a political controversy about a hybrid network that was under discussion in the early 1980s. The hybrid network would have covered only communities with more than 250 households in its first years. The political compromise then reached was that rural and remote parts of the country should have the opportunity of creating social experiments with information technology so that they would be prepared for the introduction of the hybrid network to their area at a later date. An interministerial committee managed the experimental programme, called the TMU programme (in Danish: Tvær Ministielt Udvalg).

In the legal preparation work for the hybrid network there was also a governmental working group which reviewed international experience. This working group concluded that the international experience did not include any knowledge about user needs, or social, human and environmental aspects. Thus they recommended that a Danish experimental programme should focus not only on the technical aspects but also on the user-oriented aspects of the projects (Cronberg 1990: 18–19). In the final law, passed in February 1988, the platform for the experimental programme is found in §12. From this paragraph we learn that social experiments, or pilot projects, should develop and test technology and assess its consequences in small, rural communities. But this is not a very significant definition of social experiments.

Just about the same time the European Commission's FAST programme had agreed upon a definition of social experiments. It says:

> Social experiments with information technology are specific forms of implementation of IT:
> *   in which the primary aim is to establish new forms of social organ-isation using information technology;
> *   in which the activities and the resulting socio-technical products can be used as models for a more widespread – though necessarily contextually-modified – implementation of similar IT systems;
> *   and in which, to this latter end, independent researchers describe and evaluate the implementation process concerned and its results.
> . . . social experiments qualify as '*participatory workshops*' if all the parties involved in, or influenced by, the development of the IT system concerned, participate on an equal footing in decision-making with regard to the social organization and application of the IT system in question.
>
> (Jæger and Qvortrup 1991: 37–8)

In this definition the emphasis is on 'new form[s] of social organisation' and social experiments as 'participatory workshops'. What is also remarkable is that it includes the requirement that social experiments should be evaluated by independent researchers and disseminated to provide lessons for other projects. This aspect was also a part of the first Danish experimental programme. I will return to this discussion later.

Clearly an authoritative definition of social experiments does not exist. If we go to other scientific traditions we will find clear definitions of, for example, a medical experiment or a physical experiment. These experiments are built on the ideal of natural science and here the experiment tries to reduce the complexity to a state were there is only one variable left to test. We could call this 'the reductionistic experiment'. On the contrary we have what Olsen (1998) calls 'the complex experiment', which 'instead of a limited set of variables is working with complex social contexts and instead of control groups is working with public discussion and treats the concept of a laboratory as a protective space for the actors involved to be sheltered from the press of the surrounding world'[5] (Olsen 1998: 33, my translation).

It is to make this distinction clear that I call it a 'social experiment'. I am not talking about a controlled experiment in a scientific way just as I am not talking about a pure technical experiment. I am talking about experiments where social interaction is a very important part of the experiment and where the context is playing a crucial role. In the SLIM study we defined social experiments as follows:

> By this we refer to experiments based upon the direct involvement of citizens and groups in open ended exploration of how technologies might be designed and developed to fulfil social need – driven by a democratic concern to involve ordinary citizens as actors in development, and to meet kinds of need that may otherwise be overlooked by commercial provision.
>
> (Jæger *et al.* 2000: 32)

To this definition I would like to add that the social experiment is always located in some specific setting. In the first Danish experiments (and also some latter experiments) this was a very important part of the experiments. One of the main targets was that the experiments were meant to be a driving force for regional development. But, this is not the case for all experiments.

In a social experiment it is not important whether the technology in question is completely original or that it is a kind of generic software. What is important is that the technology is new in that particular local setting or new to the group of citizens involved. It is also important that the actors themselves regard it as an experiment. This means that the activity has a beginning and an end and very often it also means that the activity is funded by somebody outside the activity. I will develop this argument later.

Theoretical understanding of social learning

Before I go on to describe what we have learned of all these social experiments I will draw in some theoretical thoughts about how we can understand social learning. As already mentioned I draw heavily on the work done in the SLIM study.[6]

The starting point for defining social learning in the SLIM study was to focus on three elements:

* the way in which technology is designed and developed
* how the technological offerings are taken up within society
* the development of the broader context of regulations, policies and so forth that set the 'rules of the game' (William *et al.* 2000: 97).

This distinction between different kinds of social learning became visible when using different sources to understand the concept. From economic studies of productivity we picked up the concept of 'learning by doing'. This idea describes how workers develop a more efficient and productive way of employing technology through experience. The knowledge which is a result of this kind of learning is often difficult to describe because it is contingent and tacit. But it is possible to read out of the volume of the production.

Evolutionary economists have emphasised the importance for suppliers to get access to the knowledge users develop in learning by doing. This has led to the learning economy approach,[7] which emphasises the institutionalisation of linkages between suppliers and users through the development of channels of communication, shared codes of conduct and conceptualisations. In the SLIM study we have called this 'learning by interacting'. During the study it also became clear that national regulation policies also play a crucial role in the societal uptake of a technology. To describe this we developed the term 'learning by regulating'.

To study these different processes of social learning the SLIM study has drawn on theoretical concepts developed within different scientific traditions. The concept of innofusion (Fleck 1988) was adopted to emphasise that technology is shaped not only in the process of innovation but also in the process of diffusion. But this concept does not pay attention to how artefacts become incorporated within practices and acquire their meaning and significance. Thus the SLIM study also had to draw on work from cultural studies and studies of technologies in everyday life. Here we found the concept of domestication (Silverstone and Hirsch 1992) usable in the SLIM framework.

Domestication emphasises how a household needs to 'tame' the artefact when it is taken into the home from the outside world. To domesticate an artefact is to negotiate its meaning and practice. Both action and meaning are important. William *et al.* (2000: 103) describe it like this:

Artefacts have to be:

- acquired, either bought or in some other way made accessible
- placed which means that they are situated in a physical, symbolic and mental space
- interpreted to be given meaning within the household or a similar local context of identity as well as symbolic value to the outside world
- integrated into social practices of action.

It is of course questionable whether such concepts developed to describe processes in enterprises or private homes are applicable to a study of how a technology is taken up within other spheres of society. I will not discuss the definition of a society here, but it is obviously something other than an enterprise or a home. When we apply the concept of 'learning of doing' we are not able to test the learning process in society in the same way as it is possible to test it in an enterprise. The SLIM study has decided to transfer the concept to a broader context because we found it useful to explain what we found in the case studies, but of course it is still debatable whether it is possible to do so.

It is relevant to raise the same question about the broader use of the concept of domestication, which is developed to explain processes in private homes. The SLIM study decided to use this concept in a broader way because it gave meaning in the analysis of processes in local communities, school classes and so forth. To sum up the theoretical framework developed in the SLIM study to understand social learning, it may be said to distinguish between different learning processes as learning by doing, learning by interacting and learning by regulating. The concept of innofusion questions the understanding of technological development as going on in separate phases. Even when the artefact is ready for diffusion there are still processes of innovation going on when the users are taking up the technology. The concept of domestication highlights the learning processes the users are going through when they tame the technology by bringing it into the daily practices and give meaning to the artefact.

Social experiments can be a valuable source of knowledge to understand social learning. If we have in mind the three elements the SLIM study was focusing on at the outset we see that social experiments have been a useful source for social learning concerning the way in which technology is both designed and developed. By examining how the technology is taken up in the society and how the broader context helps to set, for example, 'the rules of the game', the TMU programme provided knowledge about the way in which technology is designed and developed. One of the main conclusions of the TMU programme was that technology was designed and developed further when it became a part of a social experiment (Cronberg 1990). Several of the experiments listed in Table 10.1 have given significant knowledge about how ICTs are taken up within the society. Within these experiments we can find many examples of how different groups of users have started to use the technology, just as we can find examples of how technology is interpreted in local contexts and how users have given the technology meaning and a symbolic value. A social experiment can in itself be understood as the broader context around the innovation of the technology and in that way 'set the rules of the game'.

Lessons from ICT experiments and other projects

In this section I will focus on the lessons learned from different experiments and projects. I will mainly focus on experiments and projects that concern the use of ICT but where it is fruitful I will draw in experience from some other programmes. It is obvious that it is impossible to compare the substance of the results across different sectors. Results from an experiment with disabled people is of course not comparable with results from an ICT experiment. But concerning the experience with processes in an experiment and the mechanisms in the social interaction during the trial period, it is possible to compare the experience.

This selection of lessons learnt from social experiments is a subjective selection. There are a lot of other lessons learnt from the experiments, but these are what I find most important. Other researchers would, maybe, have focused on other lessons.

Lessons about social learning

It is obvious that the Danish government expects some results when it invests all this money in social experiments in different fields. It was one of the rules of the game that the experiments were expected to lead to innovations, changes, new products, new practices or new methods. When we look at the experiments as a learning process it becomes clear that the people who have been involved in the experiments have learned a lot. This was actually one of the main conclusions of the evaluation of the TMU programme (Cronberg 1990 and 1991). If the sixteen experiments in this programme were to be evaluated solely on their objectives, most of them would have been classified as failures. But the evaluation could identify a row of learning processes which had not been expected and thus not described as a target.

This finding raises the question of what a successful experiment is. In a traditional evaluation you would answer that a successful experiment was one that fulfilled all the objectives established at the outset of the experiment. But experience from many experiments shows that most experiments are set very broad objectives. For example, one of the experiments in a rural area funded by the TMU programme wanted to create more workplaces; create more public and private services; and create more education and cultural opportunities in the local community. In other words, they wanted to stop the regression they experienced mostly as a result of the structural changes in farming (Jæger *et al.* 1990). In hindsight we can see that it was naive to believe it was possible to stop this regression with a small experiment with ICT. None the less, it was the objective of the experiment.

If the evaluation, instead of focusing on the objectives, focused on the learning processes the outcome would look quite different. As Cronberg writes in the evaluation of the TMU programme:

> While the successful innovations indicate the future directions, many of the learning processes are related to the *failures*, the unsuccessful experiments revealing conflicts and lacking innovative potential. The social experiments have exposed rivalries between various employee groups (for example in the municipal administration) or uncovered conflicts between the tenants and the housing corporation. While many of these conflict-ridden social experiments are closed down today, the learning processes related to them are very instructive.
>
> (Cronberg 1991: 21)

In the SUM programme success was very much identified as a matter of making the experiment permanent. At the time of the planning of the SUM programme there had already been some early experiments. An evaluation of these early experiments had concluded that, even though some of them were very innovative and had discovered new methods for solving social problems, they were never adopted by the local administration (Adamsen *et al.* 1990). The people involved in the experiments had learned a lot but the lessons from the experiments were confined to these individuals; they were never adopted by the local administration and thus an opportunity for organisational learning was lost. Thus one overall target within the SUM programme was to make the experiments permanent as a part of the organisation of the local administration (Flex and Koch-Nielsen 1992).

This target was fulfilled for only half of the experiments in the social field (Fiske 1995: 50). There are several explanations for, this which I will consider later. Fiske (1995) calls this an 'instrumental' way of using the experience from the experiments, but he also identifies another way, which he calls a 'conceptual' way of using the experience. In the latter the experiment is closed down in the locality where it was tried out, but while it was running it succeeded in showing that it was built on a good idea or concept. Other local communities took up some of these ideas and implemented them in their local setting. Maybe they did not do it in exactly the same way as in the first experiment but they were building on the same concept.

Lessons about evaluation and dissemination of experience

To enable others to learn lessons from this experiment it was important to identify issues which were not bound by experience of the local context. This is what an evaluation of independent researchers mostly does. As mentioned earlier, research-based evaluations are a central part of the EU's definition of a social experiment in the FAST programme. Research-based evaluations were also a central part of the TMU programme just as they were in the SUM programme and other governmental programmes in the 1980s.

As described earlier, experiments have become mundane and as a consequence of that many activities are not being evaluated by independent researchers. Today only activities which are labelled as an experiment are evaluated in this way. Consequently there are a lot of activities which are not evaluated, or if they are the evaluation is carried out internally or by some professional consultants. Not even the ten spearhead municipalities (see Table 10.1) were evaluated by independent researchers. They were a part of the national ICT policy but were not systematically evaluated. The National Association of Local Authorities in Denmark has followed the ten projects and reported (National Association of Local Authorities in Denmark, 1996 and 1997) but there is a big difference in these two reports compared with the reports published by the researchers following the TMU programme. The research based evaluations are much more systematic in their approach, they are based on a theoretical understanding, they are aware of the importance of the methods used just as they are more sensible of how far it is possible to conclude. I doubt if an evaluation of the TMU programme carried out by consultants would have found the very important results about processes of social learning.

When a lot of experiments are not evaluated the consequence may be that nobody outside the experiment will know about them and the experience is not likely to be shared. This is not necessarily a problem. If the activity has fulfilled its target and has led to some local learning processes you could ask: What more could you expect? However, in the governmental programmes it has been a clear policy that the experience from the experiments should be diffused to other local communities. In these programmes it was regarded as a waste of resources if the experience was not diffused because then everybody had to 'reinvent the wheel'. This is also the policy of the EU where evaluations and research are supposed to discover 'best practice' and diffuse knowledge of them. The SLIM study questions this policy. Through careful empirical work the study concluded that lessons learnt from local experiments are very dependent on the local context and hereby extremely contingent, which makes it very difficult to generalise the experience and transfer it to other localities. The final report says:

> There are significant problems about the transferability of these kinds of knowledge: where such knowledge is tacit and difficult to formalise and communicate more broadly; where such knowledge is highly contingent to particular circumstances and stages of innovation; raising questions about whether and how it may be possible to extrapolate and apply this knowledge in other circumstances.
>
> (William *et al.* 2000: 14)

The conclusion is that what is transferable is more likely to be knowledge about change processes instead of correlations between specific factors and outcomes. Such knowledge about change processes may also include knowledge about methods and concepts. These are lessons which are possible to generalise and thus possible to transfer to other communities.

However, the identification of lessons through an evaluation is no guarantee of the dissemination of knowledge. In a case study of the digital city of Copenhagen several people highlighted some problems in structuring the information (Jæger 1999). These problems were exactly the same as Kommunedata's experiment with online service (see Table 10.1) which had identified these difficulties almost ten years earlier. When asked about this earlier project, the respondents replied, 'Which experiment?' They had never heard about either the experiment or how it had solved this particular problem! Consequently, whilst not suggesting that evaluations and the dissemination of their findings are futile, we still clearly need to be critical about the effectiveness of the dissemination process.

In the SUM programme the dissemination of knowledge from the experiments was given great emphasis. It was a part of the rules of the game that twenty local 'communication units' were funded and placed all over the country. The evaluation of these units concluded that they did have a function, but the most efficient way of disseminating this kind of knowledge was through the existing personal networks (Jæger 1992).

Another question concerning evaluation is the question about what kind of evaluation is being used. There is a rich body of literature discussing evaluation, which I will skip here but I will argue that evaluations of social experiments are much closer to the tradition of action research than to other traditions of science. In this kind of evaluation the social experiment is the start of departure and the evaluation or research is attached to it, while in the scientific or medical experiment the research is constructing the experiment (Olsen 1998). But action research is also a broad concept. In the evaluation of the TMU programme there was a group of researchers from different universities and research institutes who followed the experiments. This group of researchers developed a new variant of action research called dialogue research (Storgaard 1991). Dialogue research takes its point of departure as a critique of action research. At that time action research was criticised for focusing too much on the project and forgetting to contribute to the scientific society. Dialogue research defined a position where the researcher does not take a direct part in the action or project but has a close dialogue with it. At the same time the researcher is supposed to have a dialogue with the wider scientific community.

In a new (and smaller) experimental programme on older people's use of ICT (see Table 10.1) we take this one step further. In this programme we, as researchers, want to have a dialogue with the six social experiments in the programme. We establish a forum where all the experiments take part in a dialogue with both the researchers and the rest of the experiments. By creating this forum we hope that the dialogue will result in a continual evaluation of the single experiment where both the researchers and the other experiments give responses to the experiment. If the dialogue becomes a success it will create a learning process where all the experiments can learn from each other and the research will be just another input to the learning process (Jæger *et al.* 2000). We still do not know if it will happen, but it is our goal.

Lessons about locality

As described earlier, locality is a part of my definition of a social experiment. A social experiment simply has to take place in some kind of local setting. The emphasis on locality is obviously different in each experiment but it emphasises that the local context is an important part of each experiment. In the TMU programme the idea of creating telecottages was taken up in experiments in different local communities. One of the findings in the evaluation was that this same concept resulted in different outcomes in the different local communities (Jæger and Qvortrup 1991). The only explanation is that the context plays a crucial role in social experiments; thus the local community, where the experiment takes place, is of significant importance also for the evaluation.

This finding is also the background for that part of the definition of social experiments where I emphasise that the technology which is going to be tested in the experiment does not have to come directly from the drawing board of the designer. The same technology can result in different outcomes if it is tested in different local settings. It is not only in experiments with ICT that locality is of importance. Also in the field of social policy the local setting is crucial. Fiske (1995: 38) includes in his definition of social experiments that an experiment can be a complete copy of an experiment from another locality but it is still an experiment because it is new to the locality. He also describes how the same concept for solving social problems can change when another local community is taking up the concept.

Lessons about technology

In the TMU programme one of the significant lessons was that the technology was not ready when the experiments started. It turned out that there was a huge gap between the visions and the technological reality. In the planning of the experiments suppliers of technology had given the impression that 'only imagination would set the limits' but when it came to the reality the technology did not work (Cronberg 1991: 16). Thus it demanded the technical skills of the people involved in the experiments to get the technology to work.

If we go back to the discussion of the definition of social experiments, we saw that the European ACTS programme distinguished between different types of trials. This distinction is supported by the lessons from the social experiments with ICTs. There is certainly a big difference between trials designed to test new prototype components or systems and social experiments. This leads to the conclusion that different types of experiments lead to different kinds of learning. Technical feasibility studies (or technical trials) lead to knowledge about the technology in question and includes much learning by doing. Commercial trials result in knowledge about the possibilities of the product in the market and include learning by interaction, while social experiments primarily lead to knowledge about user-needs in a local setting and how they domesticate the artefact.

The process of domestication is especially interesting when the technology in the experiment is ICT. The SLIM study showed that even standardised and generic software could be turned into new applications when it is utilised in new settings. This is special for ICT because it is still such a new technology where we have not yet discovered all the possibilities of the technology.[8] Even in a situation where the designers thought the technology was ready for introduction to the market, the uncertainties were so big that you could in fact still call it an experiment (William *et al.* 2000).

However, referring to my own definition of social experiments, I would like to conclude that technology has to be more 'finished' or 'stabilised' in a social experiment than in a technical trial. Social experiments are not a perfect setting for testing technology directly from the drawing board. Novelty of the technology can be a barrier in a social experiment because it demands considerable technical skills, which are not always present in the locality, or because it makes the people running the experiment very dependent on technical help from the supplier.

Another lesson from the experiments is that technical support is of great importance. Today most projects are carried out in organisations where technical skills are available but you cannot take it for granted. In some places, especially rural and remote areas, technical skills are still a scarce resource. A couple of years ago a study of a small Danish island (Storgaard *et al.* 1997) revealed how dependent the whole island was on one single man. He was a Mac computer dealer, and when he moved away from the island all the Mac users on the island lost their technical support. Sometimes it is a question of the right technical skills being available. In the case of the digital city of Copenhagen there were technical skills available in the organisation but no skills around using the Internet as an online service for the citizens. In this case the webmaster became dependent on the technical skills of IBM providers (Jæger 1999).

Lessons about organisational changes

Another important lesson is that ICT experiments often make visible how technology and organisation are linked together. This was already one of the lessons from the TMU programme (Cronberg 1990, 1991) but it has also been a lesson from many of the following experiments. In different experiments and projects concerning the development of public electronic services for citizens it has become obvious that developing such a service also results in some organisational changes. For example, in Kommunedata's experiment with online services they simply reproduced existing administrative information structures. The result was that the users could not find the information because its structure used a different 'logic'. In the middle of the experiment the information was re-structured to suit the users' needs, and the evaluation at the end of the experimental period showed that the new structure had completely changed the users' assessment of the service. They were much more satisfied with the new version. But re-structuring the information resulted also in a re-structuring of the organisational arrangements (Jæger and Rieper 1991). If this organisational re-structuring is not possible to realise then it is very difficult to re-structure the information in the electronic service (Jæger 1999).

Another lesson learnt from different experiments is about the relation between the experiment and the organisation behind it. All experiments are rooted in some kind of organisation. It can be a company, a local administration, a political organisation, a social movement or something else. Lessons from earlier experiments show that the relation between the experiment and the organisation behind it is of significant importance. If this relation is not clear to all participants it can sometimes be the reason for conflicts. Many experiments have run into conflicts about who has the competence to make decisions. Who is the 'owner' of the experiment and who has the competence to change the objectives or the target group? In the evaluation of the TMU programme we talked about 'local rivalry' to describe situations where the conflicts were so fierce that it sometimes led to uncertainty about the future of the experiment (Cronberg *et al.* 1991).

As mentioned previously, only half of the SUM experiments were concerned with improving local administration even though it was a highly desirable goal. The explanation for this is to a large extent that the experiments did not have a clear relation to the organisation behind the experiment. Many of the experiments, which were initiated by social movements or volunteer organisations were not aware of the relationship to the local administration. They did not manage to build up a relationship that made the organisation want to adopt it (Fiske 1995).

Finally, I will mention a very important lesson from all kinds of experiments, and that is the role of the project manager. He or she holds a key position in the experiment. The role has many names. In the social field it is called 'the facilitator' or 'the entrepreneur'. In the SLIM study the role was identified as 'the intermediaries'. There are (at least) two central elements in this role: the ability to create networks (social networks among humans) and the ability to focus on the central theme in the experiment. The ability to create networks indicates the very big task if it is to bring different people together and convince them of the importance of the experiment. This ability is necessary to get an experiment funded and running. In ICT experiments it is the use of technology that is the central theme. In experiments in the social field it is the method for solving social problems (Fiske 1995). In the SLIM study the roles of intermediaries were identified in places such as cybercafés. Here the intermediaries played an important role in domesticating the technology for the users (William *et al.* 2000).

Conclusions and questions

The foregoing selection of lessons from the social experiments shows that we already know a lot about social learning processes. It is obvious how social experiments create a frame within which social learning can take place. Actually, one of the rules of the game is that social learning is expected in the experiments and the outcome of the learning is expected to be disseminated to other localities. It is also obvious that the people involved learn a great deal. They learn how to make experiments: building networks which support and fund the experiment and at the same time they learn a lot about the technology by doing or using it in their particular local setting.

The lessons from the experiments also show that it is not only between users and suppliers that we can talk about learning by interaction. The people involved in the experiments also interact with a lot of other people. For example, it is very important to interact with the organisation behind the experiment – at least if the experiment wants to be a permanent part of the activities in the organisation. This example tells us that our theoretical framework is still lacking some elements if we are to understand fully the processes of social learning. Here it could be useful to draw on theories of organisational change: for example, the approach of neo-institutionalism, which explains organisational learning as building new experience into routines that determine the actions in the organisation (Levitt and March 1988). Also the concept of domestication points to the importance of creating routines around the new artefact. These routines are not inscribed in the artefact, just waiting to be discovered: it is more likely that different routines will emerge in different social settings. This similarity raises the question of whether organisational theory could add some value to the SLIM theoretical framework.

Another question is how social learning processes are influenced by the changes in local administration. At least when we are talking about experiments in connection with the local administrations this question is important. Earlier I described this transition as a move from the traditional hierarchy organisation towards a network where the border of the organis-ation is not clear at all. I also described social experiments as a part of that transition. Experiments have become a part of the everyday life of the local administration and thus a part of the network. If this is true it raises the question of how we can understand social learning processes in networks. The SLIM theoretical framework does not pay any attention to this question and thus does not give any theoretical concepts for understanding social learning under these conditions.

Thus the overall conclusion in this chapter is that today we have learnt many lessons about social learning from experiments with ICT, but we still have some questions we cannot answer with the present theoretical framework. To develop the theoretical framework further must be a task for the future research in this field.

Notes

1 Social Learning in Multimedia (SLIM) was a research project running from 1996 to 1999. It was funded by the European Commission DG XII Targeted Socio-Economic Research (TSER) programme. The project was led by the

University of Edinburgh and had participants from Belgium, Denmark, Germany, Ireland, the Netherlands, Norway and Switzerland.

2 Kommunedata is a large company that supplies software to most of the Danish municipalities. 'Kommune' is the Danish word for municipality. It has status as a private company but is a co-operation between most of the municipalities in Denmark, and its board of directors consists of mayors from different municipalities.

3 In 1994 the government made a coherent policy for the field of ICT called: 'The Info-Society year 2000' (Dybkjær and Christensen 1994). It was followed up by a series of action plans in the next years. In 1999 the policy was renewed and now called 'The Digital Denmark' (Dybkjær and Lindegaard 1999). The Danish ICT policy is described in Jæger and Hansen 1999a.

4 The address of the homepage is www. distancearbejde.dk (in Danish).

5 Here Olsen refers to Kurt Aagaard Nielsen (1996): *Arbejdets sociale orientering: en undersøgelse af forholdet imellem arbejdslivsdemokrati og mulighederne for bæredygtighed i industrielle moderniseringsprocesser* (Copenhagen: Forlaget Sociologi).

6 A much more coherent and detailed description of the theoretical framework is to be found in William *et al.* 2000, ch. 5.

7 Here the SLIM report refers to E. S. Andersen and B.-Å. Lundwall (1988), 'Small national systems of innovation facing technological revolutions: an analytical framework', in C. Freeman and B.-Å. Lundwall, eds., *Small Countries Facing the Technological Revolution* (London: Pinter), pp. 9–36.

8 This discussion is further elaborated in Jæger 1997: 100–1.

Chapter 11

Change agency and women's learning

New practices in community informatics

Anne Scott and Margaret Page

Introduction

With ongoing government promotion of informatics and the new communications technologies, there are growing pressures on the community sector to change its working practices – and thus to keep up with the changing social, economic and political context in which the sector is operating (PAT 15 2000). This has particular implications for women's organisations, which, in common with black organisations, have always been particularly poorly resourced, and for which there are specific issues concerning access to, and usage of, ICTs. Thus, while under-resourced people and organisations are continuing to address issues of great social and cultural importance, they face serious questions regarding the sustainability of projects, working practices, organisations and workers' energy.

Moreover, community informatics initiatives relating to women must address a broad set of cultural obstacles that go beyond simple problems of access. Women's relationships with new technologies have historically been mediated by problematic assumptions relating to the gender of 'expertise' (Cockburn 1981, Cockburn and Ormrod 1993). Technologies have often been constructed as masculine and/or non-social, amid expectations that the practices of women are, almost by definition, non-technological (Wacjman 1991, Cockburn and Ormrod 1993). Saskia Everts argues that new technologies can provide opportunities for meeting unfulfilled gender needs (Everts 1998: 11–12) or they can (and often do) lead to socio-economic changes threatening women's employment opportunities, health and safety, control over particular sectors of production and/or independence. Many of these consequences are unintended and unforeseen. These issues have also been raised with specific reference to women's use of new communication and information technologies (Green *et al.* 1993, Spender 1995, Kramarae 1988, Bergman and Van Zoonen 1999, Adam and Green 1998).

In this chapter, we address the question of sustainability by asking the perhaps more fundamental question of how to create an environment which enables women's and community organisations to sustain themselves.

Drawing on experiences arising from the Women Connect project, we argue that 'learning communities' offer an approach with the potential to transfer, sustain and develop the best of good practice developed by community organisations, drawing on the potential offered by ICTs. We do not attempt a full description of the results achieved by Women Connect member organisations through their use of ICTs;[1] we will instead focus on processes by which they collaborate within the Women Connect network.

Technological innovation, like the learning of new skills, involves a co-construction of both artefacts and the social environment in which they will be embedded and used (Callon 1991, Latour 1993, Everts 1998). Community informatics practitioners will thus need to attend to the social, cultural and organisational contexts in which new technologies are to be developed, accessed and used. These contexts are not static. They are currently evolving very quickly, as they integrate new practices, new contexts of practice and new technologies. Thus, both in the fast-moving area of information and communication technology (ICT) and on the constantly shifting ground of community sector practice, sustainability will depend upon adaptability. For actors within women's organisations and community projects this means an ability to deliver results which meet the challenge of diminishing resources – to develop new practices while maintaining core values and aims and, in relation to ICTs, to assess how use of ICTs might help them to meet their organisational goals. Appropriate technologies can be achieved only *in practice*. It is our argument that sustainable technologies are *processes*; they are not products.

A specific type of 'skills' learning is thus needed, which incorporates a means of dealing with ongoing change, while remaining sensitive both to the context of practice and to the values driving that practice. Attention needs to be paid to process in order to sustain and build capacity to deliver results. The concept of learning communities provides us with an approach for meeting this need; an approach which allows us to reconcile tensions between diversity and inequality, to facilitate the mutual development of appropriate practical innovations, and to sustain the change agency which facilitates a 'bedding down' of new practices within organisations.

Women Connect's starting point was recognition of the effects of under-resourcing on women's organisations. The project set out to enable women's organisations to collaborate, in order to tap the potential that ICTs have to increase their capacity to meet their goals – and to deliver results to women in diverse communities. In its first phase the project set out to create a 'learning community' – encompassing the members of diverse women's organisations – to facilitate *collectively* the creation of a sustainable, feminist, ICT practice. This practice would not use the Internet uncritically, but would generate content and new tools adapted to the needs of its members; it would 'use and shape the Internet' for clearly defined purposes: to enable women's organisations to deliver results which met their organisational goals and were consistent with their values (Page and Scott 1999a). It is our argument that funding models that require working to short-term product-orientated outcomes, which predominate within the voluntary sector in the absence of core funding, actively inhibit the development and maintenance of learning communities such as that created within Women Connect.

In this chapter, we[2] start by describing the model developed by Women Connect in its first phase. Drawing on experiences from the project, we then introduce the idea of learning 'in community'; in particular we will suggest some benefits, to women, offered by this approach. Our next section addresses some conceptual problems raised by the use of the word 'community', analysing – in particular – its use in the community informatics and community-development literatures. After distinguishing between our usage of the terms 'network' and 'community', we address some issues raised when creating communities that encompass diversity and difference. We proceed to lay out an epistemological basis for our notion of 'learning community', and then draw on several feminist theorists to explore problems raised by the process of change agency.

In conclusion, we return to our starting point – the problem of sustainability. Learning communities offer a valid approach for sustaining innovation and development in a fast-changing techno-social context. Current funding models, however, do not encourage the creation of such communities. The predominance of pre-defined outcome and/or product-driven funding – combined with an absence of core funding for basic infrastructure within the voluntary sector – has tended to reduce organisational stability and unallocated space and time which can facilitate the creation of learning communities. We need a new conceptual and epistemological basis for the provision, funding and maintenance of voluntary-sector ICT projects.

The Women Connect approach

Women Connect, run by a consortium made up of the Community Development Foundation (the lead partner) and the Library Association, is the first UK-based informatics initiative of its kind, and the first catering specifically for women's organisations. In its first phase the project incorporated twenty women's organisations spread throughout England. These included two national networks; three women's refuges, seven women's centres, an older women's project, and three health information centres. Five of the women's centres catered mainly for women in ethnic-minority communities. Others had special projects catering for lesbians, younger women and women with disabilities.

Over the course of its first phase of twenty-three months, Women Connect aimed to create a supportive learning space to enable women's organisations to plan for effective use of ICTs, to take forward their organisational goals, and to gain the practical skills and equipment they needed to put these plans into action. Member organisations were offered a framework for developing effective ICT use within their organisations, consisting of agreed responsibilities and tasks. Each member organisation was asked to draw up a work plan, setting out its own learning and practice goals for achievement within the lifespan of the project. Women Connect provided equipment, group and on-site training, and networking tools and opportunities. Project co-ordinators aimed to generate exchange and collaboration between member organisations within the network, using both face-to-face and electronic communication. The aims and desired outcomes of Women Connect Phase 1 are summarised on the 'learning wheel' (Figure 11.1). The project website www.womenconnect.org.uk contains a full description of working methods, project roles, achievements and outcomes.

During Phase 1, member organisations identified substantial practical benefits in their use of ICT, and the value which membership of the Women Connect learning network had for them as they took their first steps with these technologies (Moggridge 1999). The project co-ordinators established links with related women and community ICT projects, working closely with an external evaluator,[3] and project advisers, to identify and conceptualise innovative aspects of the practice developed by member organisations. They disseminated project results through community ICT and women's networks, and published a guide for women's organisations using the Internet (Page and Scott 1999b). With the help of consortium partners, they sought to ensure that resourcing ICT for women's organisations was profiled and placed on the government policy agenda – both by contributing to the research carried out by Policy Action Team 15, for the British government's Social Exclusion Unit,[4] and by organising a high-profile conference, at the Department of Trade and Industry, in November 1999. Funding for a second phase, of three further years, has been secured; plans for this phase of the project will be posted on the Women Connect website.

Learning ICT 'in community'

We suggest that 'learning communities' such as that developed in Women Connect Phase 1 can contribute to the sustainability of informatics innovation in the voluntary sector. By this term, we mean a community within which to engage in a joint process of learning and developing purposeful use of ICTs. This kind of community does not create or sustain itself; it must be facilitated. Members – whether individuals or organisations – must be adequately resourced to allow participation. Such a community is not static, and does not depend on an essentialised, or pre-given, commonality amongst its members. Rather, 'learning community' is a social space, physical and/or virtual, within which users are invited and enabled to engage in a shared learning process, while respecting the diversity of their knowledge base. They are encouraged to set their own learning goals, and to support one another in

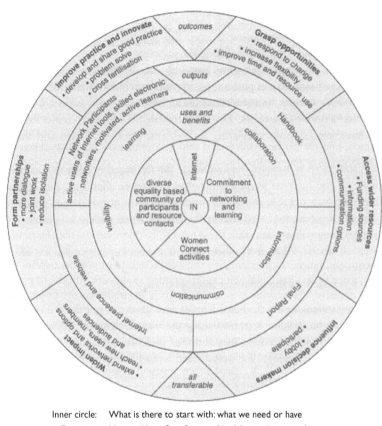

Inner circle: What is there to start with: what we need or have
First ring: Uses and benefits of networking/electronic networking
Second ring: Measurable changes
Outer ring: Longer-term outcomes (changes) for women's organisations within and beyond the initial network

Figure 11.1 The learning wheel

meeting them, in an environment that offers a holistic, action-orientated approach. Our notion of 'learning community' draws from action learning[5] and collaborative inquiry[6] in its approach, and builds on the experience of Women Connect.

This ideal environment has been described to us[7] in different forms repeatedly by women learning how to use ICTs, and by women providing training or Internet access in women's ICT projects or women's centres (Page and Scott 1999a).[8] At a seminar organised by Women Connect for Policy

Action Team 15, participants explained their need for trainers who understood the complex sets of obligations in their lives, and were able to accommodate them. Flexible approaches to learning, environments allowing self-defined learning goals (Women Connect 1999a) and practical support such as transport and childcare were considered. The need for adequate resourcing of women's organisations, to enable them to sustain their participation, was stressed by member organisations. The need for a supportive learning environment has been voiced particularly by members of communities whose needs are not addressed by traditional approaches to learning – women, and members of black and minority ethnic communities (Day and Harris 1997). Some of these needs have been noted in recent UK government funding and policy initiatives (DEE 2000, PAT 15 2000).

There is evidence that many women can benefit from a 'feminist' approach to learning and empowerment (Butler and Wintram 1991; Belenky *et al.* 1986). Such an approach asserts that women have specific needs in relation to their learning process, and that these need to be addressed as they learn how to use ICTs. This has been illustrated in our discussions with women at recent conferences. In accounts[9] of their approach to online discussion, our experience is that many women express caution. Some are attuned to potentially negative interactions, and are more likely to emphasise the importance of closed discussion lists, focused moderated discussion and quality facilitation, in order to encourage participation. Many women simply do not take to the idea of sharing views and opinions with people they do not know, and cannot identify, in open spaces over which they have no control.[10] A lack of confidence experienced by some women with regards to ICT usage was identified by Green and Keeble (2000). Perceived lack of ability also proved to be a barrier to learning for Women Connect members; many assumed, for example, that other network members would 'know more than me'. These negative self-judgements were identified by some participants as a block to participation; in the context of the learning community they were addressed through discussion and shared activity.

Descriptions of training with pre-defined outcomes, and with approaches and environments which did not specifically address internalised barriers to ICT usage, were contrasted unfavourably by Women Connect members to training which adopted a more women-friendly approach (Page and Scott 1999a). Similarly, participants in the women's centres researched by Eileen Green and Leigh Keeble described a sense of safety and relaxation in these spaces, encouraging them to undertake activities they had not previously considered (Green and Keeble 2000). Although the aims thus seem to be clear, mechanisms need better articulation; *how* are we to create a supportive environment for learning ICT? How are we to enable women to learn from each other within this environment?

It is our argument that learning communities must be actively created and sustained; this requires certain relational and political skills that can by no means be taken for granted. By 'political skills', we mean that an understanding of gendered and raced power relations is required – with an ability to take into account how these restrict access to, and inform processes of, cyber-communication. The assumption that new technologies should be embedded within existing social relations fails to address gendered power relations; real-life spaces are often exclusionary (Green and Keeble 2000). The relational skills we are describing would seek to challenge exclusionary interactions, and would enable participants to work creatively with these power relations. These skills could also be called 'community building' – but from a perspective of participation based on inquiry, rather than a rigid set of rules. Inquiry in this sense is understood as holding open the tension between individual and community in order to contribute to the development of both, towards participation (Reason 1994). This requires individuals to develop skills that enable them to bring to the surface, and to negotiate, power dynamics and inequalities. In doing so they must be aware of how inequalities relate to social differences including race, gender and class, and of how these differences may be reflected in the situated knowledge which each brings to the learning community. These differences are likely to be profound and complex, and must be acknowledged and respected if notions of community – and of participation – are not to be deeply flawed (Whitmore 1994, Butler and Wintram 1991, Harding 1991).

The concept of 'community'

What do we – *did* we as Women Connect project co-ordinators – mean by 'learning community' or 'learning network'? When we designed the project we had a vision of what we wanted to achieve. This was described in our mission statement:

> Women Connect aims to use the Internet to build a sustainable community of women's organisations and resource contacts who are working in diverse communities and fields, and a commitment to learning and networking across different areas of experience and expertise. We set out to enable women's organisations to use and shape the Internet to benefit women.
>
> (Page and Scott 1999a: 3)

While the process and activities for creating this 'sustainable community' were defined by our funding conditions, the community itself was to be based on a shared commitment to learning and networking across differences of constituency; of social identity, and of knowledge base. It was to be co-created through a process of mutual exchange and interaction.

As we[11] write this chapter, we wonder: just what *is* this notion of 'community' Women Connect has been working with? The concept of 'community', as seen in various relevant literatures, is far from straightforward. According to Crow and Allan (1994: 1), 'community' is a term that can be used as shorthand for a broad range of intermediary social structures standing between the private sphere of the home or family and the impersonal institutions of the wider society. This definition, of course, raises as many questions as it answers in relation to a technology which is *itself* contributing to a redefinition of the concepts of 'public' and 'private'.[12] In this section, we will be describing our usage of this term in relation to the community informatics and the community-development literatures.

Within community informatics discourse, there is sometimes a tendency to assume that if the Internet is a new kind of public-communications space it must therefore produce idealised 'new communities' (Jones 1995: 11).[13] In these cases, 'Community' functions as a normative term – with connotations of naturalness, stability, mutual support and benefit – as well as an idealised, exclusive, group identity (Suttles 1972, Cohen 1985, Stacey 1974).[14] However, notions of community based on pre-given commonality can operate in a static, essentialist manner. Changing identities, shifting perspectives and new developments may seem to put the commonality grounding such notions of community at risk, thereby threatening a community's continued existence.[15] The spokespeople for essentialised communities often turn out to be older, wealthier and more powerful men; as a result, assumptions that a community has a stable, unified and 'authentic' identity can act very destructively in regard to women, ethnic or sexual minorities and other marginalised groups (Macey and Beckett 2001, Mellor 1992). In reflecting on the experience of Women Connect, and in discussing boundary conditions for our[16] shared conceptualisation of a 'learning community', it became clear to us that notions of shared identity or shared interests missed the mark.[17] We needed a different means of understanding this concept.

A second assumption found in the less sociologically informed community informatics literature is that on-line communication can sometimes be enough, in itself, to create shared interests or attachment and thus to lead to 'virtual' community (Rheingold 1993b, 1994, Quaterman 1993).[18] The content or purpose of this communication can thus be treated as, literally, immaterial. Implicit in this is the assumption that the making of 'community' does not require material commitment, and that communities are beneficial even though their activities may be of little practical consequence (Jones 1995). This assumption has been strongly criticised (Aurigi and Graham 1998) and may, we suggest, support static, essentialised and normative understandings of community.

In her recent study of online lesbian communities, Nina Wakeford analysed interconnections between the active creation of 'community' and that of 'identity'. With eligibility to join an online communication group based on lesbian identity, communications provided a means of actively re-creating, reinventing and (re)affirming the identity of individual members within the online community (Wakeford 1998). These dynamic conceptualisations are grounded in agency – 'doing community' – and in the process, in the defining of self-identity in relation to others. This description of community as something produced rather than given – constituted through interaction – is one that we need to introduce into the debates within community informatics. It allows us to name issues of power as they emerge within interactions, and thus to highlight women's 'gendered' experiences within virtual communities. These crucial concerns must be addressed if we are to develop a sustainable and democratic community informatics.

The community development literature is equally ambivalent about definitions of 'community'. Gabriel Chanan, writing from the Community Development Foundation, points out that activists and policy-makers rarely specify what they mean by the terms 'the neighbourhood' or 'the community' – or what basis they have for assuming it has certain characteristics or capacities (Chanan 1989). Acknowledging that the word 'community' is used widely with varying meanings, community development research and writings generally do not focus on what community *is*; rather, they use the term as shorthand for forms of intervention designed to empower people, who may be living in a given locality or holding a shared set of interests, to take collective action to achieve a greater degree of control in social, economic and political issues that affect them (AMA 1989, Chanan 1989, 1992, 1999, Gilchrist 1998). 'Community' is often used as an adjective, as in 'community involvement', with connotations of homogeneity and common interest that may disguise differences and conflicts.

What we know of as community development in the UK has been influenced by different political strands, each of which carries its own values and histories (Twelvetrees 1998). In the 1960s and 1970s, for example, activism for radical social change, associated with the civil rights movement, inspired some community activists to promote self-organisation in local communities, and to seek to open political decision-making to wider participation. In the 1980s and 1990s, feminist and anti-racist community activists and workers drew attention to divisions within local communities, and to the need for self-organisation by women, black and Asian people (Curno 1982, Dominelli 1990, Ellis 1989, Ohri and Manning 1982). This awareness is now reflected in the more radical community-work networks and professional organisations (Gilchrist 1998, Harris 1994).[19]

The term 'community involvement' is now increasingly used by governments in relation to a range of specific policy initiatives (Chanan *et al.* 1999). However, the terms of involvement, the scope and nature of the potential benefits and the agendas on – and positions from – which members of excluded communities are invited to participate are by their nature contentious and open to challenge.[20] Participation is likely to be beyond the reach of organisations that lack basic resources to sustain their activities; this is likely to be the case for organisations in deprived communities, and for women's organisations which are not currently recognised as a priority by funders (Riordan 1999).

Clearly, then, use of the term 'community' continues to be saturated with political agendas. If 'communities' are to generate their own goals, we must ensure that diverse voices are respected and acted upon. If we are in the business of building communities – virtual or face-to-face, spatial or interest-based – we must continue to ask: 'community for whom?', and 'on what value base?' (Gilchrist 1998, Mulholland and Patel 1999).

Current writings about the job of the community-development worker describe a process – and a related set of skills – for building relationships and networks, making possible processes of empowerment and encouraging forms of self-organisation which support services and opportunities for democratic participation. The aim is to facilitate widening participation in local democracy in its broadest sense (Harris 1994, Chanan 1999, Gilchrist 1998). As advocates for resourcing community development point out, this activity is often not valued or widely understood, except by those directly involved; yet as Gabriel Chanan argues it is the unseen basis for social life – a 'background buzz of activity' which underlies more formal types of involvement (Chanan et al. 1999, Chanan 1999).

Learning community or learning network?

At the start of this Women Connect project, the project co-ordinators used the words 'learning network' and 'learning community' interchangeably. In retrospect, considering differences between the two seems a fruitful way to think about the conditions needed for sustainability by women's and community organisations.

In Women Connect Phase 1, the project co-ordinators understood learning *community* to be about creating a space in which members or partners would actively engage with each other, face to face and online, generating and transferring learning and good practice. This exchange would provide context and purpose for learning how to use ICTs. 'Learning community' meant, for the project co-ordinators, a space within which members of women's organisations would build relationships based on practical exchange, in a context of shared values and specific organisational goals. Within this space they would inspire and sustain each other in developing ICT usage, and introducing new practices within their organisations. Each participant would speak from her situated knowledge, developed in relation to the different communities of women that her organisation served; through a process of cross-fertilisation, exchange of good practice and of approach would take place.

Network, by contrast, referred to relationships between the organisations that came into membership – and from which we, as project co-ordinators, hoped to create a learning community. It referred both to a state that preceded the sense of shared enterprise we set out to develop, and to the interests and concerns which its members held in common, and set out to explore, as women active in women's organisations. In this sense, 'network' might be defined as a space within which individual members are invited to take resources to strengthen and add to a repertoire of a *pre-defined* set of practices, for *pre-defined* purposes. In this case it would refer to a single dimension of Women Connect's outcomes – the changed practices of its individual organisations – without reference to the *process* of shared learning through which these new practices were generated and inspired.

For our[21] purposes then, it seems that 'learning networks' and 'learning communities' vary in the location of their trajectories of change. Within a learning 'network', this trajectory remains with individual members and with the communities from which they have emerged. A learning 'community', however, aims to develop a *shared* trajectory of development, and in the experience of Women Connect this seemed to be crucially dependent on the existence of shared projects, obligations and/or goals. We might relate this back to our earlier discussion of the term 'community', as employed within the community informatics literature. Members of a community *do* have some degree of commonality, but this need not lie in a static identity of physical location, interests or 'attachment'. It might also be dynamically created, emerging through commitment to a shared project. The difference between learning 'network' and learning 'community', for our purposes, seems to lie squarely in the fact that members of a *community* have a common trajectory. Communities have an intentional quality, as phenomenologists use the term.[22]

When the project co-ordinators embarked upon the Women Connect Phase 1 project, they did not know exactly how their vision of a 'learning community' would be taken up by member organisations and how it would work in practice. 'The proof of the pudding is in the eating'; it would depend on the quality of participation of members as well as the conditions and mechanisms offered by the project. Member organisations were asked to nominate a primary participant, who would attend network events. Initially, these individuals came primarily to find an extra resource for their organisations. Their primary identification was with their own organisations; a commitment and motivation to identify and contribute as members of the new network or community had to be built, and this required time as well as material resources from members. Moving from learning *network* to learning *community* required an ability and commitment to work across difference: to use the diversity within Women Connect positively and creatively. This raised a further set of challenges around identity, power and diversity, which we will explore in the next section.

Realising 'community': commonality and difference

The number of member organisations invited to join Women Connect Phase 1 was limited by both time and budget. This forced project co-ordinators to address some difficult questions: what did we[23] mean by 'women's organis-ations'? How did we understand 'diverse'? Did we mean 'feminist', and, if so, should this be self-defined? If not, how wide were we prepared to go? We brought with us our values and experience of working on women's equality issues in progressive local authorities – as well as our experience as feminist activists[24] – and we wanted this to be our starting point. We wanted diversity of membership around a core commitment to promoting women's equality and to learning and networking across differences of experience, knowledge base and practical expertise. We wanted to create a network of organisations serving diverse communities with different priorities and working practices. The purpose of the network was to enable women's organisations to use and shape the Internet to benefit women; to support, train, advise and equip member organisations to develop skills in using the Internet and networking – for communication, information, visibility, collaboration and learning.[25]

Audre Lorde has argued that 'community' should not involve a shedding of our differences, or the pretence that differences don't exist (1984: 11–12):

> Advocating the mere tolerance of difference between women is the grossest reformism. It is a total denial of the creative function of difference in our lives. Difference must be not merely tolerated, but seen as a fund of necessary polarities between which our creativity can spark like a dialectic . . . Within the interdependence of mutual (non-dominant) difference lies that security which enables us to descend into the chaos of knowledge and return with true visions of our future along with the concomitant power to effect those changes which can bring that future into being.

In Women Connect, we deliberately created a 'feminist' network that incorporated differences – of race, ethnicity, class, age and sexuality – particularly in relation to the constituencies served by member organisations. Member organisations were selected to meet a matrix of criteria; in addition to differences of constituency these included a mix of regions and rural and urban localities; different degrees of familiarity with using ICTs, and access to equipment; local and national groups. This raised challenges, which interlink with the creation of 'learning community'.

As noted above, the notion of 'community' requires some commonality and/or shared perceptions– at least to the extent that it is possible to engage in shared projects and to work towards shared goals. Social difference, however, can be about more than simple diversity; it can also incorporate *inequality* – many 'differences' are rooted in histories of social domination (Plumwood 1993, Hooks 1990, Frye 1983, Haraway 1986, Albrecht and Brewer 1990). Thus, as Uma Narayan has argued (1988: 34), 'good-will is not enough' when working across difference. An appreciation of the historical (re)constitution of inequality through access to power, resources and various kinds of capital (Skeggs 1997) is also required. Members of differently located social groups may see the world in strikingly variant ways; these differences are rooted in their embodied experiences of life in a society constituted by inequality – and they lead to a difference in *knowledge*. Members of oppressed groups 'have epistemic privilege when it comes to immediate knowledge of everyday life under oppression . . . They know first-hand the detailed and concrete ways in which oppression defines the spaces in which they live and how it affects their lives' (Narayan 1988: 36). These differences in knowledge and perception *must* be addressed in the process of creating a learning community – for they provide the raw material from which new, mutually held, understandings may be created.

I[26] remember the anxiety I felt when preparing to present our vision at our launch seminar, and the rather sceptical response I anticipated from some of our feminist sisters: Who were 'we' to invite 'them' to join us in this space? What would 'they' have to gain from joining with other organisations and with us? My anxiety arose from a paradox. We were offering them an opportunity to join together to create something new; yet in order to obtain funding we had pre-defined the product – the learning community – as a process which members were required to sign up to. The term 'learning community' was not easy to sell to busy organisations accustomed to working to clear service goals. Joining was a leap of faith – a commitment of resources – and inevitably made for a mixture of motivations.

Problems raised at the launch seminar focused on the management of diversity and equality – issues that are at the heart of the concept of learning community. How could we ensure adequate returns for the investment of time and energy made? Another problem was voiced by some women from black feminist organisations: how could we assure them that they would not end up being ripped off – again – by white women putting them in an educator role about anti-racist practices? What would they have to gain? Why should they commit to working at a pace, and to a timetable, which could not accommodate scarce resources and the demands of servicing a poorly resourced community? The question asked by some – 'how can we be sure that the community will offer us something and not just take time and energy from us for no return?' was inevitably an issue for all of us. By definition, it referred to an outcome that could not be guaranteed in advance; although project staff could, and did, commit to addressing these problems, solutions would need to be collectively negotiated.

Evaluation indicated that the relationships that these women built within the learning spaces created by Women Connect did play a key role in enabling them to learn how to use ICTs, and in sustaining them in motivating their colleagues to adopt new practices in their organisations. To achieve this they needed to overcome resistance to the changes which new ICT practices brought: limited energy and resources, the comfort of established practices, the defence of existing power and relationships and so forth. Evaluation also indicated that individuals valued highly the opportunity provided by the networking and training events to access each other's practice and knowledge (Moggridge 1999, Page and Scott 1999a). Since the project ended, some member organisations continue to access each other's expertise to increase their own capacity to work with women in specific communities. A health centre in a rural area for example has approached a women's centre working primarily with Asian women, to develop health-information materials targeting Asian women, for use by both centres.

In retrospect, it is easy to see how much more we had assumed than we realised in designing the project as a learning community. We discovered that learning communities need a period of time to develop, and that members need time to generate their own learning goals. These, in turn, need to relate to the practical goals of their organisations. Each individual involved needed to find her own sense of purpose and fulfilment, and to do this in the context of the interaction with other members of the learning community, at face-to-face or online events. At the same time, she needed to remain focused on finding a practical application for her learning within her organisation. This had to be negotiated with her colleagues as well as related to the collectively held goals in the learning community. The process was complex, and relied on negotiation and commitment at three levels:

- individual participants in relation to peers and colleagues in their member organisations
- individual participants within the Women Connect learning community
- individual participants, with support from Women Connect project co-ordinators, in relation to the management of their member organis-ations, who in turn had to satisfy the conditions set by their funders.

It was the creative mixing of these different perspectives which gave our learning community its effectiveness, but which also made it difficult to establish *as* a community.

'Difference' can be conceptualised as a 'problem' within discourses of 'community' and, in fact, it has to some extent been discussed as such within this chapter. It is our argument, however, that the very differences that can make uncomfortable the 'doing of community' can also facilitate the emergence of these communities in a new form – as *learning* communities. In his work on psychodynamic group processes, Wilfred Bion argues that creative groups are those that are able to articulate and integrate destructive dynamics in order to address an agreed set of tasks (Bion 1961). By contrast, dysfunctional groups remain in the grip of unconscious destructive dynamics – one form of which is an idealisation of a false unity or 'oneness'. We would argue that learning communities infused with a sense of unproblematised 'community' may be unable to identify barriers to learning based on false harmony and consensus. In order for members to learn from each other, they need to engage with differences of social position and power; these will be embedded in their knowledge base (Harding 1991, Haraway 1991, Stanley and Wise 1993). It is the ability to maintain the tension between diversity and shared values which creates and sustains a learning community.

In her research with women working across religious and ethnic divisions, Cynthia Cockburn (1998, 1999), has drawn on Nira Yuval-Davis's concept of 'transversal politics[27] (Yuval-Davis 1997, 1999) to describe a particular kind of democratic practice which can 'affirm differences without being transfixed by them, and can look for commonalities without being arrogantly universalistic' (Cockburn 1999: 88–93). Cynthia Cockburn shows how women from communities in conflict are able to engage and disengage with difference in ways that allow them to sustain their alliances without denying the histories and conflicts which divide them. She illustrates how transversal politics can encapsulate a way of working which respects the irreconcilability of certain differences. This approach allows us to engage with the open space between subject positions, without thereby losing the materiality and embodiment of each group member's experience.

The idea of learning communities bears similarities to this approach. It requires us to step over borders that, in Gloria Anzaldúa's words, 'define the places that are safe and unsafe . . . that distinguish *us* from *them*' and to enter 'that vague and undetermined place . . . in a constant state of transition' (1987: 3) that Anzaldúa (1987) has termed the 'borderlands'. In the next section, we draw on recent feminist theory to begin conceptualising this process.

Learning in the borderlands

Many technology-training programmes in community informatics conceptualise knowledge as context-independent. It is seen as something abstract – acquired by individuals, held until needed and then employed within particular contexts. In mainstream epistemologies, reliable knowledge is often seen as that which has been garnered in an orderly and methodical manner, according to an agreed set of rules. Objective, propositional 'facts' are seen as the stuff of knowledge (Code 1995, Adam 1998). Within this approach, as Maria Lugones has noted, *competence* rules supreme. She argues that 'Agonistic [world] travellers fail consistently in their attempt to travel because what they do is to try to conquer the other "world"' (Lugones 1997: 157). As noted in our 'learning in community' section, this approach contrasts sharply with many women's stated preferences in relation to ICT training.

Lugones's term, 'world-travellers', points towards a different, more dialogic, approach to learning – an attitude that can leave us open to reciprocal engagement and surprise.

> This is a particular metaphysical attitude that does not expect the world to be neatly packaged, ruly. Rules may fail to explain what we are doing. We are not self-important, we are not fixed in particular constructions of ourselves, which is part of saying that we are open to self-construction. We may not have rules, and when we do have rules, there are no rules that are to us sacred. We are not worried about competence. We are not wedded to a particular way of doing things. While playful we have not abandoned ourselves to, nor are we stuck in, any particular 'world.' We are there creatively. We are not passive.
>
> (Lugones 1997: 158)

This metaphysical attitude is not something that one can create alone. Lugones emphasises that it is not a trait of 'individuals'. It is a quality of interaction, rather, that emerges in a context where individuals feel at home and validated within a particular 'world'. Lugones (1997) also describes the way this characteristic can be lost in the transition from one community to another. The achievement of 'playfulness', then, might result from creative intermixings of commonality and difference within learning communities. It cannot, however, be achieved if the inequalities in power involved in working across difference are not addressed.

Within Women Connect Phase 1, face-to-face activities and visits were crucial parts of the process of change. At these events, relationships were built and renewed. It was through these relationships that objectives were set, progress reviewed and encouragement given – all of which were vital to sustaining participation. This is not to say that we could *not* have addressed various issues online. Different skills would have been required on both sides, however, to replace the non-verbal interactive dimension. It would have required a different level of confidence, trust and motivation. In the early stages of the transition to new practice, face-to-face interaction seemed to play a crucial role. Members were inspired by face-to-face networking events to develop new practices, often in the face of considerable resistance from colleagues and in very challenging workplace environments (Page and Scott 1999a). The relationships built at these events played an important role in sustaining the online interactions that developed later, as did relationships with project co-ordinators and trainers who made regular visits to member organisations.

There is an important point here, and one that it would not do to under-estimate. A playful approach to learning is, inherently, a communal and grounded activity. Taking epistemological chances is easier to do in a context where the risk is shared. Sharing risk, moreover, is more easily accomplished where relations of trust have been built face-to-face; where community of place has been linked to cyber-community. If we accept this, it has implications for our conceptualisation of 'knowledge'.

Lorraine Code (1995: 144–53) develops the socially devalued concept of *gossip* as a way of thinking about the creation of new knowledge. She describes a film in which a suspicious death has occurred in an isolated farmhouse. While the sheriff and his assistant are engaged in an orderly, methodical but ultimately fruitless search for evidence that will implicate the dead man's wife, their two wives are collecting some items the imprisoned woman needs, tidying up the kitchen – and gossiping. Through an engaged, emotionally interested, discussion of the domestic details they notice as they are working, of their memories of the imprisoned woman's childhood and of the links they see and feel with their own lives, they are able to reconstruct a narrative of brutal domestic violence which was ended when the woman murdered her husband. In the process, these two women overcome an initial lack of trust associated with their own differences in status, build a new solidarity with each other and with the imprisoned woman, and decide to conceal what they know from their husbands.

This is knowledge that has arisen within relations of mutual trust and shared activity. It has not been collected in a methodical manner; in fact, it seems to be completely spontaneous. It has not been 'taught' in the traditionally understood sense of that term. It has arisen in relationship, through dialogue motivated by an emotional engagement with something outside itself. Although it is deeply rooted in a particular context, its power comes from the fact that it both draws on, and contributes to, a wider understanding. This knowledge is *responsible*; it is accountable to the community which gave it birth. It does not develop quickly, and it cannot be produced to order. Most importantly, perhaps, it allows the people who produced it to take a risk, to step outside their usual roles, practices and expectations. This is community knowledge, which can be used for the purposes of social change. This is knowledge – both reliable and useful – which is not composed of individually owned, abstract, propositional facts. What is most necessary for its development is the provision of a safe space in which dialogue can take place and relationships of trust can develop. This is the type of knowledge, we are arguing, which can be produced within a learning community.

Change agency: travelling between worlds

When we reflected on the experience of Women Connect, we realised that creating a learning community was more complex than it had originally looked. The practices the project had wanted to embed looked deceptively simple; in practice however they implied a series of commitments to change agency roles. In some cases, for example, changes in working relationships within member organisations had to be negotiated. How did members work with these ambiguities and tensions?

As discussed earlier, the lead contact of each member organisation in Women Connect had to negotiate change at several different levels: with her colleagues, with the Women Connect community and with the management of her organisation – who were also answerable to their funders. These challenges are not specific to women's organisations, or to the voluntary sector. They are faced by people of all sectors who take part in the multi-agency partnerships that are increasingly common within the 'mixed economy'. Participants engage in a group activity that generates new thinking and practice in a space outside their organisation, and are then faced with the challenge of introducing the results in some practical initiative within their 'home' organisation. Women Connect member organisations had one nominated person to attend network events, and, while many of these individuals had changed by the end, they did form a cohesive group that enjoyed meeting together. They found it difficult, however, to inspire hard-pressed colleagues to learn new practices – or to want to communicate with other members of the network – when they had not had a chance to meet them or to gain a sense of the membership as a whole.

How was the tension to be mediated between the 'learning community', created at training events and networking days, and the other 'worlds' in which member organisations were to use these new skills? Strategies had to be devised to maintain a balance between demonstrating 'added value' for the organisations in their own terms, and generating challenge and change in how these were interpreted.

Specific challenges for Women Connect members related to the under-resourcing of the women's voluntary sector (Riordan 1999). The project was designed to create an environment that sustained and encouraged processes of exchange and learning. However, the environment in which member organisations had to operate was itself in constant flux; during the short life of the project, member organisations lost and found funding, changed staff and were always overstretched and under-resourced. Member organisations had scarce resources – often only one computer for the entire office as well as for Internet usage – and issues of relationship were in some cases negotiated and expressed through the physical positioning of the computer.[28] While Women Connect could offer conditions conducive to learning and exchange at its events, members had to take this back into their organisations, and to gain support from colleagues in working out practical applications. In an environment where survival of the organisation, and the resisting of increased workloads, were often the top priority it was not easy to motivate colleagues to make time to learn new practices and to change the way they worked. The short time-scale in which Women Connect had to deliver results meant there was little scope to adjust the pace of learning to the needs of member organisations.

Feminist literature on difference has tended to focus on differences of identity between women in social rather than organisational contexts. In this chapter we have discussed the concerns raised by black women's organisations in relation to their participation in the learning network. Once the network was established, the focus of participants' discussion was on learning ICT usage, in the context of the activities and purpose of member organisations. The primary focus was on ability to learn ICT usage, and differences in ability to learn, and to apply this in organisational contexts seemed as relevant as differences of power relating to social identity. How these differences intertwined to influence participation within network events was not explored directly, and did not emerge explicitly as an issue. Participants addressed social-identity differences in relation to the practical needs of specific communities served by their organisations. Power differences associated with role within member organisations also emerged; those participants with volunteer status in their home organisations had less power to effect changes in work practice than those employed as staff; administrators had less power than project-managers. Within the network and in member organisations these differences were balanced by different levels of ability to use ICTs, and did not in themselves shape relationships between participants.

There were differences in member organisations' participation in network events, and these related both to the perceived value of participation, and a primary priority of providing direct service to women, in a context of inadequate resources.[29] It is likely that, over a longer length of time, differences between individual participants would have emerged more explicitly as an issue for participation. However during the short life of the project,[30] the focus for individual participants at learning and networking events remained on shared experience and common goals, in the context of learning to adapt and develop uses of ICT for the delivery of services to women in the specific communities served by each of their organisations. In this context, project evaluation indicated that individuals valued highly the opportunity provided by the networking and training events to access each other's practice and knowledge (Moggridge 1999, Page and Scott 1999a). Since the project ended, some member organisations continue to access each other's expertise to increase their own capacity to work with women in specific communities, as was the case in the Asian women's health project. This would have positive outcomes for women in communities served by both centres.

As Maria Lugones argues (1997), we inhabit various 'worlds', and may even inhabit more than one world at the same time. In each world, inhabitants interpret what they see in particular, shared, ways. They live in shared ways and have shared sets of practices. This conceptualisation bears some similarity to the theoretical framework that Bev Skeggs elaborated (1997) in her discussion of the constitution of subjectivity through experience. Drawing on Bourdieu (1986), she describes *recognition* as one of the means by which experiences are named, marked and interpreted, and by which individuals come to occupy particular subject positions (1997: 29):

> This enables a shift to be made from experience as a foundation for knowledge to experience as productive of a knowing subject in which their identities are continually in production rather than being occupied as fixed . . . This recognises that knowledge is situated, is produced from social subjects with varying amounts of cultural capital, located in a nexus of power relations.
>
> (Skeggs 1997: 28)

The recognition of experience depends on a great deal more than the possession of some abstract criteria for what may count as valid knowledge. It arises from the tacit assumptions that grow out of a habitus (Bourdieu 1986), a set of skills and practices (Dalmiya and Alcoff 1993) and/or a historically grounded discourse (Foucault 1974). This leads to the conclusion that knowledge is generated, recognised and acted upon within epistemological communities (Nelson 1993), or within what Lugones has called 'worlds'. In asking participants to leave the 'world' of their home organisation behind, and to enter a new group which would have, or build, a new set of practices and a new type of perception, we were asking them to become – to some extent – what Lugones has called 'world-travellers' (1987).

The first priorities of Women Connect's members were often to use new-found skills within their local context – their own organisations and local networks. It wasn't easy to find things to say online to other Women Connect members – to know what was worth sharing or what they could gain – although at face-to-face meetings this wasn't a difficulty at all. This point was made in a different way in workshop discussions at our final conference; women said they found email and e-conferencing most useful when it was employed with defined groups of members and for specific purposes.

World-travelling is never safe, nor easy. As Gloria Anzaldúa writes, 'the coming together of two self-consistent but habitually incompatible frames of reference can cause *un choque*, a cultural collision' (1987: 78). In taking that step, the 'traveller' needs a tolerance for ambiguity. She must learn to shift out of habitual modes of thinking – to adopt a perspective that includes rather than excludes. She must sustain contradictions, and turn ambivalence into something else (Anzaldúa 1987: 79). 'She is willing to share, to make herself vulnerable to foreign ways of seeing and thinking. She surrenders all notions of safety, of the familiar. Deconstruct. Construct' (Anzaldúa 1987: 82).

In organisations where, owing to staff shortage, volunteers were made the lead contact in relation to Women Connect, they often took on greater leadership roles in relation to staff and other volunteers. The skills they had learned and were being asked to pass on implied changed work practices for others, while their change agency role implied changes in their relationship to colleagues. For example, one volunteer organised a rolling training programme for staff and other volunteers in order to pass on skills she had acquired at Women Connect training events. Another volunteer initiated the use of email for volunteers whose hours at the Centre meant they otherwise rarely met; this resulted in improved communication with each other as well as with the Centre organiser.

In our introduction we argued that, in an area as fast changing as community informatics, sustainability depends upon adaptability and innovation. This, we have argued, can be facilitated within a learning 'community' that crosses lines of difference. Skills in change agency are required – the ability to take understandings arising in one 'world' and use them to instigate change in another.

> the future will belong to the mestiza. Because the future depends on the breaking down of paradigms, it depends on the straddling of two or more cultures . . . We are the people who leap in the dark, we are the people on the knees of the gods. In our very flesh (r)evolution works out the clash of cultures. It makes us crazy constantly, but if the centre holds, we've made some kind of evolutionary step forward.
>
> (Anzaldúa 1987: 81)

In practice, all the member organisations not prevented by funding or internal crises did develop new practice – each at a pace adapted to their own context and circumstances. New practice was taken back and developed in local networks. Email increasingly replaced other forms of communication, while collaboration was facilitated by the exchange of documents and information. Those individuals in each member organisation who took part in Women Connect face-to-face events enjoyed meeting, sharing their work and exchanging good practice; they energised and encouraged each other. And over and above the goals of learning how to use ICTs, they enjoyed the opportunity to meet as a network of women's organisations.

Conclusion: resourcing community informatics

The 'information society' might be conceptualised as a powerful techno-economic network (Callon 1991) which is creating a new social reality. Drawing on the work of Bruno Latour, Susan Leigh Star has described the way heterogeneous interests can be pulled together into 'mini-empires', enrolling both human and non-human actors into new techno-social networks. Once stabilised (Star 1991), these networks begin to shape our social landscape, grounding each and every social action and movement. She (re)names as 'politics by other means' (Haraway 1986) the process by which – their once divergent parts disciplined – these new networks are made stable and, seemingly, irreversible. Within these networks, new sets of physical and social conventions are established which, being unstable for non-members, also create new forms of marginality (Star 1991).

Women without ICT knowledge and access – particularly women who are not white, middle-class and professionally employed – may find themselves living marginal lives in this new techno-social environment. Women Connect's starting place was recognition of the effects of under-resourcing on some groups of women – and on the organisations that exist to meet their needs. These organisations must survive in a fast-changing context, where new practices, conventions and organisational forms – collectively known by the shorthand term 'the information society' – are developing and are affecting every aspect of their activity. In a context of increasing need, and amid greater competition for declining resources, the value to women's organisations of widespread communication, good information and effective publicity has never been greater. Yet, for a variety of reasons, the support needed to make effective use of ICT has not been forthcoming for women's organisations. To paraphrase Saskia Everts, new technologies can be used to meet unfulfilled gender needs – or they can change the social context in a way which brings about perverse and destructive effects for marginalised groups (Everts 1998: 11–12).

Women Connect was designed to address this gap, and it achieved a substantial degree of success in its aims (Page and Scott 1999a). When the project co-ordinators asked members to refer back to the goals they had set, they frequently encountered resistance; members anticipated failure and being negatively judged. In nearly all cases, however, their achievements had outstripped the goals set. In feedback from project members, and in the project evaluation (Moggridge 1999), members stated that their participation in a learning community *had* helped them sustain new ICT practice. By the end of Phase 1, substantial results had been achieved for member organis-ations and for the project as a whole. Substantial obstacles to the development of new practice also emerged in this evaluation, however many of these were related to a lack of resources – to shortages of time, space and money, and to difficulty in obtaining core funding.

Staff and volunteers in women's organisations simply do not have spare time to learn how to use ICTs, and they will not be motivated to take time out from other activities unless training is designed in a tightly defined and focused way, for purposes of clear benefit and relevance to themselves (Women Connect 1999b). Individual women, as well as women's organis-ations, needed a longer time-span to learn and adopt new practices; they needed time to accommodate flux and change in their circumstances. Rigid timetables with predefined deliverables were off-putting to members, while a pre-set timetable could not address the diversity of interests and applications which motivated women's learning (Women Connect 1999b; Page and Scott 1999a).

Members stated that belonging to a network of women's organisations, with shared commitment, *had* motivated them to learn; face-to-face contact was essential when embarking on cyber-communication. There are few spaces for women's organisations to meet; Women Connect provided members with precious networking opportunities with others sharing their values and concerns. However, a balance had to be struck between diversity perceived as useful and that perceived as useless; where members felt they had less common ground with other members, they found it harder to make time or release staff to attend network events – particularly when this was competing with service delivery.

Drawing on the Women Connect experience, we have argued in this chapter that online communities need to be built, and that this requires political courage, as well as active facilitation. Notwithstanding the ambiguities and contested values which surround the word 'community', it is our argument that 'learning community' can be a useful description for the sustainable, organisation-orientated approach we are advocating. Learning communities are dialogic, and are grounded in face-to-face interactions as well as cyber-space communication. Such communities work with the reality of gendered power relations, aiming to challenge and to change them. To achieve this, high-quality facilitation is needed, encompassing both political and relational skills. These skills are often the province of women, and are traditionally undervalued in organisations (Fletcher 1998). We have argued in this chapter that *now* is the time for community informatics to mainstream this 'feminist' approach, working to achieve sufficient resources to make this possible.

In spite of the potential of learning communities, the manner in which community-informatics projects are generally funded makes it difficult to create and sustain the conditions in which they can be created. Voluntary sector funding bodies often attach conditions to their funding, requiring guarantees of some pre-determined 'product' which can be delivered to an agreed format and time-scale. Short-term funding, linked to specific projects, and a lack of adequate core funding, makes it difficult for organisations to maintain the stability and security needed for effective innovation. The creation and maintenance of a learning community seems to us to be *actively* at cross-purposes with this product-driven model; learning communities are processes, not products, and they are inherently open processes at that. We need a conceptual basis for the voluntary sector funding of ICT projects which addresses these issues.

In conclusion, we would like to return to women's all-too-common experience of marginality in relation to new technologies.

> By experience and affinity, some of us begin not with Pasteur [the scientific inventor], but with the monster, the outcast . . . We have usually been the delegated to, the disciplined. Our selves are thus in two senses

monstrous selves, cyborgs, impure, first in the sense of uniting split selves and second in the sense of being that which goes unrepresented in encounters with technology.

(Star 1991: 29)

To be a cyborg (Haraway 1985) is to be inherently, unavoidably, caught between worlds. Cyborgs cannot be easily defined. Multiple rather than singular, they resist closure. It is our argument that, within a learning community, this openness and vulnerability can be turned into a strength.

Notes

1 For a full description of these, see the Women Connect Phase 1 report (Page and Scott 1999a) and website: www.womenconnect.org.uk.
2 'We' in this instance refers to the co-authors of this paper, Margaret Page and Anne Scott. Margaret Page is one of two joint project co-ordinators of Phase 1 of the Women Connect project. Marion Scott, the other joint project co-ordinator of Women Connect Phase 1, contributed to this chapter by commenting on draft text. In writing this paper, we have struggled to find a form that articulates these three different contributions to the paper. This process has illustrated the challenges of finding a language which reaches across the borders of academic/practitioner concerns. We have used the terms 'we', 'us' in ways which seek to acknowledge both the different knowledge bases from which we each draw in making our contributions, and the areas in which we have developed a shared language or conceptual practice for collaboration. When the terms 'us' or 'we' are used in relation to the practice of the Women Connect project, it refers to Margaret Page and *Marion* Scott, the co-ordinators of Women Connect. When it is used in any other context, it refers to Margaret Page and *Anne* Scott, the co-authors of this chapter.
3 Anne Moggridge; see her report (Moggridge 1999).
4 This was one of eighteen Policy Action Team (PAT) reports compiled by the Department of Trade and Industry's task force on social exclusion; it focused on putting ICT resources into 'deprived areas' (PAT 15 2000).
5 Action learning – an approach increasingly used in management and professional education – is the development of new practice through reflection on action. Action leaning is often facilitated, and takes place in a structured group setting with others over a period of time. Feedback is given by group members in order to generate new perspectives, and members are encouraged to test out these new perspectives in practice. For a practical handbook, see McGill and Beaty (1992).
6 For a synopsis of the discipline of human and action inquiry, see Reason (1994).
7 Margaret Page and Marion Scott; see note 2.
8 See, for example, the description of the holistic approach to the learning process taken by Manchester Women's Electronic Village Hall (Day and Harris 1997) and the workshop reports from the Women Connect conference (Women Connect 1999b).
9 See for example reports from women who took part in the Women Connect conference, November 1999, on the Women Connect website, www.womenconnect.org.uk.
10 This preference for moderated online spaces may be related to the greater vulnerability of women to online harassment or 'flaming' (Herring 1994, Brail

1996, Herman 1999). In addition, some studies have shown that men tend to dominate online conversation, even when the topic under discussion is more closely related to women's interests (Kramarae and Taylor 1993, Ferris 1996).

11 Margaret Page and Anne Scott, in post-project reflection. See note 2.

12 We are currently seeing a redefinition of the spaces for engaging in social and political action. One can now engage in 'public' action from the most private of physical spaces. The group Women Living Under Muslim Law, for example, is using a closed email discussion list to bring intimate issues relating to sexuality, domestic violence, female genital mutilation and reproductive health into the 'public' sphere (Alshejni 1999, Harcourt 1999).

13 Community sociologists often distinguish three broad types of communities: communities of locality, communities of interest and communities of 'spirit' (Crow and Allan 1994, Schuler 1996: 3). The underlying assumption in each of these definitions is that 'community' should be used in reference to people having something in common – whether relating to a geographical area, a set of interests or identity. In fact, the term 'community' is said by Paul Hoggett to have its origins in Tonnies's late nineteenth-century notion of *Gemeinschaft*, which referred to the development of social bonds based upon similarity (Hoggett 1997a: 4). There are, of course, other ways of typing or defining communities – some of which are quite sophisticated. See Jones (1995) and Albrow *et al.* (1997) for accounts of these which make particular reference to the ways this term is now being redefined in relation to ICT.

14 Douglas Schuler, for example, opens the first chapter in his influential book on electronic community networks (1996) with a quotation, by Ed Schwartz, asserting that communities incorporate three elements: shared values, unity and intimacy. This normative approach assumes that homogenised communities are, inherently, a 'good thing'.

15 See, for example, Schuler's discussion of the contemporary 'decline' of community (1996: 4–8).

16 Margaret Page and Anne Scott.

17 In fact, what comes across in some of the more sociologically informed research is the heterogeneity and diversity of communities, even when they are identified as 'traditional' – i.e. working-class and place-based (Hoggett 1997b).

18 As Howard Rheingold puts it, 'Virtual communities are cultural aggregations that emerge when enough people bump into each other often enough in cyberspace' (1993b: 57).

19 See, for example, the Standing Conference on Community Development Charter, reproduced in Harris (1994); see also Gilchrist's discussion (1998) on working with divisions within and between communities.

20 These issues were raised by women who took part in the consultation seminar organised by Women Connect for PAT 15; see note 4.

21 Margaret Page and Anne Scott.

22 Intentionality has long been considered by phenomenologists to be one of the more important marks of mental life. As Jean-Paul Sartre noted, this need of consciousness to exist as 'the consciousness of something other than itself' is what Husserl called intentionality (Sartre 1992: 389). Thus, it should not be understood as a characteristic or a trait, rather, it falls into a particular logical quality – that of direction to, or relation to, content. As Val Plumwood notes, intentionality involves a 'going-beyond' that which is given (1993: 131). This is the process by which purpose is dynamically (re)created within an ongoing life trajectory.

23 Throughout this section, 'we' refers to Margaret Page and Marion Scott. See note 2.

24 Margaret Page had worked with women's and feminist organisations and networks as a local authority community worker, freelance consultant, and action researcher; Marion Scott had worked in consultation with women's organisations on a wide range of women's equality and policy issues as head of a London local authority women's unit, and had been active in feminist networks.

25 See Figure 11.1.

26 The 'I' in this case belongs to Margaret Page.

27 This concept has been developed by Nira Yuval-Davis, as an extension of an approach being used among Italian feminist activists (Yuval-Davis 1997). For more discussion regarding this new approach, see the recent special issue of *Soundings* (summer 1999).

28 In one organisation the computer's position changed several times as different staff members developed an interest in using it to find websites relevant for their advice work. In another organisation – a women's refuge – staff had to prioritise office work, refusing access to children and their worker, and limiting access by residents. They are now fundraising for more computers.

29 This did have an uneven impact on the participation of individuals – although all member organisations were at different times faced with funding crises which inhibited participation. For example, two member organisations could not participate in network events when all staff were needed to run the services. One of these was a Centre serving refugee women, the other a centre for women in a rural area

30 Over a period of twenty months, four face-to-face network events were held.

Part III

Electronic empowerment and surveillance

Chapter 12

Social capital and cyberpower in the African-American community

A case study of a community technology centre in the dual city

Abdul Alkalimat and Kate Williams

Introduction

This chapter is about the community technology centre as a new organisational basis for democracy and social inclusion in the information society. We present a theoretical framework and an empirical case study, concluding with some reflections on democracy and cyber-organising.

Background

Historical inequalities condition new social developments.[1] In virtually every society at the dawn of the twenty-first century, polarities of income, class, colour and space are translating into a digital divide.[2] This divide is between those who can access and use phones, computers and the Internet and those who cannot. There are economic, cultural and also spatial dimensions to this divide, because, for example, the lower-income inner-city community is excluded structurally and physically, living in unmarked but well-defined neighbourhoods with different or fewer resources.

Digital-divide measures usually focus on individual or household access. However, the digital divide also involves social applications of technology and the content of networked information. Government surveys provide the most authoritative data to date on access. United States government statistics indicate 1998 household rates of access as: telephones 94.1 per cent, computers 42.1 per cent and Internet use 26.2 per cent. At the highest income levels (annual household income of $75,000 or more) computers are in almost 80 per cent of the households, with little difference between Blacks and Whites at this income level. But on the whole the digital divide is also a colour divide. In their latest study, the US Department of Commerce stated, 'The digital divide has turned into a "racial ravine" when one looks at access among households of different races and ethnic origins.'[3]

In addition to home and work, people access computers and the Internet in public settings including government institutions (such as libraries and schools), commercial enterprises (such as copy shops and private business

Table 12.1 Community technology centre associations: Toledo, Ohio and US

Excerpted Mission Statements	
Local Coalition to Access Technology and Networking in Toledo (CATNeT) Founded 1996 22 members	... to contribute to the empowerment of low-income citizens and community-based organisations by providing or facilitating access to the technological tools that are more routinely available to our community's more affluent citizens and organisations.
State Ohio Community Computing Centers Network (OCCCN) Founded 1995 39 members	... dedicated to expanding access to technology in Ohio's low-income communities ... Supports the efforts of centres that provide free public access to computers and the Internet for members of their communities.
National Community Technology Centre Network (CTCNeT) Founded 1990 400+ members	... provide opportunities whereby people of all ages who typically lack access to computers and related technologies can learn to use these technologies in an environment that encourages exploration and discovery and, through this experience, develop personal skills and self-confidence. ... offers resources ... [to] facilitate telecommunications, print, and in-person linkages enabling members to benefit from shared experience and expertise. ... a leading advocate of equitable access to computers and related technologies; it will invite, initiate and actively encourage partnerships and collaborations with other individuals and organisations that offer resources in support of its mission; and it will strive, in every arena, to bring about universal technological enfranchisement.

schools) and other venues making up the public sphere.[4] We call this public computing. The community-technology centre (CTC) is a generic name given to a computer lab open to the public. Especially with recent government and private funding, CTCs are multiplying. They have formed into associations, often funding related, at the local, state and national levels. Toledo, Ohio, the location of this study, is typical, with three associations at work, sometimes in co-ordination.[5]

The actual development of public computing labs far exceeds the membership of the various associations. Preliminary results of a census of public computing in Toledo indicate numbers exceeding 120, and generally for every competitive funding opportunity applicants far outnumber grant recipients (Williams and Alkalimat 2001).

Theoretical framework

Our general research focus is on community-technology centres in urban poor communities, especially communities of colour. Our specific research question for this chapter is this: How does social capital structure power in a community-technology centre (CTC) and influence its programmes and effectiveness for local residents?

Historical context

This research question is anchored in theoretical concerns about how the organisation of society establishes the context for and conditions the sustainability of the African-American freedom struggle. We are interested in how public computing can play a role in this freedom struggle. This struggle has been the theme of the Black experience, involving the dialectical interplay of social forces internal and external to the Black community. This dialectic is sometimes hidden under the ideological banner of nationalism versus integrationism, but the objective dynamic is that all organisations and movements of the Black freedom struggle use resources from both internal and external sources, as well as facing obstacles from both. The success of an organisation or movement depends on its resources being more powerful than the obstacles it faces.

Thus the two concepts of community and power are the main foci of the scientific literature that sets the context for our research question. Citing this literature, we formulate a theoretical framework for the case study and provide the basis for interpretation of our results.

The African-American community is rooted in a history of struggle (Alkalimat *et al.* 1986). It came into being as the result of the global expansion of capitalism by means of four centuries of the slave trade. It has experienced three fundamental historical stages: slavery, tenancy and industry. Each of these stages has ended and transitioned into the next on the basis of disruptive processes: the Atlantic slave trade, the emancipation process from slavery and the mass migration from the rural agricultural south to the urban industrial north. Beginning in the 1970s, another disruptive transition became apparent, as suggested by the new concepts used to describe the crisis: unemployment became structural and permanent unemployment, homelessness emerged, stagflation, etc. The economic expansion and political expansion of democratic inclusion that lasted from the Second World War through the 1960s was ended and a reversal began (Figure 12.1).

In his study of the Black middle class, Landry (1987) suggests a conceptual map of decades. The 1950s was a decade of expanding economics but an absence of reform politics. The 1960s ushered in reform politics on top of economic expansion, and the Black middle class grew and advanced. In the

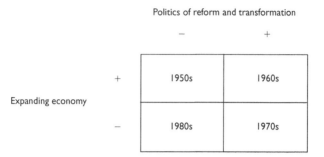

Figure 12.1 Structural Parameters for Black middle-class advancement, 1950–90

1970s, reform politics continued but the economy stalled, the Black middle class held steady. The 1980s, with neither an expanding economy nor reformed politics, was another decade of relative incremental growth for the Black middle class. This meant that the 1960s saw an unprecedented and short-lived growth of the Black middle class.

Community context

The 1970s and 1980s also produced unprecedented poverty in the inner cities of the United States. Wilson advances three concepts that sum up changes in the social organisation of Black community life during this time: social buffer, social isolation and concentration effect (Wilson 1987). These concepts capture the crisis facing Black people being marginalised through the birth process of the information society. Wilson states his argument:

> I believe that the exodus of middle- and working-class families from many ghetto neighbourhoods removes an important 'social buffer' that could deflect the full impact of the kind of prolonged and increasing joblessness that plagued inner-city neighbourhoods in the 1970s and early 1980s . . . Thus, in a neighbourhood with a paucity of regularly employed families and with the overwhelming majority of families having spells of long-term joblessness, people experience a social isolation that excludes them from the job network system that permeates other neighbourhoods . . . The social transformation of the inner city has resulted in a dispro-portionate concentration of the most disadvantaged segments of the urban Black population, creating a social milieu significantly different from the environment that existed in these communities several decades ago.
>
> (Wilson, 1987: 56–8)

As a result, the last quarter of the twentieth century gave rise to a new Black middle class and a new impoverished class.

The old Black middle class contained entrepreneurs, service professionals and farmers. The new Black middle class has almost no farmers, and the service professionals have become overwhelmingly employed by the state. Over 70 per cent of Black women with college degrees and 50 per cent of Black men with college degrees work for government (Landry 1987: 116–22). This process started during Reconstruction after the Civil War, when government employment was the main avenue open to Black upward social mobility. It continues today, as affirmative action applies only to employment in the state and in those private firms with government contracts.

While charting the main feature of what he calls the 'network society', Castells analyses unprecedented urban poverty on a global scale. He argues that the new impoverishment and social exclusion is a systemic feature of this period.

> This widespread, multiform process of social exclusion leads to the constitution of what I call, taking the liberty of a cosmic metaphor, the black information holes of informational capitalism . . . Social exclusion is often expressed in spatial terms. The territorial confinement of systemically worthless populations, disconnected from networks of valuable functions and people, is indeed a major characteristic of the spatial logic of the network society.
>
> (Castells, 1998: 162, 164)

Elsewhere, applying this analysis to the United States, he describes the informational city as a dual city.

> By dual city, I understand an urban system socially and spatially polarised between high value-making groups and functions on the one hand and devalued social groups and downgraded spaces on the other hand . . .The power of new information technologies, however, enhances and deepens features present in the social structure and in power relationships.
>
> (Castells 1998: 27)

In this context we apply the concept of social capital to the inner-city African-American community.[6] Social capital, contrasted with physical capital (for example machines) and human capital (for example education), describes the social relationships, expectations, obligations and norms that facilitate productive human activity.[7] Putnam measured US social capital over the twentieth century. Collecting longitudinal data on American participation in all sorts of organised groups, he found that since roughly 1960 there has been an across-the-board decline in social capital. His thematic metaphor is that people used to bowl in organised leagues, and now are 'bowling alone'.

Putnam makes a distinction between bonding social capital, relationships within a group, and bridging social capital, relationships that link a group with others. These two types of social capital together make up the social capital of any given social group:

> Bonding social capital is good for undergirding specific reciprocity and mobilising solidarity. Dense networks in ethnic enclaves, for example, provide crucial social and psychological support for less fortunate members of the community . . . Bridging networks, by contrast, are better for linkage to external assets and for information diffusion . . . Moreover bridging social capital can generate broader identities and reciprocity, whereas bonding social capital bolsters our narrower selves.
>
> (Putnam 2000: 22–3)

The distinction between bridging and bonding social capital plays a particular role when a community lacks key resources, for instance, money:

> among the disadvantaged, 'bridging' social capital may be the more lucrative form. All told, people in economically disadvantaged areas appear to suffer doubly. They lack the material resources to get ahead, and they lack the social resources that might enable them to amass these material resources.
>
> (Putnam 2000: 32)

Discourse

The concept of the public sphere has been debated since its historical exegesis from European intellectual history by Habermas (1989), Calhoun (1992) and Negt and Kluge (1993). The public sphere is a social ecology for relevant discourse that shapes policy, public opinion and the dominant intellectual themes of an era.

Dawson critiques Habermas in such a way that we can connect Putnam to our focus on the dual city (Dawson 1994). Habermas concludes that the public sphere of capitalist society is a bourgeois phenomenon, but Dawson utilises a concept from feminist theory to argue that the Black community has always had a 'subaltern counter-public' as the social basis for resistance: 'An independent Black press, the production and circulation of socially and politically sharp popular music and the Black church have provided institutional bases for the Black counter-public since the Civil War' (Dawson 1994: 206). After articulating an analysis of the same economic transformation discussed by Landry, Wilson and Castells, Dawson states: 'the ideological and political restructuring that accompanied this transformation was decisively accomplished in the 1980s by a number of extraordinary conservative regimes including those of Margaret Thatcher, Helmut Kohl and

Ronald Reagan' (Dawson 1994: 213–14). He then asks what continues to be a relevant research question in and after the same period discussed by Landry, Castells and Wilson: 'The question before us becomes, what is the basis in the 1990s for restructuring an oppositional subaltern public in the aftermath of a rightist backlash of historic proportions' (Dawson, 1994: 215). In sum, our approach to community examines the dual city (Castells) for social capital (Putnam) in the socially isolated Black inner city (Wilson) to produce a Black counter-public sphere (Dawson) by means of a community-technology centre.

Social movements

Morris analyses the institutions that the Black counter-public relied on during the civil rights movement in a case study of the Montgomery, Alabama, bus boycott movement in the 1950s led by Martin Luther King (Morris 1984). He employs an 'indigenous perspective' use of resource mobilisation theory to define the Black movement: 'Resource mobilisation theory emphasises the resources necessary for the initiation and development of movements. They include formal and informal organisations, leaders, money, people, and communication networks' (Morris 1984: 279). Landry describes how the Montgomery movement was: 'led by a young middle class minister, Martin Luther King Jr., but was sustained by poor Blacks of the city, domestics, garbage collectors, and unskilled laborers as well as Blacks of other classes' (Landry 1987: 71). Landry's data on this broad-based mobilisation supports Morris in arguing the primacy of internal resources.

Morris anticipated Putnam's distinction between bonding and bridging social capital:

> The basic resources enabling a dominated group to engage in sustained protest are well developed internal social institutions and organisations that provide the community with encompassing communication networks, organised groups, experienced leaders, and social resources, including money, labor, charisma, that can be mobilised to attain collective goals . . . The significance of outside resources, in this view, lies in the help they can give in sustaining movements. However, our evidence suggests that they are not a causal determinant.
>
> (Morris 1984: 282–3)

Cyberpower

Jordan advances the notion of cyberpower and identifies three interrelated regions of cyberpower, 'the individual, the social, and the imaginary' (Jordan 1999). Cyberpower – the effect of online activity on power – can be measured and mapped. We use three definitions of these types of cyberpower:

- *individual*: gaining skills and connections for oneself
- *social*: gaining skills and connections for a group
- *imaginary or, as we have renamed it, ideological*: gaining skills and making connections in order to advance the imaginary: a vision, a movement, an ideological purpose.

Jim Walch (1999: 23) argues for a research agenda in this area:

> A new, 'wired' political community is emerging, a net-polis. The contours and nature of this political community are only in formation, nebulous. The task of research is to study what is happening, why, and what possible patterns might emerge. A major concern – for politicians, scholars and citizens – is maintaining democratic values in cyberspace: equal access, responsibility, representativity, public control and accountability.

There is an emerging research literature on the community technology centre. Researchers with the Educational Development Centre have documented that users of CTCs gain computer-related job and job-hunting skills as well as advances in the areas of employment, learning, increased confidence and sense of community (Mark *et al.* 1997, Chow *et al.* 1998, 2000). Breeden *et al.* found that CTCs are popular with all ages, provide a wide variety of benefits and offer management and sustainability challenges to their operators (Breeden *et al.* 1998). The Department of Commerce has published three dozen case studies of CTCs funded by their Technology Opportunities programme (formerly TIAAP) (Department of Commerce 2000).

Somewhat in advance of the nationwide spread of CTCs, a sequence of studies by Bertot and McClure (with others) quantified the continuing expansion of public computer access across the nation's public-library outlets.[8] Lentz *et al.* (2000) observed computer users at seven CTCs and public libraries and found that environmental factors such as layout and staff behaviour can structure access to technology in ways that sometimes discourage users. From a background of building and studying community networks as well as CTCs, Bishop (2000) outlines design recommendations for technology literacy projects in low-income communities: a community-wide approach, reliance on native talent rather than outsiders as staff, working through existing human networks for outreach and adopting a 'discovery' approach to educational goals.

CTCs elsewhere in the world can also be found in the research literature. Relating to evaluation, Hudson (2000) has proposed a tele-centre typology, which includes a range of services (phone, fax, computers, Internet, print matter, training, copying, design and research services) reflecting the developing world's simultaneous leap into all forms of telecommunications. In the UK, the PAT 15 report, issued by one of the Policy Action Teams reporting to the government's Social Exclusion Unit, reviewed progress in community technology to date and recommended that by April 2002, 'each deprived neighbourhood should have at least one publicly accessible community based facility to complement any home access' (PAT 15 2000: 6). Gurstein (2000b) and Loader (1998) are among those who have identified community informatics as a strategy whereby information technology helps develop communities as well as individuals.

The global construction of the Internet has led to cyberpower as a tool in the fight for human survival and freedom. Marginalised and socially silenced groups have used information technology to build support and global media attention (Dyer-Witheford 1999). Such groups are found in East Timor, Nigeria, Congo, Yugoslavia and South Africa. Three particular examples illustrate high levels of bonding social capital utilising information technology to escape social isolation and leap into connectivity with a global abundance of bridging social capital.

First, *Wilmington, North Carolina* (Mele 1999). Faced with a demolition/reconstruction plan that threatened their apartments and their community, residents of the Jervay Place public housing project purchased Internet service for computers already in use in a resident training centre and expanded their library-based research to include listserv participation and email communications and the publication of a well-received Jervay website. With the help of online contacts, they produced a counter-plan for redevelopment of the housing project in the interest of current residents and negotiated their way into the planning process.

Second, *Chiapas, Mexico* (Cleaver 1998, Ronfeldt and Martinez 1997). Upon the implementation of NAFTA, the Zapatista National Liberation Army came out of the jungle to take over a series of towns in the state of Chiapas and make indigenous voices heard at the national level. Friends and reporters posted news about the Zapatistas on the Internet, and more than a dozen support websites and listservs were set up, in various languages. Once the Zapatistas and their allies began to use the Internet directly, they were able to mobilise seven thousand people from around the world to two conferences held in Chiapas and in Spain and to continue to provide 'counter-information' side-stepping local news blackouts.

Third, *WTO* (Vari 2000, Tabb 2000). The 1999 WTO protests in Seattle were the results of email mobilising, and the Seattle Independent Media Centre posted on the Web moment-to-moment reports on the demonstrations and the police response. The resulting global visibility fuelled subsequent protests, workshops and teach-ins. Indymedia.org, which received 1.5 million hits during the week in Seattle, now has thirty local spin-off sites. A16, which organised counter-events to the Washington DC IMF/WTO/World Bank meeting, can perhaps best be described as a networked movement centre, with listservs, web pages linked to those of co-operating organisations, online donation mechanisms etc.

Our general theoretical model is summed up as:

Social capital → Community technology centre → Cyberpower

Our thesis is that the social capital invested in a community technology centre determines its role in the community and the continuing freedom struggle. Community-technology centre outcomes will be expressed in cyberpower. The overall question is whether social capital and cyberpower are creating a new Black counter-public in the information society.

Method

This study is an example of what the African-American psychologist Kenneth Clark (1989) called involved observation. In his study of a social-action agency in Harlem, New York, he played two roles simultaneously, executive director and researcher. He recruited another social scientist to help him debrief and escape the blinders of his own subjectivity. This is very different from the detachment required of participant observation. The two authors here are volunteers and board members at the centre involved in planning and implementing programmes. We have used our two viewpoints to triangulate towards objectivity. We have also discussed this analysis with staff, volunteers, and other board members.

In addition, we made use of the centre's archives, benefiting from co-operation with the centre as a whole. The archives include 18 linear feet of papers in files and binders and a number of electronic documents. Part of our work was assembling and inventorying this material for the centre: minutes and handouts from board and staff meetings, financial records, day-to-day programme records and programme plans and reports. It is testimony to the care taken from the beginning days of the centre that staff preserved these records. We also conducted interviews with key participants. In turn, we discussed research findings with board members, staff and volunteers, whose input only helped improve the study.

Historical narrative

The object of our case study is the W. J. Murchison Community Centre, a centre which today carries out tutoring, community gardening, support for other community groups and most of all computer classes and open computer time. The centre has seventeen PCs and is located at street level on a smaller arterial street in African-American central Toledo, Ohio. The community garden is one block away, across from Martin Luther King Jr Elementary School. Half of the computers are networked to the Internet. An average of two hundred people use the centre each month, and more than 170 have user IDs for which they paid $5 annually, $10 for families.

According to the 1990 US census, 70 per cent of households in the surrounding area live at or near federal poverty levels and 70 per cent are female-headed. Ninety-seven per cent of residents are African-American. The area has lost population over the last forty years. Many of the mostly wooded houses, built around 1900, are boarded up. The city has also torn down abandoned houses. Inhabited houses may be broken down or freshly painted and carefully maintained. Yards may be overgrown with weeds or rich with flowers and trimmed hedges. The community is also dotted with vegetable gardens with greens, tomatoes and an occasional stand of corn.

Nine churches are located within half a mile, more beyond that radius. These churches serve both community residents and people who live in the generally more affluent and newer African-American communities to the west, many of them with ties to the old community. Hair salons, little stores selling candy, soda, junk food and beer, and 'big box' auto-parts stores, dominate the local economy. McDonald's is the morning coffee spot for older men in and from the community. The absence of a grocery store has been a political issue for some time.

Interstate 75, a major highway linking the southern and northern United States, slices the Toledo Museum of Art away from the community. The museum does not conduct any outreach in the area, although the founder, Edward Drummond Libbey, a local glass magnate, stipulated that admission to the museum was to remain always free, and built a wing that has long housed art classes for the general public, classes which many older white Toledoans remember fondly.

In 1998, in a well-publicised move against drug dealing, Toledo's mayor declared martial law on a side street next to the centre. The police moved in and set up guard stations limiting people's access to their homes and preventing guests from visiting. This prompted a brief debate. After a few months the city removed the concrete barriers and martial law was lifted. In 2000, the federal government allocated over $4 million to gentrify parts of the area, continuing a nationwide pattern of depopulation preliminary to a (real or promised) return of the middle class to the central city.

Stage one: church

Bishop W. J. Murchison is pastor of nearby St James Church, which he founded in 1967. A retired construction worker and contractor originally from Alabama, he and his wife Sister Dorothy Murchison live six blocks away from the centre. She sings and has for many years organised youth choirs at St James and across Toledo. She is also known for her grassroots fundraising: bus trips to nearby outlet malls, gospel concerts, birthday calendars, banquets and especially her 'brownies' funds (pennies).

In 1992 crack cocaine swept through the area, snatching up many vulner-able individuals of all ages and settling into buildings that became crack houses. For Bishop, who had always emphasised the church's ministry to youth, this recalled Ecclesiastes 3: 1–8, especially 'A time to plant, and a time to pluck up.' He experienced a vision, which was to found a community centre. As he puts it, 'We were about to lose a generation.'

With crack tearing through the families of his own congregation, it was natural to draw together a group of church members to implement his vision. His own niece Deborah Hamilton, saved since her mid twenties, was among the group; her husband Gary was staying clean after a recent run-in with crack. Bishop also recruited a younger minister, Dr C. E. Reese to administer the effort. Remembering the early days of the centre, Sister Murchison references another Bible verse, Proverbs 18: 29: 'Without a vision, the people perish.'

In 1993, partly because drug-treatment agencies had already set up nearby, the group decided to focus on prevention – agreeing in one early handout, 'If the mind is replete with substance of the positive nature, then the need for further stimulus becomes a moot point.' Dr Reese outlined the centre's first mission statement: 'Awareness . . . Education . . . Outreach'. The centre's programmes got under way in the basement of St James Church.

Programmes consisted of counselling, job preparation and computer skill training. By 1994, there were two donated Wang word processors. When both computers were in use, participants practised keystroking on keyboards hand-drawn on particleboard. This work was driven by their religious faith and loyalty to the programmes of the church, and their hunger for education and advancement.

In 1994 Dr Reese left Toledo, and the board asked Deborah Hamilton to become the executive director. Members recall four reasons: she had a college degree, she knew how to use computers, she had served as secretary of the board and she was a staunch member of the church.

Guided by Mrs Hamilton's self-study on organisational development, the board became a fundraising committee. In the tradition of the Black church, a series of projects kept bringing money in, several hundred dollars at a time, and the organisation always had close to $2000 saved up. An effort to recruit a grant writer began, and in early 1995 a volunteer began to work with Mrs Hamilton on a Community Development Block Grant proposal.

By February 1995, the board was so encouraged by the programmes and the fundraising that, when Bishop suggested for a second time that for $100 the centre could rent part of a small building he built and owned on Lawrence Street, it agreed. Moving out of the church was a marker of the start of a second stage in the life of the Murchison Community Centre.

Stage two: state

Although it was rejected, the 1995 CDBG grant submission, done in communication with the responsible city agency, was a learning experience for the centre. What the centre began to learn was how to jump through the hoops set by the state, the government bureaucracy. Once the funding started to flow – $44,000 in 1996, $25,000 in each of 1997, 1998 and 1999 – it dwarfed the funds raised through the social networks of the board members, i.e. church members, and defined the terms under which the centre operated for the next stage of its life.

For example, the second mission statement of the centre made no reference to the first, and was developed by Mrs Hamilton and a centre volunteer with the aim of fitting the requirements of the CDBG grant application process. Within a year this volunteer joined the staff of CDBG and was assigned for some time as the CDBG liaison to the centre. Since then, she has continued to look out for the interests of the centre and provide valued unofficial advice.

CDBG is a programme established in the 1980s when so many 1960s Great Society federal funding streams to impoverished communities were cut off. In their place, President Reagan and Congress directed a much smaller amount of funds through the Department of Housing and Urban Development to be doled out by city and county authorities according to federal guidelines. Thus CDBG provided federal funds, but local officials directed the flow.

Another example of an external authority setting the agenda for the centre came when Mrs Hamilton and a few others were working into the wee hours one night on another government grant proposal. They were stumped when it came to writing a needs statement, and read the suggestion: 'conduct a needs assessment of your community such as by means of a survey.' They had never surveyed the community. The grant process used the same language of 'needs assessment,' so the idea of conducting a survey took hold.

In fact, most of them had been raised or had raised their own children in the community, but the exercise of a survey captured the attention of the centre for several months. The board settled on twelve questions, and eventually 116 surveys were gathered. It is not clear what use was made of the information, gathered in response to external bureaucracies rather than as an outgrowth of the centre itself. Echoing the critique of John Kretzmann and John McKnight, the questions themselves portray the community as a collection of needs rather than a collection of resources that can be mobilised (Kretzmann and McKnight 1993).

When the local CBDG office rejected the centre's 1995 proposal, it further recommended that the centre should partner with a start-up Community Development Corporation. CDCs were again a product of the 1980s, which saw an epidemic of homelessness. By the 1990s in Toledo, CDCs had carved up the inner city and were taking the lion's share of CDBG funding. This money subsidised them in building and occasionally renovating small areas of inexpensive housing, and then selling with great fanfare.

The neighbourhood had been mostly left out of the 'gold rush'. Roosevelt Revitalisation Corporation and the centre, in these tracts, were to partner and submit one proposal for 1996. This process again took attention away from the grassroots fundraising that the board had been focusing on, but the joint proposal was funded and stage two was really under way.

Within two months of the grant period, Roosevelt proved unready to start work. Mrs Chestnut, now representing CDBG, recommended that the two organisations should split, with the centre getting the funds, because programmes were already under way and governance well established. Roosevelt would go back to the drawing board. A new term, leverage, came to the board as Mrs Chestnut explained why the city had funded the centre. The funds ($44,000) were to be used to lever other dollars, so that the centre would not remain 90 per cent CDBG-funded. The city, the board learned, had funded the centre, first as part of the now-suspended Roosevelt partnership, second, as a fresh effort in census tracts 25 and 26 (which no doubt covered a CDBG gap) and, third, because the grant focused on job development.

Not only did the CDBG office recommend policy directions, but also they required a complex of procurement, personnel, programme and financial policies, procedures and reporting that the centre had to master. One of the most onerous was the process of reimbursement. The monthly activity reports were to include every document produced that month plus a quantitative and descriptive report on each area of programme activity. These reports were required before a monthly cheque was sent. Then, every expenditure had to be documented, every cheque copied, and submitted monthly to CDBG. Several weeks later a cheque would arrive for all approved expenses. Disputed or incompletely documented expenses would be delayed one month or more. In order to provide service the centre had to obtain a line of credit, which it did, with the personal assurance of Bishop Murchison and his construction-business track record.

Financial administration became particularly difficult given that the payroll and all book-keeping was being done by an older member of the church who was in bad health for more than a year, making any change a sensitive matter. By October 1998 the indebtedness ballooned to more than $11,000.

As a result of the reporting requirements, programmes were documented as never before, and a monthly number, reflecting the number of people participating in centre programmes, was reported. The total number hovered around fifty-five per month during 1997–8.

As soon as the first CDBG grant began, three new board members were elected and an assistant director and programme co-ordinators, all working part-time, were hired. The terms of the grant did not allow for a full-time salary for Mrs Hamilton, so she continued to work a full-time day job and volunteer her time to the centre, taking occasional payments that just about equalled her travel and incidental expenses. The new individuals were either not members of St James or were more loosely tied to the church; the staff members, only one from St James, worked during the day or after school hours rather than in the evening when the board met, so the close personal ties that the board had used to keep the centre together began to loosen.

The role of the board changed during this time. What had been an active fundraising committee became a bureaucratic group that approved policies and financial reports. Meetings were held almost weekly over 1995 and early 1996; then monthly meetings became the norm. Near-perfect board-meeting attendance also became a thing of the past. The 1997 strategic plan, for instance, was the result of only four of twelve board members attending a session with a paid consultant and a representative from the city's plan commission. These two people wrote up the strategic plan.

Accompanying this shift, staff rather than volunteers carried out programming during this time. For example, a children's programme that started out with arts and crafts with one volunteer followed by a rap session with another, Mr Hamilton, was converted into that same volunteer doing arts and crafts as paid staff, with various 'guest speakers' following the arts and crafts. With the programme carried out as a job rather than a church youth mission, speakers were often unskilled or absent, and the effect on the kids was not nearly as powerful, because there was no ongoing relationship with any adult outside of the arts and crafts leader. Eventually the programme was arts and crafts only, with the modest supplies and skills of the staff member, who worked days as a security guard.

Computer classes continued over the years, with different projects to buy or get machines donated. The board investigated but then declined to pursue a 1996 opportunity to apply for $80,000 from another CDC to build a computer lab. The reason noted in the board's minutes was 'not enough room'. That same night the board adopted a slogan for the centre: 'Knowledge is Power'. It is a curious reflection of the balance of power in the organisation: the conservatism of staff, succeeding in nixing a plan to bring in computers which they did not know how to use, and the determination of the St James members. Donated computers were sought in lieu of the $80,000, and the organisation connected with a more gradual citywide effort to bring computers into the community known as CATNeT.

CATNeT – the Coalition to Access Technology and Networking in Toledo – formed as a collaboration between the University of Toledo's Urban Affairs Centre and a local subsidised housing agency related to the Catholic Church; this agency had won a US Department of Housing and Urban Development Neighborhood Networks grant to build labs at six apartment complexes. With only one donated computer materialising for the centre over the first year of the connection, Mrs Hamilton could not make it a priority to attend meetings, which were held during her workday.

Stage three: university

In early 1998 a University of Toledo (UT) Africana Studies course called the Poverty Seminar invited Mrs Hamilton to speak. The seminar was discussing the question of 'ending poverty once and for all', and made a special effort to look for ways to use computers and the Internet to end poverty and to bring participants up to date on the Web, email, etc. The Murchison Centre attracted students' interest as a site teaching computers in a low-income African-American community.

Soon after Mrs Hamilton visited the seminar, the seminar organised a 'Day of Dialogue' on 'Ending Poverty versus Ending Welfare' and recruited centre staff to host an event. More than five hundred people attended three panel discussions held that day. The locations – a soup kitchen in the Black community, a local farm workers' union in the Latino community and the largest auditorium on campus – attracted a wide variety of people and helped to bond the organisers – the Africana Studies programme – and the Murchison Centre.

Summing up the event, the seminar decided to approach the Murchison Centre about a partnership. The seminar would start meeting at the centre and in exchange would contribute some volunteer time to the centre and its programmes.

While the students collected data about the community, the seminar helped the centre in a number of ways. Most of these were summarised in a written letter of agreement between the director of Africana Studies and Deborah Hamilton:

- computerise accounts and train staff in Quicken
- design and help pay for a newsletter
- provide after-school tutoring for elementary schoolchildren
- send student techs to troubleshoot and teach computer classes.

Work on the accounts led to some work on grant proposals, and a university representative joined the board of the centre. Data gathered and discussed in the seminar, together with the tutoring experience, led to a focus on mathematics and the proficiency tests.

During this time the programmes of the centre that the university was not involved in dwindled to a point where the assistant director complained that the centre was being used by just three families, as a babysitting service. A gap emerged between the more middle-class staff, who themselves worked other jobs or were looking for other work to supplement their part-time work at the centre, and the people from campus, who were 'fresh legs' and brought from the seminar process a sense of mission similar to the church founders. Different from the paid staff, the university group aimed to partner with poor people rather than deliver services to them. The university group was also more diverse: Blacks, Asians, Whites, multiple faiths, experience with national social movements against racism, AIDS, nuclear weapons, environmental pollution and the death penalty, and 1960s, Gen-X, and hip-hop in personal style.

The community research by the students turned up the fact that almost no local elementary students were passing the math proficiency tests, and everyone recognised that math skills are a ticket to high-tech, high-paying jobs, where African-Americans are underrepresented. Moving past the original partnership, UT and the centre launched a programme of practice testing and tutoring, taking place in the centre, in the school and on the university campus. A similarly oriented summer youth programme followed. The centre's assistant director distanced herself from the partnership without participating in any meetings and soon left the centre, but Mrs Hamilton continued to hold the university volunteers in high regard, because of the focus on computers, the resources coming into the centre and the education she was getting along the way. One component of this was a group trip to the Black Radical Congress in Chicago, which was her first exposure to Black Power as a movement.

The Black Radical Congress gathered together Black academics and social activists to rally African-Americans who were critical of the mainstream efforts of elected officials and the conservative orientation of the Million Man March, which opted for atonement rather than activism to change state policy. The main tool used by the BRC in creating this counter-public has been and continues to be the Internet via listservs discussions involving fifteen thousand subscribers.

The university's seminar approach carried over into programme management. Work was evaluated in meetings that included staff, volunteers and parents. For instance, after discussing various approaches to discipline, the group developed an axiom: 'Discipline is a result of engagement'. In other words, policing kids who are not interested in an activity was not effective. The kids had to be drawn into an activity that would absorb their attention, the way video games did at home or learning PowerPoint did at the centre. This would have to involve reasoning with children and making a convincing case for whatever activity was at hand.

Both administration and programming at the centre were changing, but not only as a result of the university involvement. Bishop Murchison was pressing on with building a new centre across the alley from the old one, and it was finished in June 1999. He invited the director of Africana Studies to give the keynote address at the grand opening, a gathering of more than three hundred people in front of and inside the new centre. The Bishop had designed the facility with a distinct room for a computer lab, and small grants finally came in to allow the centre to fill the lab with eight new computers. Slightly used computers were donated by UT, as were volunteer time and a student worker who kept the PCs up and networked. The centre also hired three part-timers at wages lower than the earlier staff: two Africana Studies graduate students and a computer-savvy father from the neighbourhood who had joined the practice proficiency testing.

In August 1999 the board acknowledged the changes in the centre's programmes when it added the phrase 'community based cyberpower' to the mission statement and added 'strengthening the nearby school' to the centre's goals and objectives. Over the next year the board voted in three people who came out of the new activities. One of these was an information-technology staff person at the University of Toledo and the other two were grandmothers who got involved along with the grandchildren they were raising.

Fifteen hours a week of computer classes, tutoring in the schools, and practice math tests became the programming. The number of people served monthly climbed steadily from roughly fifty-five to more than 250 by early 2000. Parents – predominately grandmothers raising grandchildren – were recruited into the tutoring and testing activities and began to help make decisions and implement programmes.

Several of them had computers or wanted computers, and an electronic discussion list was implemented via the online service e-groups. With a free electronic discussion list via www.egroups.com and two donated computers placed temporarily at grandmothers' homes, four people from campus and four from the community were able to stay in touch and make decisions. An average of sixty-two messages were posted per month. One-third of the messages came from the non-university list members, who were not accustomed to typing or to broadcasting their ideas. A breakthrough came when one grandmother succeeded in using e-groups to assign out tasks for a barbecue. This was done from her home without any direct assistance from others.

The centre's computer classes ranged from elementary (Adult Basic Computing) to advanced, particularly when a new UT course, 'The Black Church', set a requirement for students to build a web page for a local church. Cyberchurch, as it came to be called, evolved into a mainstay offering at the centre. One of the students stepped forward to teach it.

This did not come without struggle. Board members representing local agencies within the government bureaucracy kept aloof from the centre. One expressed strong disagreement with the centre's programmes. Elements at King School became defensive about new forces in the PTO and attempted to steal the PTO election. A controversy broke out over a passage in a report published by the centre, a passage that one grandmother ultimately labelled a 'wake-up call':

> Year after year . . . the King Cougars win the city basketball tournament. Last year the team was undefeated, 28–0.
>
> Also last year, no 4th or 6th grade King student passed all five proficiency tests. Nine per cent of 4th graders and 7 per cent of 6th graders passed the math test.
>
> But with support and study, King students can excel in math just like they do in basketball. The test scores show how much the entire school (students, parents, teachers, administrators, and community) has to change to meet TPS's [Toledo Public Schools] stated goal of 75 per cent passing.

Table 12.2 Historical stages of the Murchison Centre, 1992–2000: facilities, budget, partners

Stage	Facilities	Budget	Partners
Church (1992–5)	St James Church basement, 1520 Hoag Street (July 1992)	Under $4,000 per year, raised by grassroots fundraising projects: $1,000 or more in account	Roosevelt CDC (local start-up)
State (1995–8)	1610 Lawrence (February 1995)	Average $30,000 per year, 90% from CDBG: line of credit briefly tops $11,000	CDBG, Lucas County Human Services Department, CATNeT
University (1998 to present)	1616 Lawrence (July 1999)	Average $35,000 per year, primarily grants, contracts, grants, user fees, small donors	University of Toledo, PASS charter school, Toledo GROWS, OCCCN, CTCNeT

A crisis came in spring 2000 when the CDBG grant proposal was twenty minutes late and as a result, rejected. The centre's testimony before the city council – delivered by the director of Africana Studies – did not change matters. The centre drew strong approval from long-time liaison workers at CDBG, who had read the detailed monthly reports and saw the centre's tremendous growth trajectory. New people were brought on to the board and are at work raising funds.

As of now, the watchword at the centre is 'sustainability,' both in terms of funding and in terms of people. The university forces brought a movement mentality to the centre, which supplanted the relatively careerist or workaday orientation of stage two. The state edged out the tight group of ideological St James Church leaders of stage one. The goal is to move firmly into a stage four, where the broader community itself is in the driver's seat at the Murchison Community Centre. At that point St James Church, the state and the university will all have to move into new supporting roles. The centre is now an island of connectivity in the community; as it moves forward it will be poised to become just one station on the modern underground railway, one node on a network into the information-society promised land.

Analysis

The historical narrative of the Murchison Centre is summed up in Table 12.2. Each stage is named after the form of social capital making the critical contribution in the life of the centre at that time. This has been a cumulative process, so at present there are four kinds of social capital on the board: church and community (bonding) and state and university (bridging) social capital.

As noted above, this pattern of social capital is highly suggestive of a broader pattern that has been repeated at various stages of Black community development and the freedom struggle. Innovation takes place on the basis of initiatives generated within the Black community. The state steps in, either to stop what is new or to reconfigure it in line with agency specifications and funding requirements. This process suggests a process of spontaneity followed by institutional co-optation. For instance, in 1964 the Mississippi Summer Project initiated by the Student Non-violent Co-ordinating Committee (SNCC) started a network of 'Freedom Schools' to intervene in the early childhood development of poor children. In 1965 the federal government took this project as inspiration for a federal programme called 'Operation Head Start'. In this case a state bureaucracy replaced a movement.

Several scholars have studied the intervention of the state to block the new tactics of the 1960s civil rights movement. Doug McAdam (1999) found that the state was interested not in advancing the movement but in preserving 'public order'. Piven and Cloward (1979: 231) found that 'in the wake of the student sit-ins and the freedom rides the Kennedy administration attempted to divert the civil rights forces from tactics of confrontation to the building of a Black electoral presence in the South'.

The difference in the case of the Murchison Centre is the continuity of leadership. Throughout the history of the Murchison Centre, continuity ensuring the stability and growth of the centre has rested on its founder, Bishop Murchison, and its founding institution the church, which has supported the third continuity in the form of Mrs Deborah Hamilton. Mrs Hamilton has been executive director, mostly without pay, since 1994. Bishop Murchison has attended 94 of 107 total board meetings of the centre.

Attendance at meetings is a solidly documented empirical indicator of social capital. Putnam bases his social capital argument on a decline in attendance: 'In short, in the mid-1970s near two-thirds of all Americans attended club meetings, but by the late 1990s near two-thirds of Americans never do' (Putnam 2000: 61).

In Figure 12.2 we present data on attendance at board meetings from 1992 to 2000. Board attendance is aggregated by the background of the board member and charted from 1992 to 2000. There is a general pattern consistent with our conception of three stages, basically 1992–5, 1995–8, 1998–2000. Overall there has been a sharp decline in the relative importance of attendance by board members representing bonding social capital. Church members have been replaced by the state and the university. Part of this is subtle, as three board members are both church members and government employees. One of these individuals works as a claims examiner for the Ohio Bureau of Employment Security; another is a security supervisor with the Lucas County Department of Human Services (the welfare department).

The mission statement of an organisation is a good indicator of its ideology. As noted above, the first Murchison Centre statement reflects church language

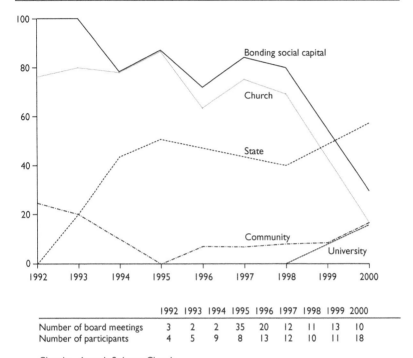

	1992	1993	1994	1995	1996	1997	1998	1999	2000
Number of board meetings	3	2	2	35	20	12	11	13	10
Number of participants	4	5	9	8	13	12	10	11	18

Church: Attends St James Church
State: Works for government agency
University: University student or faculty
Community: Private sector employment, lives in area served or is participant in programmes
Bonding social capital: church, lives in area served or is participant in programme

Figure 12.2   Social capital: attendance at board meetings by institutional affiliation,
1992–2000, as percentage of total, by year

along with the grassroots slogan of 'Awareness, Education, and Outreach'.
The second statement speaks the language of bureaucracy, but the slogan
'Knowledge is Power', also adopted during stage two, expresses the orientation of Bishop Murchison and St James Church, reflecting the historic
Black commitment to education and to struggle. Stage three brought a new
concept from the technologically oriented poverty seminar: community-based
cyberpower.

> Prevention is designed to focus upon [the] central city [with] Axiology/
> value . . . Metaphysics/reality . . . Epistemology/knowledge Awareness
> . . . Education . . . Outreach.
>
> (Stage 1, church – May 1993)

Knowledge is Power

(Stage 2, state – October 1996)

Our mission is to educate, counsel, and provide the necessary training to alleviate the problems of underemployment, drug/alcohol abuse, peer pressure, and violence. We are committed to enhancing the overall social and economic growth of the neighborhood residents in our service area.

(February 1997)

Knowledge is Power

(Stage 3, university – continued usage)

Our mission is to educate and provide community support to alleviate the problems of underemployment, drug/alcohol abuse, peer pressure, and violence. We are committed to enhancing the overall social and economic growth of the neighborhood residents in our service area. Our main tool for change is community-based cyberpower.

community based cyberpower: community empowerment and organising using computers and the Internet.

(August 1999)

The board and its changing ideological orientation connect with the programme activities of the centre and related participation. Figure 12.3 charts attendance at different programmes from 1997 to 2000. Computer-related programs begin to grow in mid-1998 with the technical support and teaching input from campus. Tutoring and practice testing in co-operation with parents and the university began in January 1999, but figures were not incorporated into monthly reports until October 1999. This in itself is a reflection of the bureaucratisation of the centre, to the point where new developments were not swiftly incorporated into reporting. Reporting was seen as solely for the state and not for internal records. University volunteers had a big impact on mobilising the community to participate. Demarcation between stage 2 (state) and stage 3 (university) is visible.

A closer look at the centre's programme offerings – computer classes and otherwise – allows us to identify the cyberpower that emerged from the social capital and other inputs that went into the centre. Cyberpower was an outcome, but also, we will see, a further input into the centre.

Individual cyberpower

As soon as the centre acquired computers, adult beginners were taught to use the computer, to type, and to produce résumés. Once educational games were available on CD-ROM, children came in to do that as part of tutoring. By

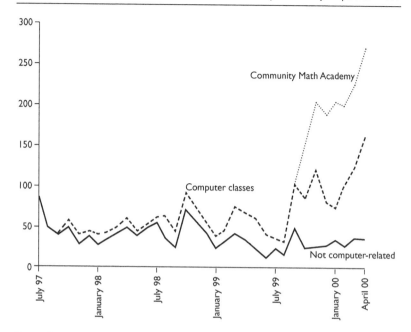

Figure 12.3 Social value: monthly participation in Murchison Centre programmes, July 1997–April 2000, in number of participants per month

1999, when computers had modernised and more computer-savvy staff and volunteers were on hand, these jobs and/or school-related classes grew more sophisticated. By 1999, adults were learning Adult Basic Computing (Windows and Wordpad), Word, Excel; children were using CD-ROM games but also learning Kids Basic Computing, Word, PowerPoint, and being guided through using educational websites.

The individual power that resulted was seen in adults' job-skills development and job-hunt successes, their individual mastery over the software. It was also seen in their moving to teach others, either the student sitting at the next computer or a whole room of students, as they moved from learning to teaching a class. At this point individual cyberpower becomes social cyberpower.

Social cyberpower

Long before 'community-based cyberpower' was part of the Murchison Centre mission, it was in evidence. The first sign of this was in 1994 when Mrs Hamilton explained her 'field promotion' from board secretary to executive director. 'I had been to college and I knew computers.' At that point computer knowledge was seen as something to be shared with the community. According to Mrs Hamilton, the board at that time was looking for her not just to word-process letters but to teach others.

When the Community Math Academy began in January 1999, a local father began to volunteer at the monthly practice proficiency tests. When attendance at these was taken, it included not just name and phone but also email. His email address was piesqd@[. . .]. Pi is the ratio between the diameter and the circumference of a circle. Asking about this creative screen name, other volunteers learned that he was a UT student, a working engineering technician and, for the neighbourhood, an early adopter of computers. Within a few months he volunteered to teach the evening Word/résumé-production class. Soon after he was promoted to computer lab manager. He computerised attendance records so that the monthly quantitative reports were produced by Access instead of by pencil and paper.

The Community Math Academy itself was a product of and a generator of social cyberpower. As we have said, students in the UT Poverty Seminar had found the Murchison Centre's computer lab in an online listing on the CATNeT site, and the partnership that resulted came from the shared attitude that computers were a key to Black community empowerment. Where the seminar managed to show its participants the Web and perhaps get a few people HotMail accounts, the Community Math Academy went further, using e-groups to cement its volunteer leadership core and thus build social cyberpower. This involved some private computers as well as some loaners that went into people's homes, although they then decided to return the loaned computers and get their own more powerful units. In addition, centre staff and volunteers' contacts with school officials were by email instead of phone or letter-writing, which was either unsuccessful or cumbersome.

A year after first inquiring about it, the Community Math Academy was able to make use of the school's computerised automatic phone message system to notify parents about the practice proficiency tests. In this way the voice of the newly elected King PTO delivered a message to six hundred King families. Just as with the loaner computers from the university, this board of education system was a case of bridging social capital and bonding social capital investing together in building the centre's programmes.

Perhaps the pinnacle examples of social cyberpower are the two classes, Cyberchurch and Cyberschools, which began in 1999 and 2000 respectively. Here, though, we cross over once again, as social cyberpower becomes ideological cyberpower.

Ideological cyberpower

The university brought to the scene the language of the digital divide, the Black liberation struggle and the community technology movement. This language expressed, clarified and advanced what the centre was already doing to some extent. The ideology of community uplift using computers, rooted also in the concept 'Knowledge is Power', was elaborated in the day-to-day work, the plans and the mission statement of the centre. Embedded here was an ideological orientation towards the community as a set of assets as well as needs, best evidenced in the last sentence of the mission statement developed by the Community Math Academy (emphasised below). The goal of 'ending poverty once and for all' was an early critical ideological issue.

> The Community Math Academy aims to improve the math skills and change the math attitudes of young people in central city Toledo. We see math as an academic subject and a tool for social transformation. We see math as part of ending poverty once and for all.
>
> The academy is a project of UT, the Murchison Centre, and King School. We join with children and their parents to conduct educational activities in the school, the community and the home. *Parents are the leaders of the academy because parents love their children and, more than anyone, determine their futures.*

Operating as it did over the Internet as well as through face-to-face meetings and sessions, the Community Math Academy programme was itself an instance of ideological cyberpower. But two classes, Cyberchurch and Cyberschools, began in 1999 and 2000 respectively and also illustrate the ideological cyberpower generated through the centre.

Cyberchurch emerged as an assignment in a university course on the Black Church. When each student went to complete a website for a local church, they came to the centre to build their site. This class then took on a life of its own, with word of mouth bringing more students, one student stepping forward to teach it, and more skills and web space being applied. The course assignment originated as an idea that the director of Africana Studies sold to the instructor for Black Church. The instructor, a local pastor and high-school guidance counsellor, had pastored in various Toledo churches for twenty-seven years, and provided his church space to the local Black Panther chapter when it formed. While the website building assignment in his course was a burden to him at first – he was asking students to do something he hadn't done – one day after hearing a lecture by the director he told him, 'I've heard you talk about this "e-Black" many times, and I always agreed. But now I really, really get it! I have it so much on my mind that I'm thinking of taking out all the pews in my church and using folding chairs, and getting in some computers. It can still serve on Sundays but can be a lab the rest of the time.' His plans began to unfold.

The ideological content of this form of cyberpower is the vision that, if the Black church is online, then a good portion of the Black public sphere can be kept intact as our personal, cultural, political and spiritual lives move into cyberspace, as more and more Black people get online. If the Black church is intact, then the Black liberation struggle has that important institution, with all the social capital embedded therein, to rely on.

While Cyberchurch was a class that expresses the dynamic combination of university social capital (bridging) and church social capital (bonding) within the context of the centre, Cyberschools had a slightly different origin. It originated from a combination of university social capital with community social capital (bonding), again within the context of the centre.

Murchison's Community Math Academy project put the centre and its volunteers, especially the university students, in close proximity to King Elementary School. The CMA, especially the involved parents, who were all grandmothers, attended the school's PTO meetings, seeking more parent involvement. CMA volunteers worked in the schools as classroom teacher aides and after school as tutors. As a result, new officers were voted in as PTO leaders.

The King PTO had two members who were a couple with one son in the school but had been unable to organise parents to do more than bake sales and an annual book sale. The Murchison Centre began to do outreach to get more parents to the PTO meetings. Thus the annual election brought in a full slate of PTO officers with new energy and a plan to build the library up, participate in practice proficiency testing and so on.

Cyberschools was begun to support these parents and others like them. Like Cyberchurch, it meets one night a week. Cyberschools sessions are dedicated to two things: organising to get more families to practice proficiency tests, and helping local PTOs get their plans and contact information posted on to web pages devoted to their schools and their families, plus email.

PTOs across the country have web pages and use email to keep parents in touch and organised. But these PTOs do not often appear to be in the Black community. With computers moving into homes and workplaces, anyone can take advantage of the Internet to organise. Not only that, the websites that Cyberschools takes people to explore include the Toledo Public Schools, the teachers' union, the University of Toledo, the Ohio Board of Education (which posts information about schools, testing, standards, the Ohio 4th Grade Guarantee (no fourth-grader failing the reading test will be advanced to 5th grade) and more. So the Internet is a source of information as well as a communication tool used by parents to impact children's experience in public schools. Parent involvement is proved to be perhaps the deciding factor in student and school success.

Implications

We are now able to elaborate further the theoretical framework emerging from our analysis. We will move beyond the particularity of this case study to conceptual implications for our general research focus, community technology centres in urban poor communities, especially communities of colour. First we will concentrate the lessons of this case study into several propositions that in turn can serve as guidelines for further research. Second, we will discuss the implications of this research for the public sphere, especially the Black counter-public sphere.

The first point is that these centres are social organisations, and therefore part of the structure of social relations in a community. This understanding requires a paradigm shift from the current dominant trend to study individuals who pass through the centre, to the centres themselves as social units.

A second point is that the digital divide has to be understood as a community attribute, part of a broader phenomena called public computing. The digital divide as community descriptor can be determined by how extensive and effective are the local organisations, which provide and promote public computing.

A third point is that the CTC as community organisation is the locus for the concentration of resources. These resources can be conceived as different forms of capital:

* *physical*: buildings and equipment
* *human*: staff
* *financial*: budget
* *social*: social background and ties of board members and the organised partnerships of the organisation.

A fourth point is that social capital is the key. Bonding social capital is the fundamental resource that makes something belong to a community. Without this form of community wealth and legitimacy the organisation is an artificial construct. Bridging social capital is essential in acquiring temporary resources and external support. Whenever bridging social capital is dominant, the organisation is in crisis and in danger of dying or being transformed as an extension of external interests rather than the interest of the original community and its bonding social capital.

A fifth point is that the investment of these resources produces a social value, cyberpower. There are three forms of cyberpower:

* individual cyberpower: new human capital
* social cyberpower: collectives engaged in cyber organising
* ideological cyberpower: ideas and policy promoted by individual and social cyber power.

A sixth and final point is that the success and sustainability of a centre is a function of whether point five loops back and feeds into the capital resources of the organisation. The organisation produces bonding social capital or it fails the litmus test of success and sustainability.

On the basis of these six points it is critical to raise the issue of democracy and social inclusion of people who are living in the social isolation of the poor part of the dual city. The existence of a democratic system is not merely the actions of individuals at the polls. Democracy requires informed citizens who are socialised and live in a complex set of overlapping social networks. Each network is an interest group, and multiple memberships mean multiple interests, sometimes congruent and sometimes in conflict. This complexity is the basis for democratic discussion and compromise. We argue and compromise because while we have differences with others, on other issues we share common interests.

Building sustainable democratic equality in the information age means more than how many individuals are online. The key is to stabilise and support people working with information technology in the form of social organisations rooted in the legitimate social capital of the community. The key is to invest all forms of capital to produce social capital for the socially isolated inner city Black poor. In turn, this investment should be utilised to produce Black cyberpower. Powerlessness, especially the lack of cyberpower, is anathema to democracy in the information society.

Notes

1 In an earlier publication we discussed continuing social inequalities in the information revolution. See Alkalimat, Gills and Williams (1995).
2 See the URLs for the Department of Commerce and the Benton Foundation.
3 Department of Commerce (2000), p. 4.
4 See Bertot and McClure (2000) for the use of library computers to access the Internet; Williams (2000) presents data on Internet service being provided by libraries in Ohio.
5 See URLs for CTCNeT, OCCCN and CATNeT.
6 Orr (1999) presents a useful case study of Black social capital in a historical study of Baltimore school reform in which he discusses bonding and bridging social capital as intergroup and intragroup relations of Blacks and Whites.
7 For definitions and literature review on social capital see Resnick (2000), Feldman and Assaf (2000), and Putnam (2000).
8 Bertot and McClure (2000). Previous studies were released in 1994, 1996, 1997 and 1998.

Chapter 13

Online forums as a tool for people-centred governance

Experiences from local government in Sweden

Agneta Ranerup

Introduction

This chapter focuses on whether local-government initiatives to provide a virtual public sphere have functioned as a tool for people-centred governance. More specifically, the chapter discusses the results of a comparative study of all the online forums that have been implemented on loca-government websites in Sweden. There are two main arguments that inform the study. First, the chances are higher that information technology in the form of, for example, online forums will have democratic effects in situations where they are used in connection with existing political institutions such as local government (Buchstein 1997). Second, this research on virtual political public spheres is grounded on very concrete and factual experiences in contrast to more theoretical discussions (Brothers 1999, Buchstein 1997). As a consequence, we are in a position to determine the actual use of online forums and reflect on their value.

People-centred governance

In this study we have chosen to investigate how local-government organis-ations use the Internet to enhance democracy because 'it is at the local level that citizens most directly experience service provision, and act as direct participants in the democratic process' (Musso *et al.* 1999: 3). In this chapter, online forums will be seen as an example of a tool aimed at people-centred governance. Our description of various kinds of reforms aimed at people-centred governance is intended only to serve as a background to more concrete discussion of experiences of online forums. Furthermore, we will not, like Musso *et al.* (1999), investigate the use of municipal websites in general in relation to various kinds of governmental reform. Instead we study online forums as technology to support *a particular kind of reform*, which values a dialogue about local-government issues that includes citizens. What is 'people-centred governance', or, perhaps more appropriately, what can it be?

People-centred governance can be described as a range of measures that are taken with the ultimate aim of enlarging the role of 'ordinary citizens' in government activities. An example of such a measure is the decentralisation of services and political bodies such as local government. For example, Sweden's process of decentralisation towards local government in many cities has, among other things, resulted in the creation of local-government districts with their own councils. As a consequence 'Decentralisation has meant that responsibility for a number of elements of government – including schools, childcare, libraries and social welfare – has been devolved to a unit with a comparatively small population and geographical spread' (Ranerup 1999: 178). The main idea in this kind of arrangement is that the politicians as well as the services come closer to the citizens, and as a consequence the governance becomes more people-centred.

Another example is when citizens themselves are invited to become members of user boards at the local political level with the right to influence the many kinds of services provided by local government. Citizens might also be offered an opportunity to become part of the board of, for example, a school or a similar kind of institution (Bogason 1996). A further example is when market mechanisms are introduced in the provision of services. In this case citizens are seen as consumers, with the right to 'shop around' on the market for a certain kind of service (Bogason 1996). In Sweden, parents have been offered a choice of schools for their children, and disabled people have been given the right to choose nursing assistants to help them in their daily lives (Norén 2000).

Involving citizens in discussions in some kind of public virtual sphere is a further example of a measure that is taken with the aim of enlarging the role of 'ordinary citizens' (Musso et al. 1999). This is, of course, also the kind of measure or tool for achieving people-centred governance. The essence here is that, as described by Coleman (1999), the citizens themselves are offered the potential to participate in discussions about, for example, local-government issues. This means that the 'middle person', who otherwise is in a position to control the participation in debates through media such as television and newspapers, is being cut out. Instead, citizens are in a position to choose the agenda for discussion completely freely, or are allowed to influence it to a much higher degree. As Richard puts it, 'The decision-making model is considerably stretched. The old model of decide-announce-defend is challenged by the emergence of the citizen-as-a-partner. Networking online allows government to work closely with communities of interest. Citizens expect to be part of this dialogue' (Richard 1999: 79).

Historically, involving citizens in the decision-making process, rather than having a selected elite of political representatives in political discussions, has been defined as being problematic (Coleman 1999). In contrast, over the last two decades writers as well as politicians (Buchstein 1997, Coleman 1999) have proposed a vision of direct democracy with the help of information technology. However, as Coleman argues, debate in a virtual political public sphere, rather than simply voting using IT, is a preferred alternative vision. In addition, 'The vision of leaders and their governments actively working in collaboration with citizens and interest groups towards measurable goals is prominent in Internet-related discourse. This ideal may come from the fact that the Internet blends tools for public participation and representation in a unique way' (Richard 1999: 71).

A working definition of online forums

In a broad comparative investigation such as this the object of research must be clearly defined. We have already argued for the value of focusing on online forums in a local-government context, but we have yet to define what such forums actually are. For the purpose of this research, online forums had to meet the following criteria.

First, they had to be situated on one of the local government websites that existed in Sweden during the period of investigation (April to June 1999). Alternatively, citizens and others had to be able to access the forums by a button on a local government website.

Second, citizens and others had to be able to make contributions to the online forum through the website, as well as to read contributions made by others. This accordingly excluded other online facilities where citizens were invited to post their opinions by using email forms without being able to read the contributions made by others. In addition it excluded facilities of a more 'chat-like' character where contributions can be accessed during a very short period of time (maybe only for a few hours). Both of these alternatives had been judged as not being in line with the ideal of *deliberative* democracy (Buchstein 1997, Kim *et al.* 1999). According to this ideal, a genuine discussion, or a deliberative process between citizens and politicians, is defined as being of utmost importance. For this reason, citizens must be allowed to form opinions during a longer period of time with the help of information technology, rather than just to express them. This explains the definition of online forums given above, as well as why online 'chats' and email forums have been excluded from the investigation.

Local government websites were searched for online forums which fitted the criteria outlined. In order not to omit any online forum, or alternatively to avoid omitting one that might have been implemented during the period of investigation, all of the local governments without an online forum were contacted by mail as well as by phone. In addition, the online debate was studied through the Internet, and issues such as the right of citizens to influence the agenda for discussion were studied with the help of approximately sixty interviews with webmasters and 'infomasters'.

Topography of online forums

Traditionally, few municipal websites, digital cities and the like have provided citizens with interactive functions for discussing political issues. According to Aurigi (2000), only 10 per cent of two hundred city-related websites in the European Union investigated by him in 1997 provided facilities for online discussion. In Sweden, by 1999 15 per cent of local-government websites contained some kind of online discussion. A study of municipal websites in California indicated that only 9.3 per cent of them had functions that are similar to online forums (Hale *et al.* 1999). In other words, the participatory and inclusive potential of highly interactive and electronic environments has been ignored, with the Internet being mainly used as a platform for marketing cities. Accordingly, with online forums being still very much an exception on government sites, the experiences of such forums when they present is of interest.

In an evaluation of the deliberative capacity of political discussion groups and newsgroups on the Internet, Wilhelm (1999) introduced a conceptual framework of features or aspects that affect the political potential of virtual public spheres. He argues that there are no universal effects of online discussions, which is why the particularities of the topography regarding each virtual public sphere are of special importance. Accordingly, *topography* is a general feature or aspect that determines the effect of online conversation within virtual public spheres (Wilhelm 1999). An aspect of particular relevance in a discussion of forums on local-government websites is what has been said above about the democratic effects of online conversation. According to writers such as Buchstein, it is more likely that information technology will have democratic effects if it is used *in connection with existing political institutions*: 'Here computer democracy would be based on an already existing community and used to distribute and to collect information and to foster deliberation' (Buchstein 1997: 260). This would be a way of avoiding a scenario of supplanting the democratic process, as we know it, by an electronic process where participation is trivialised. In such a scenario, political participation is reduced to the passive and private act of registering one's own preconceived opinion on an issue (Buchstein 1997).

There are a few alternative forms of topography regarding online forums. First, there are online forums for political debates on the Internet generally in the form of Usenet bulletin boards or newsgroups (Benson 1996, Wilhelm 1999). Here the discussions are performed within a virtual public sphere without any clear connections to, for example, a city or a region. As a consequence, there are no connections to an existing political institution such as a particular local government. However, there are also discussion groups, newsgroups or online forums within digital cities such as Bologna, some of which are used for a discussion about political issues. This kind of online discussion has much clearer connections to a city or a region. Some of these online forums have a closer connection to existing political institutions such as local government, as is the case in Bologna (Tambini 1998). In contrast, in the digital city of Amsterdam there are no strong connections to such institutions. Rather, the digital city of Amsterdam focuses on the city as a whole, and its discussion groups are run by a combination of voluntary and commercial interests. It began as a grassroots initiative which has grown into a substantial, self-supporting, non-profit organisation with paid staff as well as voluntary staff (Francissen and Brants 1998).

The research in this chapter has been grounded on Swedish local-government experiences only. One reason for focusing Swedish experiences is the concrete ambitions in this country at state, regional and municipal levels not only to employ information technology to improve efficiency in the administration but also to use it to enhance democracy. A recent example is the broad commission ('Demokratiutredningen') that was appointed in 1997 with an assignment to investigate the present conditions for democracy at large, but also to investigate the potential effects of using information technology for improving democracy (Amnå 1999).

Another reason for studying online forums in Sweden is the high Internet access in this country. According to statistics from the period of investigation, in May 1999 50.3 per cent of the Swedish population between 12 and 78 years of age used the Internet actively (SIFO 1999), and the access rate is steadily rising. High access has been defined by many researchers (Coleman 1999, Tsagarousianou *et al.* 1998), as well as practitioners (Ranerup 1998), as a necessity in order to fully exploit the democratic effects of the Internet. According to this line of argument, a tool that is used for democratic partici-pation and for acquiring political information must be accessible to everyone. Limited access would be similar to a situation where the suffrage or freedom of expression applied only to some groups in society.

Focus on investigation

Design

Wilhelm (1999) described the *design* of virtual political public spheres as an aspect that very much influence their political potential. Other writers, when arguing that the design of a technological artefact creates a span of possible actions, make a similar point of view. According to this view the design of for example, an online forum both empowers and restricts the behaviour of users (Akrich 1992, Stolterman 1998). Coleman (1999) describes online deliberation as one way of 'cutting out the middle man' between citizens and politicians. This makes possible a conversation on issues chosen by those who participate. Despite this, in some of the online forums there might exist various ways of controlling the debate to avoid obtrusive language, flaming etc. (Docter and Dutton 1998). The effect of such arrangements on the freedom of expression and the participation in the debate in general is not obvious. Measures of control such as moderation can in fact be positive if they result in a debate where people do not withdraw from the discussion because of flaming and other similar kinds of behaviour (Docter and Dutton 1998). Regardless of the position one takes on this issue, the potential of affecting the issues for discussion has been seen as central in our investigation (see especially the section on people-centred governance above). One of the main aims of this research was to study whether citizens are allowed to *influence the issues for discussion* in the online forums.

Furthermore, a second very simple aspect of the design of the forums formed the focus of our interest. *The name of the online forums* is taken as an indication of whether there has been an intention that they should function as an arena for political discussion or not. In addition, the names are seen as an indication of whether they have been perceived by citizens as arenas for political discussion. To conclude, the openness of the agenda for discussion as well as the names of the forums are features of their design that are used to indicate whether they have functioned as a tool for people-centred governance.

Topicality

Above we have discussed various issues that are related to the topography of online forums. The concept of topography is of course of relevance to our study but it is not one that is employed to make a distinction between the forums. The reason for this is very simple. There are no differences between the online forums in our study regarding topography since all of them have a clear connection to local government. However when examining the concept of topicality of the forums, another important characteristic of virtual political public spheres (Wilhelm 1999), the situation is different. By 'topicality' Wilhelm simply refers to the content of the discussion in virtual political public spheres or the topics that are discussed. In our investigation of whether local-government initiatives in the form of online forums have functioned as a tool for people-centred governance, topics that might be relevant to this issue were identified. Thus, the concept of topicality will be employed through an investigation of whether *political issues actually have been discussed* in the forums. The word 'political' is here used to denote for example, economic issues, school issues, childcare issues, environmental issues, discussions about the society as a whole, information-technology issues etc. These kinds of issues are considered to be in contrast to conversations on such issues as hobbies, greetings and more 'chat-like' conversation.

This process of analysis is, at least in theory, much simpler regarding online discussion in newsgroups or bulletin boards like those we have referred to above. Both Wilhelm (1999) and Benson (1996) chose to study online discussion in forums with a specific political focus that was expressed by their names (alt.politics, talk.politics and the like). In Wilhelm (1999) the name was taken as a sufficient criterion for the discussion to be characterised as political. The online forums studied here might contain a discussion of a wide range of issues. More specifically, it is not their name but rather where they are situated and their functional design that made them the object of study.

Deliberation

Lastly, deliberation was defined by Wilhelm as one of several important features of virtual political public spheres. According to his definition, deliberation means 'Subjecting one's opinions to public scrutiny for validation' (Wilhelm 1999: 159). Accordingly, it is highly relevant to collect empirical data on to what extent the online forums have been employed to exchange views and opinions. In the previous section we described the intention to investigate the topicality of the online debate, and especially whether there has been a discussion of political issues. This might be taken as one way of evaluating the use of online forums from the perspective of deliberation. A further way of evaluating the deliberative potential is to investigate the *amount of online discussion*. This is why we will try to determine the amount of debate that has taken place within the forums, as well as to use it as a means of comparison between the forums.

Results

According to our investigation, approximately 15 per cent of the 289 Swedish municipalities have provided citizens with an online discussion forum. In the spring of 1999 forty-three local government websites had this kind of facility (Appendix 13.1). These forums will now be examined more closely regarding their design, topicality etc.

Design of online forums

The strongest indication that online forums have the potential to function as a tool for people-centred governance is given by an agenda for discussion that can be influenced by the citizens. With this as a background it is interesting to note that in all but a few of the online forums in Swedish local governments *the agenda for discussion has been completely open*. The exceptions were as follows: in the forums in one municipality (Östersund), where there was an explicit focus on discussing school issues, and in another municipality (Oskarshamn) where there was an online forum with an explicit focus on discussing where nuclear waste should be stored. In both cases the forums were implemented as a part of a project with a special focus on these issues. However, the amount of debate in these forums was negligible. In four other municipalities there were online forums with an aim to discuss issues about information technology (local-government website and the like). In spite of this policy, in two of these forums other issues were allowed as well. In all other forums the citizens were allowed to choose the issues for discussion. The only thing that limited the freedom of citizens was a notification that the appearance of offensive language and content (such as sexism and racism) would mean that the contribution was removed from the forum. However, in the vast majority of the forums (thirty-nine out of forty-three local government municipalities) the agenda for discussion was open. This means that the citizens were completely free to introduce issues for discussion as well as to ask questions according to their own preferences.

On the other hand, it is a totally different matter whether there was an intention that all of these forums should be used for a discussion about political issues. The name of the online forums has been taken as being a very simple way of indicating if this has been the case. In total, twenty-five of the thirty-nine municipalities that had forums with an open agenda had a name that indicated that they should be used for a discussion about political issues. 'Open forum' (Swedish *Öppet forum*) and 'Discussion forum' (*Diskussionsforum*) are typical examples of names that these forums were given. At the same time, some of the forums with an open agenda had names of a more neutral character. As an example, three online forums were called 'Noticeboard' (*Anslagstavla*). Lastly, eleven of the forums with an open agenda for discussion were called 'Guestbook' (*Gästbok*), something which does not in fact indicate that they were seen as an arena for political discussion. However, the open agenda of these forums as such still made it possible for the citizens to influence the issues for discussion. In other words, the citizens are in a position to use these online forums as an arena for political discussion.

In summary, a majority of the online forums had open agendas, as well as names that indicated that they could be used for political discussion. In the next section we will discuss to what extent this actually has been the case.

Topicality of the debate in online forums

Our investigation indicates that in twenty-five of the municipalities there were forums with a discussion that included issues of a more direct political character. Traffic issues (the construction of roads, public transport issues etc.) and school issues (the cuts in school expenditures etc.) were the most frequent issues that appeared in the online discussions. In addition to these issues there were a multitude of themes in the discussions, such as childcare, rural development, activities for young people, health care, libraries and cultural events, as well as the online debate itself. Moreover, in twelve of the municipalities there were forums with a discussion which focused on the local-government website itself. This discussion can be characterised as treating political issues in a more indirect manner. The local-government website is a tool that, because of its close connection to local government, as well as its democratic content (information about services and political process in local government) might be used to exercise political influence.

The rest of the forums contained a very small number of contributions, mainly because they had been opened for a very short period of time. Alternatively, they contained only contributions that can be classified as greetings or 'chat-like' conversation.

In summary, a vast majority of the online forums that have been implemented on Swedish local-government websites either contained a discussion about political issues, or a discussion of the local-government website itself.

Deliberation in online forums

The topicality, together with the amount of debate, is here used as an indicator of the deliberative dimension of virtual discussions. The median value of the amount of contributions in these forums is approximately ten per month. This means that there are, on the one hand, forums where the discussion is almost dead (one or two contributions per month), and, on the other hand, forums with a discussion of forty-five to sixty contributions per month.

All in all we are in a position to conclude that there does exist discussion of political issues in the majority of the online forums on Swedish local-government websites. However, the number of contributions can be characterised as surprisingly small. Still, there are many municipalities where citizens are given the opportunity to discuss political issues in a virtual political public sphere. Furthermore, citizens as well as politicians are, to a certain extent, using these opportunities to discuss political issues. One interesting question that might be raised with this as a background is how an online discussion with this frequency and content should be valued; an issue which will discussed in the following section.

Online forums as a tool for people-centred governance

The most significant results from our study can be summarised as follows. In a vast majority of the online forums in local-government websites in Sweden there was an open choice of issues for discussion. This potential was, in many cases, used by citizens and politicians for a debate on political issues. In contrast, the average number of contributions to these debates was comparatively small. This is of course very damaging to the hope that online forums should function as a tool for people-centred governance. However, perhaps some more pragmatic comments might be appropriate to put our experiences into perspective. First, the amount of debate in the online forums we have studied must be evaluated against the background of the size of the municipality in which they had taken place. The municipalities in our investigation have 22,000 inhabitants as a median value. It is also worth noticing that the smallest municipality has 4000 inhabitants, and the largest 736,000 inhabitants. This is an important point to remember when these experiences are compared to cities such as Bologna and Amsterdam with significantly larger populations.

Another important factor is that our investigation includes only the *active* use of the forums, or in other words the very contributions that have been posted to the online forums. However, a complete description of actual usage should also include more passive users such as 'lurkers' who do not post messages themselves (Wilhelm 1999). This is a behaviour that also can be characterised as a way of participating in a democratic process. According to Danish experiences of political discussions on the Internet, the number of lurkers might be considerably more than those who actively contribute to the online debate (Dybkjær and Lindegaard 1999). Experiences of newsgroups and message lists also indicate that this might be the case (Pepper and Clegg 1999). This is in itself is an interesting issue for further studies.

Furthermore, it has to be remembered that many other forms of participating in democratic processes are used by small numbers of citizens, with the exception of the right to vote. Despite this they are still not considered as being without a democratic value. A similar argument is made by Wilhem in a discussion about differences between people regarding their willingness to take part in political discussions: 'There will always be people who are unable or unwilling to engage in . . . discursive practices' (Wilhelm 1999: 176). In other words, online forums can never be expected to attract everybody.

Lastly, an online debate on a local-government website has, as we have argued, a special democratic value owing to its close connections with already established political institutions. According to Buchstein (1999) it is more likely that in this kind of context deliberation appears, rather than merely a passive and private act of registering one's own preconceived opinion on an issue. There are also further arguments in support of the value of an online debate in a local-government setting. A critical success factor for online debates in general is described as follows: '[We must explicitly take] into account the context in which the discussion takes place. A debate or discussion must be a logical component of a (policy development) process and must be integrated in the whole process from the beginning. Only then a discussion has a chance to be successful' (Smit and Van Boeschoten 1998: 3). This is also a feature of a local-government context, where meetings in local government councils, district councils etc. are being held regularly. But what more could be done in order to increase the size of the debate and, as a consequence, to enhance democracy?

An important phenomenon with relevance to the potential of online forums was noticed in a comparative case study of four online forums (Ranerup 2000a). Only a few of the local politicians actually had access to information technology as well as an email address that they could use in connection with, for example, the online forum. The question of access to technology, email and knowledge about the technology among *the politicians* is strategically important, and as a consequence should be in focus of further studies. Moreover, it might be a way of safeguarding the commitment of politicians and similar groups in the project. This has been defined as a critical success factor in projects aiming at using information technology in municipalities. One example is the recent 'Infovilles' experiences in Spain (Perez 1999). In these projects there were three key aims related to using the tools of the information society. First, it was hoped to produce a significant transformation of the region of Valencia in general. Second, it was aimed to reform the public administration of the cities. Finally, it was seen as a way to enhance the ways that citizens are using technology. In conclusion, these and similar projects were categorised as being 'political'. As a consequence, a deep involvement of politicians and leading civil servants was a must.

An issue of equal importance is how to engage more citizens in the online discussion. One way of doing this would be to provide citizen groups and civil associations with information technology in the same way as with the politicians above (Ranerup 2000a). This would give them the basic infra-structure for participating in the debate. Another way would be to give them the opportunity to take part in the process where the online forum is intro-duced and managed. Surprisingly, this seems to be rather unusual according to previous rather limited experiences (Ranerup 2000a). If we can show a relationship between highly connected local government politicians and citizen groups, on the one hand, and the appearance of a lively online debate, on the other hand, we could, as a second step, draw conclusions about relevant activities to be suggested in the light of this.

Online forums today and tomorrow

The open agenda of the vast majority of the 15 per cent of the Swedish municipalities with online forums indicates that they at least have a potential to function as a tool for political discussions that are heavily influenced by citizens. This also means that they have a potential to function as a tool for people-centred governance. Also, there exists some evidence in support that this actually has been the case. Approximately one out of ten municipalities in Sweden had an online forum that actually was used for a political discussion. In other words the topicality of these forums indicated that they are used in a way that is in line with people-centred governance. As a contrast, the amount of debate in the forums was at first sight comparatively small, with a median amount of ten contributions per month. In spite of this being the case, in April to June 1999 there were fourteen Swedish municipalities that had online forums with a discussion of political issues that included ten or more contri-butions per month: Berg, Tyresö, Göteborg, Härjedalen, Pajala, Sölvesborg, Hudiksvall, Ronneby, Bollnäs, Dorotea, Landskrona (closed in May 1999),

Sandviken, Mjölby and Sundsvall. In a further study we will take a closer look at the deliberative qualities of the online debate in the 'best' forums that appear in our investigation (Ranerup 2000b).

In previous sections we have made some comments that might be of relevance to put these experiences into perspective. The most important message from our investigation is that online forums are not a panacea that will automatically result in a lively debate. To what extent the debate in the online forums had a democratic effect is not obvious. This has to do with how we value the whole span of tools and forms for political activities that are in our possession in relation to their actual use. However, in the most successful municipalities in our study, steps have been taken to bring about a situation where online forums have a clear function as a tool for people-centred governance. This is, if nothing else, 'the end of the beginning' of a process of using virtual public spheres for such a purpose.

Acknowledgments

This research was funded by the Swedish Transport & Communication Research Board (KFB).

Appendix 13.1   All online forums on Swedish local government websites, April to June
1999 ('l.g.' = local government)

Municipality	Number of inhabitants	Name of forum	Choice of issues	Topicality	Number of contributions per month
Berg	8,000	Snacklådan	Free	Greetings, meetings, building permits	10
Bollnäs	27,000	Bollnäsdialogen	Free	Childcare, drugs traffic	20
Degerfors	11,000	Gästbok	Free	Chat, l.g. website	7
Dorotea	4,000	1. Cybercafé Forum	Free	Meetings, IT-café, IT	20
		2. Diskussionsklubben		Greetings, IT, rural development	4
Eskilstuna	88,000	Gästbok	Free	Chat, greetings, l.g. website	22
Finspång	22,000	Gästbok	Free	Chat, greetings, l.g. website	4
Färgelanda	7,000	Anslagstavla	Free	–	Test contributions
Gagnef	10,000	Gästbok	Free	Chat, greetings, l.g. website	14
Göteborg	460,000	Debatt	Free	Three districts traffic, independence of district, schools childcare	1. 11 2. 3 3. 2
Haninge	68,000	Diskussionsforum	Free	Libraries, playground, housing	9 (100 in one month during pre-election debate)
Herrljunga	9,000	Herrljunga kommuns gästbok	l.g. website, but in practice free	Chat, greetings, l.g. website	40
Huddinge	81,000	Tyck till om Huddinge kommun	Free	l.g. website, traffic, childcare, splitting up Huddinge	7
Hudiksvall	38,000	1. Debattforum Hudiksvall	Free	Traffic, future, construction	16
		2. Gästbok	Free	Chat, greetings, l.g. website, recreational activities	41
Härjedalen	11,000	Diskussionsforum	Free	Schools, health care, the debate, traffic	12
Krokom	14,000	Krokomsforum	Free	Greetings, chat, the online debate	7

Municipality	Number of inhabitants	Name of forum	Choice of issues	Topicality	Number of contributions per month
Landskrona	38,000	Fråga din politiker	Free	Traffic, health care, environmental issues	25 (closed in May)
Lidköping	37,000	Gästbok	Free	Chat, greetings, l.g. website	6
Lysekil	15,000	Allmänt forum	Free	Taxes, tourism	3
Malung	11,000	Gästbok	Free	Chat, greetings, l.g. website	Not available (closed in June)
Mjölby	25,000	Fullmäktige-partiernas frågeforum	Free	Schools, libraries, environmental issues	44 (opened in May)
Nordanstig	11,000	Anslagstavla	Free	–	Test contributions (opened in May)
Nyköping	49,000	Synpunkten	Free	Traffic, schools, l.g. website, recreational activities	8
Nässjö	30,000	Diskutera mera	Free	Traffic, schools, IT	8 (opened in June)
Oskarshamn	27,000	Diskussions-forum om kärnavfall i Oskarshamn	Nuclear waste	Nuclear waste	2
Orust	150,000	Insändare	Free	Traffic, schools, l.g. website	1
Pajala	8,000	Öppet forum	Free	Traffic, culture, recreational activities, economy	12
Robertsfors	7,000	Diskussions-forum	Free	Traffic	3 (opened in June)
Ronneby	29,000	1. Allmänhetens bok	Free	Chat, recreational activities, traffic, IT, l.g. website	20 (closed in June)
		2. Öppet forum	Free	(See 1)	14 (opened in June)
		3. Snacket	Free	Music, sex, sport, schools	10
		4. Byn på nätet	Free	Schools, the debate, local website	6
Sala	22,000	Gästbok	Free	Greetings	11
Sandviken	38,000	Diskussions-forum	Free	Greetings, schools, music, future	40
Skara	18,000	Tyck till	Free	l.g. website, l.g. policies	6 (opened in May)

Municipality	Number of inhabitants	Name of forum	Choice of issues	Topicality	Number of contributions per month
Stockholm	736,000	Användar-debatter	Free	Various policy issues	2 (not managed actively since autumn of 1998)
Storuman	7,000	Synpunkter på Storumans WWW-sidor	l.g. website	l.g. website	2
Sundsvall	94,000	Tyck om Sundsvall	Free	Greetings, chat, traffic, schools, l.g. website, construction	60
Sölvesborg	17,000	Fritt forum	Free	Greetings, traffic, construction, tourism	14
Trelleborg	38,000	Gästbok	l.g. website, but in practice free	Greetings, l.g. website, tourism	14
Tyresö	38,000	Tyresö debattforum	Free	Traffic, schools, childcare, environmental issues	10
Vindeln	6,000	Anslagstavla	Free	Greetings, chat, tourism	60
Västervik	38,000	Västerviks kommuns gästbok	Free	Greetings, chat, l.g. website, recreational issues	15
Västerås	125,000	Gästbok	Free	Greetings, chat	40
Åtvidaberg	12,000	E-postlista	IT-issues	IT IT	Less than 1
Älmhult	16,000	Insändarsida	Free	Greetings, l.g. website, recreational activities	2
Östersund	59,000	1. Medborgar-dialogen om utbildning 2000	School issues	Schools	2
		2. Skoldebatten	School issues	Schools	2

(l.g. = local government)

Chapter 14

Surveillance in the community

Community development through the use of closed-circuit television

C. William R. Webster and John Hood

Introduction

During the 1990s closed-circuit television (CCTV) surveillance cameras rapidly diffused into a wide range of public settings across the UK. This widespread diffusion includes the introduction of CCTV into community settings including residential areas and community facilities and buildings. CCTV is being introduced into such settings to improve safety, and to reduce crime and the fear of crime. In this respect, CCTV can be seen as the intro-duction of a form of information and communication technology (ICT) which contributes to the facilitation of community development. These systems have proved to be very successful and are consequently very popular amongst local policy-makers, politicians, residents and community leaders. Typically they are community-driven, the result of local demand, regardless of any potential fears associated with extending the electronic capabilities of 'big brother'. The objective of this chapter is to explore the diffusion of CCTV in community settings. In doing so it is apparent that the increased surveillance of communities via CCTV implies that CCTV is becoming a key part of the informated community. Moreover, as a community informatics (CI) initiative, CCTV represents the provision of an electronic service to meet local demand thereby signalling a shift to a citizen-centred approach to governance.

This chapter has two main parts. The first part discusses CCTV in the community; by exploring why CCTV can be considered a CI, by presenting evidence of diffusion in community settings, by exploring the purposes of CCTV in such settings and by discussing local demand for such systems. The second part explores some of the issues raised in the first part through the presentation of a case study based on the Greater Easterhouse CCTV system. The second part is followed by concluding remarks. The research presented here derives from two independent but interlinked pieces of research being conducted at the Caledonian Business School, Glasgow Caledonian University. Doctoral research exploring the policy processes surrounding the diffusion of CCTV in the UK by William Webster provides much of the background information on CCTV in the community, and an evaluation of the Greater Easterhouse CCTV System commissioned by Safe Greater Easterhouse and conducted by John Hood and David Ross (1997–2000) provides the material for the case study.

Closed-circuit television in the community

Closed-circuit television – community informatics?

The concept of CI focuses on the introduction of innovative technological applications, and in particular new ICTs such as the Internet or World Wide Web, for the economic and social development of local communities. The focus is thus both technical and geographical: technical because the transforming capabilities of new ICTs are seen as offering new ways of realising community development, and geographical as these technical systems are geographically embedded and developed within community settings by and for local communities. CI are thus technological applications which are in the community, for the community, demanded (to various degrees) by the community and used by the community. Typically, the CI perspective leads to an examination of how community groups are using new technology as a tool to change their local community. Of particular concern are those systems, which connect communities to cyberspace in order to reinforce existing social networks 'virtually'. The focus is usually the Internet.

The focus of this chapter is a totally different technological application, the closed-circuit television surveillance system. During the 1990s a 'surveillance revolution' has swept across the UK as CCTV surveillance cameras have been installed in a wide variety of public places (Webster 1999a, 1996). Of particular interest here are those systems which are located in community settings and are operated, promoted and financed (in whole or in part) by agencies of the state, including the democratic institutions of local governance. 'CCTV' is a widely used generic term to denote the use of video surveillance cameras and systems in public places where camera technology is linked in 'real time' to a control room containing monitoring and storage equipment. Systems in community settings are usually either small systems in community buildings with a few cameras linked to recording facilities or larger systems in public spaces which incorporate a number of strategically located cameras networked to a staffed control centre. They can be considered CI because they are:

- in the community
- for the community
- demanded by the community, and
- used by the community.

The surveillance capabilities of new ICTs mean that greater *electronic* surveillance of citizens by the state is a core element of the emerging information society and that emergent CI, based on the capabilities of new ICTs, thereby also provide opportunities for greater surveillance, monitoring and control. Consequently, the potential to 'transform' communities via CI is closely interlinked with the potential to 'survey' communities. In other words the potential to transform is also the potential to control. It is for this reason that the CI perspective should consider and account for the surveillance aspects of new technologies, such as CCTV. Although it is clear that sophisticated electronic surveillance in the form of CCTV is becoming a central part of community life, other electronic forms of surveillance are less obvious and more discrete. This raises a number of issues for the CI perspective: issues about potential threat to civil liberties, issues about communities understanding and awareness of these technologies, and issues about the intended purposes for introducing new ICTs.

Closed-circuit television – in the community?

It is now commonly accepted that during the 1990s CCTV has become a central part of daily life in towns and cities across the UK (Graham 1996, Graham *et al.* 1996, Goodwin *et al.* 1998, Bulos and Sarno 1994, Fyfe and Bannister 1996), with the diffusion of CCTV having been so rapid that it can be described as a phenomenon. Fyfe and Bannister go so far as to state that CCTV cameras are becoming as commonplace 'as telephone boxes or traffic lights' (1996: 3). As noted elsewhere, the uptake of CCTV by local authorities and other public agencies can be considered 'revolutionary' in that it has been both rapid and widespread (Webster 1999a, 1996). Diffusion beyond towns and cities has occurred in a wide variety of public locations including schools, hospitals, sports centres, railway and bus stations and car parks. Not only have we seen an unprecedented speed of installation but also a remarkable diversity of implementation across a variety of public places. CCTV is becoming a more prominent feature of local-community shopping areas, rural and residential areas, transport facilities and local community facilities, such as schools, community centres, sports and leisure centres and local car parks.

Data from the first comprehensive national survey of CCTV in 'public places' (Webster 1999a) provides insights into the extent and location of local-authority uptake in community settings. This research shows that 86.1 per cent of local authorities had installed CCTV systems in public places and a further 20 per cent indicated they intended to install CCTV into public places; 64.2 per cent stated that they intended to extend their existing systems. This data clearly shows that the vast majority of local authorities in the UK have installed CCTV systems into their public spaces and that further systems, including extensions to existing systems, are being planned. The survey also

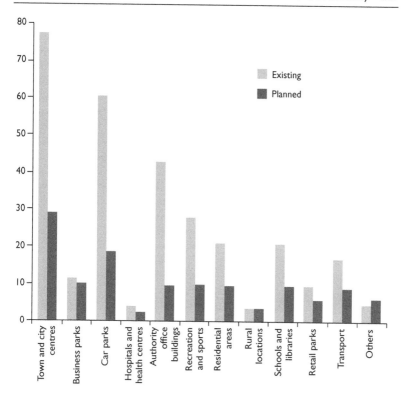

Figure 14.1 The location of existing and planned local authority CCTV systems (%)

provides data on the location of existing and planned CCTV systems. Figure 14.1 illustrates the distribution of CCTV by type of location for all those local authorities that indicated that they had installed CCTV. The chart shows that local authorities have installed CCTV into a wide variety of public locations. Whilst 77.6 per cent of local authorities have installed CCTV into town and city centres and 60.6 per cent into public car parks, between 20 and 30 per cent of authorities had installed CCTV into recreation facilities, sports and leisure facilities, residential areas and schools and libraries. Figure 14.1 also illustrates that approximately 10 per cent of local authorities were planning to introduce CCTV into residential areas, recreational areas and schools and libraries.

A closer examination of the data shows that the location of CCTV systems is also closely related to certain attributes of the sample variables. Urban authorities are more likely than rural authorities to have introduced CCTV in town and city centres, car parks, residential areas, schools and libraries, and sports and recreational facilities. London and Metropolitan authorities and those controlled by Labour are most likely to have introduced CCTV in residential areas and in schools and libraries.

In addition to existing systems, government policy announced in 1999 means that government funding of CCTV will focus on installing new systems in community and residential areas and away from areas already extensively surveyed, such as car parks and town centres. The 'CCTV Initiative' launched in 1999 is an extension of the Crime Reduction Programme (CRP) announced in 1998 and is managed jointly by the Home Office, the Department of Environment, Transport and the Regions and the National Assembly for Wales. It replaces the Home Office's 'CCTV Challenge Competition' which between 1994 and 1999 distributed over £50 million to seven hundred new schemes across the UK (Webster 1998a). Under the CRP £153 million is available for CCTV in England and Wales (a further £17 million is available for Scotland and Northern Ireland) between 1999 and 2002. The initiative was launched on 16 March 1999 by the then Home Secretary, Jack Straw, to help local crime-and-disorder reduction partnerships to combat crime and disorder and to support the regeneration of local estates with high crime rates. The first round of the initiative received 745 outline bids, of which 377 were short-listed for further consideration. To date 282 of these bids (for £49 million) have been approved awards and a further seventy-two bids are being further scrutinised. In Scotland the Scottish Executive awarded £1.865 million to thirty-four schemes as part of the 'Make Our Communities Safer' Challenge Competition 2000–1 administered by the Crime Prevention Unit. A further £1.5 million has been made available during 2001 (see Scottish Executive 2000 for details of awards).

The second round of the CCTV Initiative was announced in March 2000. In contrast to the first round and previous CCTV Challenge Competitions, this will be a rolling programme of funding, running until December 2001. In the second round 'schemes in residential areas also remain a priority – around half of the funding is expected to be allocated to housing related projects over the lifetime of the initiative . . . we are also concerned in this round with reducing crime levels and the fear of crime in rural areas and small community shopping centres, where absolute crime levels may be lower, but where the fear of crime is having a significant adverse effect on local communities' (Home Office 2000a: 2). The application prospectus is explicit in stating that the CCTV initiative will support schemes in residential areas, community-shopping areas and rural areas, in other potential 'hot-spots' including community facilities, schools, hospitals, railway and bus stations, and car parks including those servicing hospitals, residential areas, education establishments, leisure complexes and local amenities. Moreover, 'Housing bids, especially those linked to regeneration plans and other schemes to improve the quality of life for residents are being particularly encouraged' (Home Office 2000b: 6). The initiative will fund up to one hundred per cent of the capital costs of CCTV including cameras, lighting and other fixtures, transmission infrastructures, command and control systems, IT systems, and data storage and retrieval systems. Running costs are not eligible for funding. Proposals for funding must be from crime-and-disorder partnerships and be consistent with the local crime-and-disorder audits established under the Crime and Disorder Act 1998 (the Crime and Disorder Act applies only in England and Wales, although bids to the Scottish equivalent are also dependent on the formation of partnerships between local police and local authorities). It is very apparent that the diffusion of CCTV is set to continue and that recent government policy represents a shift in emphasis from diffusion in cities, towns, commercial and retail areas to diffusion in community settings.

Closed-circuit television – for the community?

It is clear that CCTV is in the community, but how then does CCTV benefit the community? These systems are being installed for various reasons including the detection and deterrence of crime, petty crime and other anti-social behaviour, to reduce the fear of crime (FOC), to improve policing practice and to regenerate localities through a technologically motivated 'feel-good factor'. The original CCTV Challenge Competition stated that the cameras 'help prevent and detect crime . . . [and] . . . also deter criminals and reassure the public' (Home Office 1994: 3). The latest CCTV initiative says that CCTV can be used to deal with crime and disorder in housing areas, burglary, racially motivated crime, public-order problems, street robbery and violence, drug-related crime, alcohol-related crime, repeat victimisation, retail crime, school-related crime and low-level anti-social behaviour (an illustrative list). In the aforementioned national survey of CCTV local authorities were asked to indicate the main objectives of the CCTV systems within their boundaries, with the intention being to identify the strategic council-wide purposes of (or the reasons for) CCTV. The results, illustrated in Figure 14.2, show that the main reasons for installing CCTV are to prevent crime, reduce the fear of crime and deter anti-social behaviour. Other important reasons, though significantly less important than those already mentioned, include detecting crime, meeting citizens' demands for CCTV and protecting public and private property. The point to note is that the introduction of CCTV is not solely about reducing crime but to revitalise communities in a variety of ways.

Closed-circuit television – demanded by the community?

One of the most notable features of the CCTV revolution is the extent to which the general public supports such systems. Part of the explanation for this is the belief that the cameras work in preventing, detecting and deterring

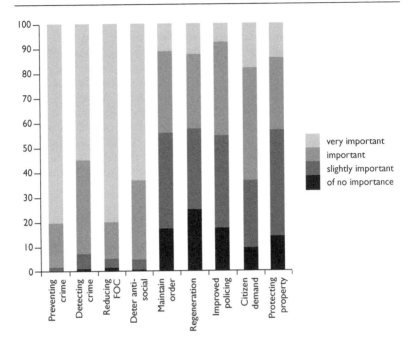

Figure 14.2 Local authority reasons for introducing CCTV (%)

crime. CCTV has been promoted against this belief and marketed to the general public primarily as a 'state-of-the-art' technological tool to combat crime. The view that CCTV actually reduces crime has been widely and successfully disseminated across society, and accordingly there is widespread support for CCTV amongst politicians, policy-makers and the general public (Webster 1999b). Scottish Office Home Affairs Minister Henry McLeish, when announcing the results of the 1998–9 Scottish Office's 'CCTV Challenge Competition', said: 'We are giving CCTV our strongest support because there can be no doubt that CCTV works . . . [and] . . . most crucially for me, CCTV helps reduce the fear of crime on the streets' (McLeish 1998: 11). Consequently, the deterministic view that crime reduction is inevitable following CCTV installation has cascaded down into the general consciousness of the population. Public perception surveys, such as those conducted by the Home Office (Honess and Charman 1992, Brown 1995) and for prospective operators (see for example Goodwin *et al.* 1998, Ross and Hood 1998), show clearly that the public views CCTV as a highly effective tool to reduce crime and the fear of crime. The view that 'CCTV works' is backed up by the continued demand from both public bodies and citizens for more systems: 'This continuing demand demonstrates again that partnerships regard CCTV as a valuable asset to strengthen their ability to reduce crime and the fear of crime, increase detection rates, and bring wider benefits, including aiding the development of communities in need of regeneration' (Home Office 2000a: 1). The overwhelming support for CCTV is unquestionable and it is noticeable how little debate there has been across society on the use and impacts of such sophisticated surveillance systems. The belief that society needs these systems has overridden any dissenting voices that question their effectiveness and impacts.

Debates about CCTV have been led and shaped by political rhetoric which has wholeheartedly supported the technology. Consequently, public discourse has focused on the success and benefits of the cameras and not on the more complex issues associated with extending the state's surveillance capabilities (Webster 1999b). Statements made when announcing recent tranche of government funding by the Home Secretary, Jack Straw, and the Deputy Justice Minister of the Scottish Executive, Angus MacKay, highlight the extent of support for CCTV at the governmental level: 'This technology has proved its worth in reducing crime and making people feel safer . . . it will greatly improve the quality of life for local residents and help regenerate some of our most vulnerable communities', Jack Straw (BBC 2000); 'Today's awards show that people are committed to making their communities safer and are prepared to be dynamic and innovative in the fight against crime,' Angus MacKay (Scottish Executive 2000: 1). At a local level, debate has been about how communities can secure the necessary funding to install or extend systems in their area. This is illustrated by three recent headlines from Glasgow's local press: 'Lack of cash is real turn off' (Mackie 2000), 'CCTV extension plan hit by funding crisis' (McAuley 2000) and 'Crime camera cash blow' (Wilson 2000). These headlines demonstrate that at a local level the main concern is finance; it is assumed that CCTV will benefit the community. Absent from the debate is any discussion about the appropriate use of CCTV, the implications of using such technology in the community, the impact on the civil liberties of the surveyed community and the changing relations between citizens and the state arising from the use of CCTV (Webster 1998b).

The CCTV competitions in England, Wales and Scotland state that awards will be made only to projects which can demonstrate a demand for CCTV and where bodies representing the community have been consulted and are supportive. Partnerships are obliged to undertake 'genuine consultation' to ascertain the views of all sections of the community affected by CCTV. A dialogue with the community via consultation is therefore a key part of securing CCTV funding and ensuring that CCTV is delivered in accordance with citizens' wishes. To gauge the extent of consultation on CCTV provision, the national survey of CCTV (Webster 1999a) asked local authorities to indicate which bodies, organisations and forums they had consulted. The results, illustrated at Figure 14.3, show that a wide range of organisations outside the authority have been consulted by most local authorities.

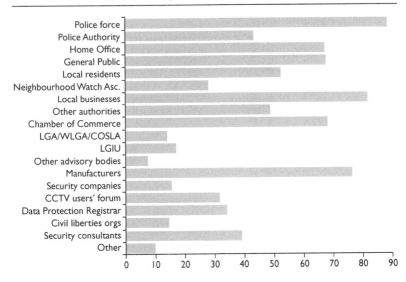

Figure 14.3 Bodies consulted about the provision of CCTV (%)

Citizen consultation was varied, with 67.3 per cent of local authorities having consulted the general public, 52.1 per cent having consulted local residents, and 27.9 per cent having consulted neighbourhood watch associations. The local authorities were also asked to indicate how they consulted citizens about their provision of CCTV: 41.8 per cent of authorities had consulted citizens through Town Centre Forums, 41.2 per cent via public attitude surveys, 27.9 per cent through Parish or Town Council meetings, and 21.2 per cent through local newsletters; 15.2 per cent indicated they had consulted citizens in other ways such as through presentations, open days, local press comments and residents' meetings. Clearly, community demand for CCTV captured by political rhetoric and local press comment is irrefutable and is backed up by public-perception surveys and extensive public consultation. The public, residents, citizens and communities want CCTV.

Closed-circuit television – used by the community?

Although it is relatively easy to argue that CCTV is in the community, for the community and demanded by the community, it is less obvious how CCTV is used by the community. CCTV is used by the community in two ways. First, systems are usually operated by, or on behalf of, local community bodies or partnerships. These bodies are usually responsible for training the operatives and making sure that they follow an established code of practice. Second, it is the local community who are the surveyed. Thus, as with the other CI applications, CCTV involves the capture, transmission and storage of information and data about the community, realised through the new configuration of technology. They are the subject of the technology in a new artificial virtual community. The key difference between CCTV and other CI applications is that the use of CCTV is involuntary, compulsory, unavoidable, simultaneous and continuous. Perhaps it is more accurate to say that CCTV is based in the community but not community-based. That is, whilst the cameras may be used by the community and generate information flows with a community content, ownership and control over the system is not community-wide but through selected public agencies.

From these discussions it is possible to see how CCTV systems can be considered CI applications implemented for the economic and social development of communities. In this respect CCTV is seen as a very successful and popular application. However, whilst CCTV is being promoted and used in this way its inherent technological capabilities mean that it is also possible for the systems to be used as a tool for ensuring social control and public order [Scientific and Technological Options Assessment Unit (STOA) 1998]. At the very least the introduction of CCTV *by definition* results in the increased surveillance of citizens and communities. The question of who benefits from the increased surveillance capability is pertinent. The configuration of a technology for community purposes does not remove the need to ask this question. Issues of ownership, control and use are central to the CI perspective; they are explored in more detail through the case study presented in the second part of this chapter. The case study explores the Greater Easterhouse CCTV Initiative, which is geographically embedded in the Easterhouse community.

The Greater Easterhouse case study

Greater Easterhouse, known simply as 'Easterhouse' was created in the 1960s, and is the largest of four peripheral council housing estates, or 'schemes', built to accommodate population overspill arising from the post-war baby boom and to facilitate slum clearance in inner-city Glasgow. Easterhouse, population approximately 35,000, is located to the north-east of Glasgow about five miles from the city centre. It has for some time been synonymous with unemployment and crime, and regarded as a breeding-ground for gang warfare. Unlike the contemporaneous, self-contained 'new towns' of East Kilbride and Cumbernauld, situated further from Glasgow, the construction of Greater Easterhouse consisted mostly of high-density municipal housing stock. However, the initial improvements in housing were not accompanied by employment opportunities, social infrastructure or basic shopping facilities. So, despite the initial optimism of its residents, significant socio-economic problems rapidly developed. Easterhouse quickly became a medium-sized town with limited recreational facilities and poor social provision.

Consequently, a range of crime-related problems developed in the community, and juvenile crime became a particular problem based on territorial conflicts in Easterhouse. Strong territoriality based on the fifteen distinct local communities, or 'sub-schemes', within 'Greater' Easterhouse has been cited by residents as a significant factor in the high levels of juvenile, drug-related and violent crime. By 1969, nearly a third of residents had sought transfer from Easterhouse (Keating 1988) and in the 1970s regeneration policies were initiated with Easterhouse recognised as a site of 'multiple deprivation'.

In the mid 1980s Easterhouse was one of the four estates to feature in the Centre for Environmental Studies (CES) (1984 and 1985) research which sought to make recommendations for the revitalisation of deprived areas. CES recommended, *inter alia*, that improvements could be brought about only by a strategic co-ordinated national partnership involving the community, relevant local authorities and central government. Subsequently, in June 1990 the 'Safe Greater Easterhouse (SGE) Community Partnership' was launched under the Scottish Office Safer Cities Programme (SCP). The objectives of the SCP were to reduce crime, to lessen the fear of crime, to create safer cities, to improve the quality of life of the community and to encourage economic growth (Carnie 1995). The SGE community partnership established under the SCP was set up to meet these objectives in Easterhouse. The SGE partnership was intended to empower local residents and citizens by giving them a voice in local decision-making; Hall (1997) refers to this approach as a new 'bottom-up' approach to community planning as opposed to the traditional 'top-down' approach. Community involvement is central to SGE's strategy for regeneration: 'For the project to be successful it is essential that from the beginning there should be close and continuing involvement of local people and agencies in setting the project's objectives, strategies and priorities' (Carnie 1996: 22). Since its inception SGE has introduced a variety of community projects primarily concerned with the reduction of crime and the fear of crime in the Greater Easterhouse area (Carnie 1996). SGE therefore represents a crucial link between the local community and the local police force: 'What we can do, and that no one else can do is act as a broker between the police, who have a responsibility for preventing crime, and the community . . . I think that the role of an organisation like SGE is to listen to what the community wants, sometimes to advise the community as to what they need and to take that to the police and try to get both sides together' (1998 interview transcript with SGE Co-ordination). The SGE Management Committee, consisting of an eclectic band of community activists, local councillors and local and national government officials, oversees the work of the partnership.

Initially SGE focused on 'target-hardening' by embarking on a campaign to improve the security of residents and local businesses. This initiative was seen as a great success, achieving a 41 per cent decrease in household break-ins (based on reported incidents between 1991 and 1994), a figure notably higher than the 24 per cent national average decrease (SGE 1997). Additionally, the fear of household break-ins fell by 7 per cent during this period (Carnie 1996). Target-hardening in local businesses led to a notable improvement in Easterhouse's main shopping centre, Shandwyck Square, which has been transformed from a 'no-go' area into a viable shopping concern. Whilst 'property crimes' such as housebreaking and vandalism have fallen dramatically over the lifetime of SGE, violent crime, group disorder and drug-related crime have continued at unacceptably high levels. Although overall crime figures fell by 36 per cent between 1991 and 1996 the crime rate was still much higher than in the rest of Scotland, 153 crimes per 1000 population compared to a national average of eighty-eight (Ross and Hood 1998). Moreover, some areas continued to be perceived as 'no-go' areas because of the continued presence of drugs and gangs. SGE decided to address the issue of persistently high levels of violence and drug-related crime by pursuing the installation of CCTV.

The Greater Easterhouse CCTV Initiative

The Greater Easterhouse CCTV Project was proposed by SGE following two gang-related murders in 1994 and the subsequent lobbying for cameras by local councillors, politicians and residents. Two petitions, totalling 2808 signatures, requesting the introduction of CCTV cameras were raised by local residents. The key objectives of the system were to 'reduce crime' and improve 'crime detection'. Other important aims were to stimulate economic growth, improve the quality of life, address the drug problem and reduce the fear of 'no-go' areas. The project has been developed over three years by a local working group comprising representatives of Glasgow City Council, SGE, Greater Easterhouse Community Empowerment Project, Greater Easterhouse Initiative and Strathclyde Police. The local communities' desire for CCTV has been matched by financial support from the Scottish Office. Under the Scottish Office's CCTV 'Challenge Competition' the Easterhouse scheme has to date secured £210,800 from two separate bids. A further 50 per cent of matched funding for capital costs has been raised by contributions from a range of local public, semi-public and private bodies, including; Blairtumock Housing Association, Glasgow City Council, Greater Easterhouse Development Company, Greater Easterhouse Initiative, Lochfield Park Housing Co-operative, SGE, Scottish Homes, Social Work Department, Strathclyde Passenger Transport, Ossory Property Investments, the Post Office, Soapworks Limited and Strathclyde Buses Limited.

The Easterhouse CCTV project was to be installed initially in three phases and was the first major residential system in Scotland. The first phase went 'live' in May 1998, quickly followed by the second phase in September of the same year. At the official launch of the system in September, Scottish Home Affairs Minister Henry McLeish said, 'I am delighted to be able to officially launch the Greater Easterhouse CCTV Initiative . . . it is an impressive project which I am sure will go some way to cutting the worrying level of crime – and the fear of crime – in this area' (Scottish Office 1998: 1). Phase one of the system consisted of nine cameras and an optic fibre loop, known as the 'Lochend Loop', to and from the control room located in Easterhouse Police Station. System operatives are civilians employed by SGE following Strathclyde Police's 'CCTV Code of Practice'. The second phase of the system has installed a further twelve cameras stretching from the police station south-west along the main Edinburgh Road. A further extension (phase three) is planned and is dependent upon the successful application for funds from the challenge competition currently being drawn up. When completed the Greater Easterhouse CCTV Project will contain a sophisticated network of up to thirty one surveillance cameras. Unlike the majority of the large CCTV systems in the UK, the Easterhouse system is primarily based in residential areas. Clearly then the system is in the community and is intended to survey the community. Furthermore, the inspiration for the system came from within the community, via the previously mentioned petitions, and is organised and managed by one of the key bodies representing the community – SGE. For these reasons the CCTV initiative in Easterhouse can be seen as a good example of a CI application.

Under the CCTV Challenge Competition awards were made to initiatives which could demonstrate a need for CCTV, a crime issue to be addressed by CCTV, a local demand for CCTV and an obligation to evaluate the system. SGE consulted a range of local bodies prior to submitting an application, including voluntary organisations, residents' groups, businesses, public authorities and the police. SGE also agreed to administer the application for funding and contract an independent evaluation of the system. Typically evaluation takes the form of a pre- and post-installation review of crime statistics and pre- and post-installation public-attitude surveys. Presented here are findings from the evaluation of the Easterhouse system conducted by Glasgow Caledonian University on behalf of SGE. Research activities carried out to date and presented here are: a pre-installation residents' street survey conducted in 1998; pre-installation semi-structured interviews with prominent community actors, and preliminary findings from a pre- and post-installation review of crime statistics in the CCTV area. This evaluation represents the first independent evaluation of a major public residential CCTV initiative in the UK.

It is reasonable to assume, following the two petitions which inspired SGE to pursue CCTV, that the residents of Easterhouse believed that CCTV would help prevent serious crime, aid the detection of crime and make Easterhouse a better place to live. This view of CCTV was however contradicted by the pre-installation interviews with prominent community activists unconnected with SGE conducted before the first public-perception survey. In general these activists took a more circumspect view of CCTV, raising concerns about civil liberties and the efficacy of the system. Despite these concerns, it was generally agreed that there appeared to be no concern in the community about civil-liberty issues. This, it was noted, contrasted sharply with the large number of complaints made by local people concerning the use of Easterhouse by Strathclyde Police as a pilot area for the deployment of officers armed with CS gas. This, they argued, shows that issues about civil liberties are a current concern in Easterhouse. Thus, whilst CS gas and CCTV are similar in that they are new innovative policing tools with civil-liberties implications, CS gas is seen as a tool used by the police against (certain sections of) the community whereas CCTV is perceived as a tool used for the community. Regardless of the technical capabilities of the system or any potential threat to civil liberties, it was felt that the local community did want CCTV and that, if all it achieved was a reduction in the fear of crime, then it would be seen as effective.

The public's perception of crime, the fear of crime and the usefulness and desirability of CCTV is to be measured in a series of public-perception surveys. The first street survey of residents was conducted in 1998 before the system became operative. It was to be followed up with a similar post-installation survey in 2000 designed to see how attitudes have changed over the last two years. Survey methodology included: the selection of the most appropriate survey points (streets) around Easterhouse; the construction of a stratified sample designed to reflect local demographics; and the construction, administration and analysis of a concise street survey. Survey methodology, responses and results are presented in more detail in Ross and Hood (1998). A number of points are relevant here. First, the data indicated that 23 per cent of residents regarded Easterhouse as a 'bad' or 'very bad' place to live, with no significance according to gender or age. The survey also identified why residents thought Easterhouse was a bad place to live. Crime, disorder and anti-social behaviour featured highly in the responses. The surveyed were asked to rate their concern for a range of crimes and anti-social behaviour perceived to be common in Easterhouse. A selection of the responses are illustrated in Figure 14.4. This shows that the residents of Easterhouse were most concerned about drug abuse (60 per cent stated that they were 'very concerned'), drug-dealing (59 per cent), gangs (37 per cent), vandalism (32 per cent) and public rowdiness (27 per cent). Looking at the data in more detail shows a statistical significance pointing to greater concern about gang and drug-related incidents among 15–24-year-olds. In addition to these concerns the majority of respondents perceived 'no-go' areas as existing: 38 per cent respondents during the day and 68 per cent at night. This fear of no-go areas was positively skewed towards the young and women. The two no-go areas of greatest public concern are covered by the first phase of the initiative, thereby suggesting a link between citizen concern and service provision. These data suggest that, for CCTV to be seen as a successful CI application in Easterhouse, it has to help address residents' concerns about drug use and public order.

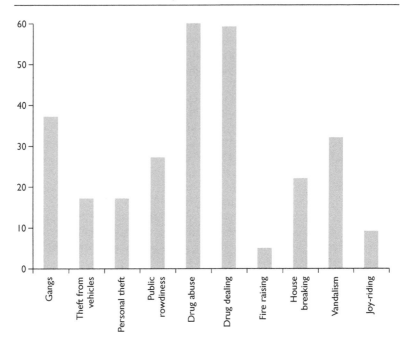

Figure 14.4 Residents' rating of crime and anti-social behaviour – 'very concerned' (%)
(adapted from Ross and Hood 1998: 514–15)

Respondents were also asked to indicate whether they were aware of the proposed CCTV installation and to what extent they supported it. Figure 14.5 illustrates the extent to which residents supported the introduction of CCTV in Easterhouse. The chart shows that, regardless of whether the respondents were previously aware of the CCTV proposals, the vast majority were very supportive: 95 per cent were 'satisfied' or 'very satisfied' with the proposed installation, whilst only 3 per cent were 'unsatisfied' or 'very unsatisfied'. There can therefore be no doubt that the public wanted to see CCTV in Easterhouse. Whilst there is strong support for CCTV, it is interesting to note that 'only' 38 per cent of the surveyed had heard of SGE and 35 per cent were previously aware of the CCTV proposals. This is perhaps a surprising finding, given that the proposals for CCTV have been presented as community-driven. Of those who were previously aware of the CCTV proposals, 54 per cent had heard via 'word of mouth' and 46 per cent from a range of formal and informal means. The post-installation survey was to be conducted in late 2000 with as many of the original respondents as possible. The intention is to see whether the residents of Easterhouse have altered their attitudes towards

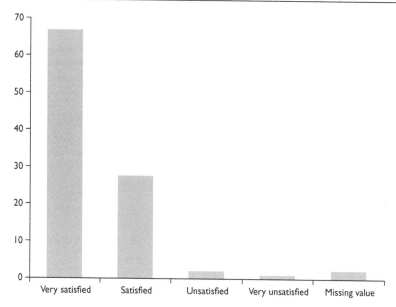

Figure 14.5 Satisfaction with CCTV proposals in Easterhouse (%)

crime, the fear of crime and CCTV. The key question would be whether they are still as supportive of CCTV after two years of its operation.

Although it is clear in Easterhouse that residents and the public support the introduction of CCTV, a number of developments in its provision question whether it is actually the community that benefits most from CCTV or whether the main beneficiaries are not actually the community but the police. Developments discussed here include the processes determining the location of cameras, the actual purpose and use of the cameras and the extent to which the cameras are meeting residents' concerns – gangs and drugs. Such developments ultimately question whether CCTV is a 'true' CI application.

In Easterhouse the location of the cameras is of particular interest. To address residents' concerns about gangs and drugs it would be reasonable to expect the cameras to be located in those areas identified as no-go areas. This would match service provision with service need and citizens' demands. Interestingly, however, this is not the case as other factors have influenced the location of cameras. The first factor is technical. In order to make the system economically feasible it was set up as a loop from the control room in Easterhouse police station. The close proximity of the police station to the loop was an important factor determining the location and spread of the cameras, and areas further afield have not been wired up. The second key factor is both political and financial. Two of the cameras in the loop were unofficially 'earmarked', where funding was secured in return for the positioning of the cameras in particular locations. Again community 'need' appears not to be the main criterion for camera location. Additionally, the positioning of the cameras has followed police advice, thereby ensuring that the cameras are located in areas most beneficial to policing needs.

The role of the police in the provision of CCTV in Easterhouse and across the UK generally raises issues about the primary purpose and use of these systems. Are they for the benefit of the community, as posited in Easterhouse, or are they actually utilised for the benefit of local policing? The local police force plays an important role on the provision and operation of CCTV. Awards for funds from the Challenge Competitions are made only to partnerships which have the support of the local authority and local police force, and where a local crime concern is highlighted. Although the police do not usually contribute financially to the capital or running costs of schemes, they do provide advice on the citing of cameras, house the control room and train the operatives. Locating the control centre in a police station (Easterhouse Police Station in this example) and directly training the operatives (who work under Strathclyde Police's 'CCTV Code of Practice') points to the use of CCTV as a policing tool, used to assist their role in preventing and detecting crime and maintaining social order. The intention here is not to suggest that a reduction in crime, disorder and anti-social behaviour and an improvement in policing are not a benefit to the community, as obviously they are; the suggestion here is that the introduction of CCTV may be to meet policing goals *as well as* community concerns.

CCTV benefits the police in a number of ways. First, CCTV makes possible a prompter response to incidents as they occur. The inherent technological capability of CCTV provides a constant accurate real-time flow of information about incidents as they evolve. CCTV is therefore a critical knowledge-based information-system of strategic importance. The information generated by the system can be used to direct police resources or not, as the case may be. Thus officers can be directed to intervene in an incident or can instead be withdrawn with the incident monitored virtually and remotely. CCTV therefore removes the need to pursue stolen cars or suspects physically as this can now be done electronically in surveyed areas. Second, CCTV systems, through their ability to store footage, are also knowledge-based 'expert historians' in that they provide footage of incidents after the event. Such footage can be used to collaborate witness statements, to determine whether or not a prosecution is viable or as evidence in a prosecution. Third, CCTV can also be used as an information-gathering device, in that it can be used covertly to monitor individuals and locations. Neyland (2000) argues that where CCTV systems are operated by the police the configuration of knowledge and information contained within the system offers benefits in three key ways. They provide:

- access to the immediate
- access to the past, and
- a greater articulation of the observable.

These benefits enable the police to realise swifter response times, better resource distribution and the prevention of unnecessary prosecutions. Ultimately these systems reduce unnecessary costs and improve efficiency within policing: 'the police have been allowed an opportunity to do less, to move less resources and people, by relying on a greater input from a new source of knowledge, the CCTV system' (Neyland 2000: 16).

Ditton *et al.* in their evaluation of the Glasgow CityWatch CCTV system estimate that the annual cost of running seven or eight cameras is equivalent to the cost of one police officer (1999: 23). Superintendent Howard Parry of Merseyside Police goes so far as to say: 'This [CCTV] system is like having twenty officers on duty, twenty-four hours a day, who take note of everything, never take a holiday and are rarely off sick' (quoted in Groombridge and Murji 1994: 2). Cost-cutting arguments, whilst valid, are often not put forward by the police as then they might be expected to contribute more to the ongoing costs of running a system. Community partnerships and local authorities on the other hand are also reluctant to push perspectives which suggest the police are the main beneficiaries, as then the system itself will be perceived as a police tool, used for the benefit of the police and not the local community. This contrasts sharply with their responsibility to defend the interests of citizens and communities: they do not want such a sophisticated surveillance and control tool – with its inherent potential threat to civil liberties and citizen–state relations – to be seen as solely police-controlled. Typically then, arguments about improving the quality of life are put forward by both the police and local authorities. These arguments are usually based on benefits derived by the community from reduced crime in surveyed areas.

Preliminary findings from a review of the crime statistics conducted as part of the Easterhouse CCTV evaluation are mixed and ambiguous. Recorded police statistics tend not to be co-terminous with CCTV geographies but are based on police 'beats'. This makes comparisons over time and between areas difficult. A longitudinal study of the statistics suggests that since the introduction of CCTV certain crimes have decreased in number while others have increased; importantly the key issue of gang and drug-related offences seem to be unaffected by the introduction of CCTV. This of course raises the question of whether CCTV has met citizens' concerns in Easterhouse. A close reading of the statistics is not straightforward as there are a number of other factors which may account for a statistical rise in crime during the period. The figures may not represent a 'true' increase in crime, but may reflect higher levels of the detection of crime, mainly achieved via CCTV. A greater detection of offences has invariably led to a greater number of arrests and subsequently a greater number of successful prosecutions. Thus, whilst crime has risen, so have detection, arrests and the number of crimes 'solved'. This has enabled the police to demonstrate improved policing performance and value for money. The statistics are further complicated by other anti-crime initiatives introduced by Strathclyde Police during the evaluation period. These include the 'Spotlight Initiatives', such as 'Operation Blade', which resulted in a greater number of arrests for carrying 'offensive weapons'.

Consequently, from a preliminary examination of crime data in Easterhouse it is very difficult to say whether the introduction of CCTV has or has not resulted in reduced levels of crime or anti-social behaviour. This is reinforced by research conducted elsewhere in Scotland (Short and Ditton 1995, 1996, Ditton *et al.* 1999), suggesting that CCTV is not a panacea for all crime challenges the perceived wisdom that 'CCTV works'. Ross and Hood (1998) argue that in Easterhouse much of the crime and undesirable behaviour is directly or indirectly related to drugs and that CCTV cannot address the drug problem on its own. For Ross and Hood there are 'unrealistic perceptions of the ability of CCTV to deal with far deeper social issues which are intrinsically associated with drug related crime' (1998: 497). If it is difficult to show that CCTV works in reducing crime, and if it is difficult to show that CCTV has effectively addressed citizens' concerns about drugs and gangs, then we have to ask: in what ways have CCTV been effective and what are the actual benefits derived from the system? We would suggest that, whilst communities do benefit from improved policing and to a certain degree from the 'feelgood factor', it is actually the police themselves that derive the greatest benefit. This argument we feel is not reflected in current public debate or discourse on the use and implications of introducing CCTV in society.

Conclusion

No exploration of CI is complete without some recognition of the role of new ICT intensive-surveillance technologies and their increasing importance to everyday life. This chapter addresses this issue by showing that new technologies associated with CI are enabling CCTV surveillance cameras to become a prominent feature of local communities. The research presented here shows that the majority of local authorities in the UK have installed and are continuing to install and extend CCTV surveillance systems into the community. Whilst currently CCTV diffusion is concentrated in town and city centres and public car parks, it increasingly also extends to other public spaces such as residential and recreational areas, schools, leisure centres and libraries. The increased use of CCTV in community settings has necessarily led to the increased surveillance of communities. Community-driven and community-supported systems such as the Greater Easterhouse CCTV Initiative are being introduced for a variety of reasons, including the revitalisation of the community itself. Whilst CI applications such as CCTV can be in the community, for the community and demanded by the community, it is overly deterministic to suggest that they benefit just the community. As we have sought to demonstrate, there are a range of reasons for the use of CCTV and a range of benefits and beneficiaries. CCTV should not be seen as a panacea for all community problems but as a tool which is socially, politically and technically constructed. Only through a closer examination of its development and use are we likely to have a better understanding of how CCTV works and who benefits and how. The CI perspective therefore needs to be sympathetic to the idea that the introduction of new ICT-based applications may have unintended, unforeseen or undesirable impacts and consequences.

Acknowledgment

The authors would like to acknowledge the assistance of David Ross and Safe Greater Easterhouse in developing the Greater Easterhouse Case Study.

Chapter 15

The techno-flâneur

Tele-erotic re-presentation of women's life spaces

Tamara Seabrook and Louise Wattis

Introduction

This chapter is a discussion of the issues surrounding women's safety and closed-circuit television (CCTV). It has two main themes: the effectiveness of CCTV in relation to women's interpersonal safety, and also the extent to which women are monitored voyeuristically by male CCTV operators. The chapter will draw on relevant literature from feminist studies, criminology and cultural studies. Empirical data will be presented to illustrate how different populations of young women within the same community perceive and experience the presence of CCTV in their everyday life. For the purposes of this chapter the community will be referred to as Townsville, a community situated in the north-east of England. In comparison to the national average Townsville suffers from a combination of high unemployment and crime levels, as well as persistent drug-usage problems, above-average teenage pregnancy levels and below-average education attainment.

The data were elicited from one of four initiatives, which was part of a three-year action-based research project titled 'Action Risk'. The initiative, on which one of the authors was the researcher, explored with young women how they experience and perceive risks that they take and/or risks that they are exposed to. The young women involved in the research were aged 10 to 16, and comprised those which attended a centre-based youth centre (sample one) and those who chose to hang out on the streets (sample two).

Although the 'Action Risk' research was not specifically focused upon CCTV, it became evident from findings that it was a recurring theme. We therefore decided that this issue was worthy of further exploration, and we accompanied groups of the young women at various intervals to the local CCTV centre where we were able to get an insight into how CCTV was operated. Our own research in this area is ongoing; however preliminary findings converge with that of Norris and Armstrong's (1999) suggestion that CCTV is utilised in a gender-blind manner whereby women are yet again subject to the male gaze: this time via the electronic eye of the CCTV camera operated in the main by men, the techno-flâneurs of modern-day society.

The techno-flâneur

Accounts given by the young women in the research demonstrated the import-ance of locality in their lives and how this is often subjectively experienced, on the basis of calculations concerning risk, danger and safety. Subjectivity refers to how individuals draw upon their own understandings and experiences in order to position themselves in relation to certain discourses or dominant ideas and norms (Crawshaw and Seabrook 2000). This can seem a somewhat abstract notion, but can be summarised neatly as Steven Pile (1996) does to suggest that within urban landscapes people live out their daily lives within a mental map of their locality rather than within their actual physical locality itself. Feminist geographers (Rose 1993, Massey 1994) have long reported the importance of how *feelings* of space and power can be located within the gendered constellations of everyday practices and language. They suggest that women, irrespective of their class, race or sexuality, are expected to look 'right' for a voyeuristic gaze which is investigative, controlling and masculine. They have criticised the masculine scientific gaze which establishes a distance by 'othering' what it sees in order to gain mastery over the image. The flâneur, a key figure in critical literature, has been cited as an archetype of the male voyeur who not only told of changes in urban modernity, but as feminists note, also told of the intersection between male power, knowledge and masculine desire. The flâneur absents himself through his eyes; nowhere is forbidden, for him to see is to know. While leisurely streetwalking he remains at an objective distance of detachment and yet imposing an order on what he sees. This creates a tension between the object of the gaze and role of the flâneur. The flâneur is constituted as a sensitive artist as well as an objective voyeur in his approach to the world. Rose (1993) argues that conflict is inherent within this masculine pleasured gaze as emotion threatens to erupt and mark the author of the gaze as a responsive feeling subject and thus less as a disinterested individual in search of scientific evidence. Pile suggests:

> The flâneur seems to be just like everyone else, but he is a spy, a tourist, a detective, a journalist, scrutinising the otherwise alien streets, reporting back on its excessive, exotic, erotic lives . . . but while he may be in the margins, he is not of the margins. It is this poet male's location *inside* and *outside* power relations that gives him access to the streets, to the crowds, to the erotic underground of city life.
>
> (1996: 230–1)

In the nineteenth century men occupied the public sphere while women, with the exception of prostitutes, were confined to the private sphere. The prostitute transgresses the boundaries of the male scientific gaze as, on the one hand, threatening and, on the other, out of place, and yet, because she is perceived as being in such a position of 'freedom', is inherently fascinating. As

Pile (1996) suggests, prostitutes entered uncharted territory and thus became visible, an image caught in the space between classes, between sexes and between looks, and for this transgression they were subject to re-presentation and intrusive and oppressive state legislation. It is this internal relationship between power, knowledge and desire that renders the male gaze as inherently unstable, subverted by its own desires for the pleasures that it fears. It is to this end that Virilio (2000) suggests that it is not exactly usage which defines space but rather vision or insight. The conquest of space proves in the end to be only images of space.

CCTV operates as the prosthetic eye of the white male operator: it is today's flâneur. It is operated in a very gender-blind manner, rendering the image of woman invisible in public space, which consequently reinforces masculine ideologies of traditional female roles. However because as we have argued masculine power, knowledge and desire are inherently unstable, it also re-presents the image as woman as 'other' to be desired and controlled. As Fiske argues: 'When it serves the interests of power to "other" those whom it monitors, the social differences between the seer and the seen will loom large; when, however, the other is to be enrolled in a temporary alliance with "us", the difference shrinks into significance' (1998: 156). We argue that the real-time image of the CCTV screen is supplanting space: the visual, the tele-erotic, takes precedence over being, and the everyday reality of women's life space is hidden in the flatness of tele-visual images and representations.

CCTV: issues and themes

CCTV: background

Surveillance of public space by cameras has been vastly expanded in recent years with the installation of CCTV as a crime-control measure in numerous locations. In 1998, the Scottish Office announced plans to award funding to the value of £1.5 million to twenty-three new schemes in a variety of locations across Scotland; these were in addition to the sixty-two schemes already in existence. In March 1999, the Home Secretary announced a new CCTV initiative as part of the Home Office's Crime Reduction Programme. Up until March 2002, £153 million will be made available to regional Crime and Disorder partnerships who submit successful bids. In the past decade, £1 billion has been spent on the actual systems and the monitoring of the cameras in the UK (Arnot 1999). Britain is a world leader in the use of CCTV, which, according to Coleman and Sim, 'has developed in the context of an increasing politicisation of law and order and recurring crime control crisis' (1998: 27). This also relates to a current attitude whereby crime is regarded as an inevitability which must be dealt with rather than something which should be understood. In a society where concern about crime supersedes worries over illness and job security,[1] CCTV is presented by its propagators as something of a miracle solution in the fight against crime. It can also be viewed as composite to wider technological advancements in all spheres of contemporary life which some authors argue has led to a society of mass surveillance (Lyon 1994, Davies 1996, Graham 1996). Consistent with this is the view that the proliferation and ready acceptance of CCTV is not due to its perceived effectiveness as a crime-control measure but relates more to its place as a technological solution in a technological age (Bottoms and Wiles 1994).

The principal objectives of CCTV in relation to crime control have been identified as detection, prevention and fear reduction (Bennet and Gelsthorpe 1996). It is also considered a central element in the revival of city-centre leisure spaces where the aim is to increase usage via the creation of public spaces which are safe and accessible for all social groups (Oc and Tiesdell 1997). However, there is considerable debate relating to the effectiveness of CCTV in terms of deterrence and crime-reduction: numerous studies have indicated its effectiveness to differing degrees but most stress that its success is not as straightforward as its supporters would have us believe (Brown 1995, Short and Ditton 1996, Ditton *et al.* 1999, Tilley 1993, Short and Ditton 1998). Those concerned with evaluating the effectiveness of CCTV conclude that it 'sometimes "works" and sometimes doesn't', and that this is dependent on specific contexts and locational conditions (Ditton *et al.* 1999). Even if CCTV could be hailed as an undisputed success, evidence suggests that it is much less effective in preventing crimes of an interpersonal nature such as assault and street robbery where camera coverage is more likely to be used as evidence (Brown 1995). This raises questions as to the usefulness of camera surveillance in relation to public-order offences and interpersonal violence and leads us to question its effectiveness when considering women's interpersonal safety. Furthermore, even when CCTV appears to be successful, the main worry is that crime may have been displaced to other locations, something which in terms of research is methodologically difficult to determine.

Attitudes towards CCTV

One of the most striking things about CCTV is the public's relatively 'benign' acceptance of its burgeoning usage. The public in other European countries is much less supportive of the surveillance of public space by cameras (Reeve 1998). This is in contrast to the UK, where CCTV appears to have been 'readily accepted' as a necessary measure in the 'fight against crime'. According to Norris and Armstrong (1999), this is due to a number of interacting and diverse factors from the western world's preoccupation with surveillance which originates from the time of the Cold War. In addition the use of CCTV complements the law-and-order discourse which developed in the 1980s and has since been adopted by all the political parties.[2]

As well as broader political trends, isolated catalytic events have contributed to the exponential growth and somewhat unquestioning public support for CCTV. For example, the part which it played in connection with a number of 'high-profile' incidents such as the murder of James Bulger and the IRA bombing of Harrods has led to its mass acceptance as a crime-control mechanism within the public's consciousness.

Numerous studies indicate a high level of public support or at least a low level of objection towards CCTV (Honess and Charman 1992, Bennet and Gelsthorpe 1996). Honess and Charman's (1992) research into CCTV in specific locations found that between 85 and 92 per cent of respondents surveyed in three separate sites welcomed the installation of CCTV. When asked about its effectiveness 74 per cent believed it to be effective in detecting crime, 62 per cent felt it to be effective in preventing crime and 63 per cent felt it would make people feel safer. Other findings demonstrate similar levels of support. A study in Glasgow found that 95 per cent of those asked were in favour of CCTV in Glasgow city centre. A study in Airdrie found that 89 per cent of respondents felt CCTV would reduce crime (Ditton and Short 1998). Honess and Charman (1992) conclude that, although people view CCTV positively (concern over civil liberties is low and estimations of effectiveness are high), these views are mediated via a limited knowledge of the complete mechanisms and full potential of CCTV. According to Ditton (1998), high levels of public support as demonstrated by survey research are problematic and can be explained by methodological flaws where the contextual positioning of survey questions affects the responses given. For example, if someone is asked if they support the use of CCTV directly after being asked about concern over crime, they are more likely to respond favourably to CCTV.

CCTV: civil liberties and the state

Grim prophecies of a dystopian vision relating to both the present and the long-term implications of mass surveillance and a 'big brother' totalitarian state have been outlined by various authors (Norris and Armstrong 1999, Lyon 1994, Graham 1998, Fyfe and Bannister 1996, Coleman and Sim 1998). Closed-circuit television and other forms of surveillance represent an actual and potential means of extreme intrusion into the lives of individuals whereby civil liberties are severely infringed upon. This point relates to the emergence of a pervasive 'surveillance society' within late modernity (Lyon 1994). This is not just about surveillance in relation to crime control; it also relates to computer surveillance by the state and other organisations. Rapid advancements within the field of information technology have resulted in a vast expansion in the collection, storage and monitoring of information on individuals. Although it is significantly different in form from other surveillance mechanisms, it can be argued that CCTV is potentially a key element within the burgeoning surveillance society (Graham 1998, Lyon 1994).

The power of the state is also reinforced by the reorganisation of crime-control to include decentralised organisations such as local authorities and private business, of which CCTV is a part. This can be understood using Foucault's notion of the 'dispersal of discipline' – whereby discipline and surveillance are administered and carried out not by a unitary monolithic state apparatus but by a variety of institutions acting within specific contexts at specific times. Crime-control has been extended to local and non-state agencies, and this has extended the power of the state in what McCahill (1998) terms the 'responsibilisation strategy'. CCTV is a central element in this strategy in the way in which it is the government who initially presents it as a measure for crime control, but it is the multi-agency crime partnerships who are responsible for running the actual systems. The dispersal of control, however, is not at the expense of the state, who can now 'govern at a distance', and centralised government becomes 'more powerful then before, with an extended capacity for action and influence' (Garland 1996, cited in McCahill 1998). According to Norris and Armstrong (1998), CCTV is the 'interface' between public and private policing, where it is controlled and operated by decentralised crime-and-disorder partnerships but is utilised by the police as part of its crime-control strategy.

Indeed, developments in criminal-justice policy and new modes of policing indicate that the power of the state has not diminished as a result of decentralisation; police powers have been increased, punitive policy has been extended and policing has become more aggressive and militarised (Fyfe and Bannister 1996). CCTV is a central and complementary device within these new modes of social control, yet it also stands alone as an autonomous mechanism which works for the state but not as a direct part of it.

CCTV and spatial exclusion

CCTV also plays a central role in the attempted revival of urban shopping centres by retailers and local authorities (Oc and Tiesdell 1998). The objective has been to promote increased usage of these public spaces, which have been in decline as a result of negative images of crime and urban decay (Fyfe and Bannister 1996). The assumption is that enhanced feelings of well-being will promote enhanced usage of these spaces for shopping and other leisure activities, where 'public space is being reconstituted, not as an arena for democratic interaction, but as a site of mass consumption' (Norris and Armstrong 1999: 8). This increased use of town and city centres as spaces of consumption is obviously good news for business and commercial interests whose principal aim is profit. Those social groups however, who do not possess the appropriate economic and cultural resources required to partici-pate within this 'lifestyle' of consumption will be excluded from such spaces. CCTV is the mechanism by which commercial businesses and town-centre management can regulate who occupies public space.

According to Fyfe and Bannister, surveillance plays an active role in the sanitisation of public space, where social groups classed as 'undesirables', such as the homeless, the unemployed, ethnic minorities and the young, can be effectively removed to make space more 'comfortable' for those who can afford to 'occupy' such spaces. Norris and Armstrong (1999) found in their research that exclusionary practices and attitudes were held by the operators of CCTV towards certain social groups. They report how operators regularly used racist language to refer to ethnic minorities whose very presence within public space rendered them automatically under suspicion. In addition the presence of certain other groups was also viewed as objectionable, not because of criminal activity but merely because they did not adhere to personas and behaviours deemed suitable within public space.

> The concept of 'otherness' is intimately bound up with views as to the appropriate use of social space and who has a right to do what in the city centre. In County Town, for instance, one group that was continuously surveilled was the town centre drunks – not because they caused any trouble but because their activities did not accord with the appropriate use of town centre space.
>
> (Norris and Armstrong 1999: 141)

This removal and regulation of 'unwanted others' from public spaces, in order that they may be enjoyed by the more affluent and socially desirable members of society, is a working reality in the city of Los Angeles (Flusty 1994, Davis 1990, Graham and Marvin 1996). Within this American city public space is no longer freely accessible to all; instead it is made up of different zones where the rich are 'protected' from the poor by walls and barriers. These 'urban fortresses' are defended by CCTV, which ensures that the poor are excluded and that they do not trespass into the spaces of the rich. Clearly CCTV is much more than a device for crime-control where it predicates much wider factors in relation to how power is administered and diffused within society and who has the right to occupy public space.

Even when we consider CCTV purely within a crime-control framework, it is still problematic. CCTV is positioned within an approach which constructs crime as a phenomenon of public space; in addition to this, previous research appears to indicate that cameras are most effective against property crime rather than crimes against the person. Consequently these factors render CCTV problematic as a device which could be of any real worth in relation to women's safety.

Young women: leisure, space, time and CCTV

'Action Risk'

Drawing on the findings from the 'Action Risk' research, it is to the everyday reality of young women and the problematics of CCTV that we will now turn.

We will discuss, first, the young women's perception of how risky their locality is and how this effected their access to space, and, second, the young women's perception of the use of CCTV. Semi-structured interviews and photography were used as research methods to gain insight into how the young women perceived their locality. This enabled them to show their locality as they see and experience it. They were asked to go into their community in friendship pairs and to take photographs of spaces that they considered being safe or dangerous. Once the photographs were developed they wrote comments on each photograph explaining why they had taken it. All photographs included in this text will show the young women's original quotes. The use of photography was particularly useful as a research method, as many of the young women were uncomfortable with traditional textual means of documentation. In considering the role risk has to play in the young women's lives and how this comes to affect their use of leisure space-time, all the young women involved in the research often presented risk as an organising principle (Bunton *et al.* 1997) of their daily experiences. That is, the young women suggest they encounter and need to manage risk on a daily basis and that this can come to determine their use of space within their own town as well as having a role in determining their other daily experiences.

Sample one: young women attending the centre-based youth club

Most of the young women thought that their locality was a dangerous place to live. They generally considered 'outside' public space to be dangerous, but portrayed 'inside' private spaces as safe. Indeed, when asked where they feel safe the girls always listed indoor spaces such as home, the women's centre, the youth club and the police station. The girls had an overwhelming and predominant fear of what might happen to them in outside spaces. This fear was particularly apparent when discussing evenings, a time which they considered to be their time for leisure. They linked this with the presence of 'dangerous men'. These dangerous men were often portrayed as men out of control in that the men's dangerous desires were a result of drug-taking, excessive alcohol consumption and uncontrollable sexual urges. These 'dangerous' men were described as maniacs, perverts, nutters, stalkers, flashers, dirty men, mucky men, paedophiles, drunken men, smack heads and druggies. They repeatedly expressed their real fears of being kidnapped, raped, murdered, flashed at and grabbed. These dangerous men were perceived to be unpredictable, which brought about uncertainty and heightened the sense of risk. Outside spaces with the physical characteristics of darkness and enclosure predominately featured in their photographs (see Figure 15.1). Badly lit spaces, boarded-up houses, alleys, a tunnel to the supermarket, parks and bushes were all perceived as potential hiding and

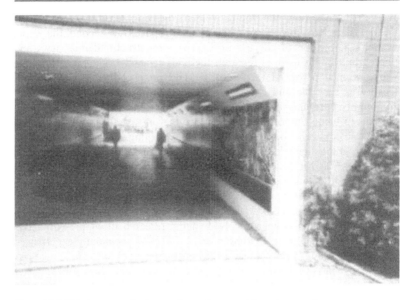

Figure 15.1 This is not a safe place to hang about at night – the tunnel

entrapment spaces. It is not an unimportant fact that many of these spaces were on routes between the girls' homes and other places they considered to be safe. Figure 15.2 shows that a tunnel leading to the only supermarket in the community was considered to be unsafe.

The effect on access to outside leisure time and space

At worst the young women felt incapacitated by their fears and anxieties which involved not going out at all on an evening.

> I'll go to my nana's after school but most of the time just go in 'cause you don't feel safe hanging around the streets. (aged 13)

> I think we should play inside instead of outside. Just in case somebody's around there, like dirty men. (aged 11)

Other young women suggested that they do play out in the evening but always stay close to home as it was too risky to venture further afield. What became evident when working with these young women was that, when asked if this knowledge came from direct experience, the majority suggested that knowledge of dangerous and safe spaces was gained from informal and formal

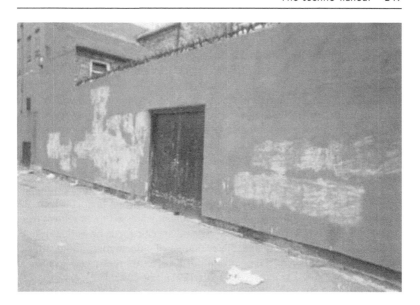

Figure 15.2 It is in the alley. It is dangerous because someone might grab you

communication networks. The girls often blurred media reports with their own experiences.

> And they were saying [the newspapers] there was em an old man and if he walked by me he always, he gets you and he kills you and all that, that's what they were saying . . . I won't go there again. (aged 12)

They recounted reports of terrible happenings in the locality gained through local gossip, from life stories of mothers, aunts, grandmothers and from the media.

> It's what people have told me and I've read it in books and newspapers and heard it on the news. (aged 11)

> Erm like my mam used to like go outside and she got raped and that by men that she didn't even know. (aged 12)

> Yes it's like, like my friend Jackie said that erm when her mam was little . . . her friend got raped and she went and tell someone and they didn't believe her, wouldn't phone the police or 'owt so like that's dangerous. (aged 14)

And they don't take you seriously [the police] or nowt. (aged 14)

Two of the girls talked about their own experience of being flashed at more than once and even though it was reported to the police they suggested that nothing came of the matter. Youth workers also told similar stories of children being flashed at near to the youth club, saying that the police never take them seriously. The British Crime Survey does not produce figures for this type of incident even though, as Burgess (1998) suggests it is a widespread and common experience in public space.

Sexual violence in particular by its very nature has marked effects upon women and their perceptions of public space (Gordon *et al.* 1980, Riger and Gordon 1981; Stanko 1987). According to Valentine (1992), women's apprehension of public spaces is heightened by various factors which she identifies as: parental fears about sexual danger expressed to daughters from a young age; the media's over-reporting and specific focus on violent crimes and rape in public places; and the exchange of information about attacks via friends and relatives. These are important factors that cause women to perceive public space as dangerous space (Valentine 1992).

The girls also talk about being harassed on the streets by staring males. It is these crimes that tend to be invisible to the naked eye, often go unreported and are often trivialised as harmless. For example, when asked, *Do you ever get stared at then and followed or anything like that by other people?*, two young women replied:

B   Just by the workies.
    Where compound was . . . I walk past through the day by myself. They stood there whispering at me, he was going, Oi blondie.
A   They just shout at you, they don't do nowt.
B   They doesn't hurt you, they just walk by, don't they.
A   Yes, they're harmless because like they're older men . . . Yes, they're bored. (aged 13 and 14)

The real fears and anxieties felt by these young women lead them to rely passively on outer surveillance rather than develop their own mechanisms autonomously. Their information is mostly mediated from informal and formal networks. As reflected in the workshops run with the young women, their knowledge on issues such as rape, alcohol, sex and drugs was very vague. This most definitely blurs the way they perceive and manage risk. They tend to use strategies that over-compensate for their heightened sense of risk, or fear of risk. They perceived technological surveillance and Neighbourhood Watch as very good, for they could make their locality a safer place. All of these girls suggest that there should be more CCTV cameras.

The cameras . . . yes there should be one next to each other. (aged 13)

Everywhere else you can think of. (aged 11)

However, the girls reported that the cameras alone would not increase their confidence as they dislike the anonymity of the watchers. They suggested that they would like to see real people patrolling the streets so that they would know who was watching out for them.

> You don't know what's going to happen to you outside but you know when you're inside you're safe and you don't, and you know who's looking after me and that. (aged 12)

> They should have cameras and that and, er, people who walk around the streets, like security guards making sure you're all right and everything. (aged 12)

> Safe places and more cam, there's been cameras put all over and more and . . . yes, and the police walking about all the time. (aged 11)

> We should have a more better place but with all the dirty men going round killing people there should be, the police should be doing something. (aged 13)

The girls were also unsure as to whether or not the CCTV worked, and there- fore it did not increase their social and spatial mobility. They suggested that community-design projects should also take their fears into account when designing areas.

> Erm, it's not [the CCTV camera], it's norm, normally like you know on the drugs street and, erm . . . I think like they should like try and like, you know build, something for us to like go on and then talk about stuff like that. (aged 11)

Darke (1996) suggests that negative identification with public spaces is further exacerbated by the masculine characteristics of the physical environ- ment, constructed on male usage patterns which transmit the message that 'the city belongs to men'. In addition, poor lighting, overgrown foliage and poorly designed public areas do not lend themselves easily to public surveillance and so can render that space problematic (Jacobs 1967, Newman 1972). Similarly, the young women believed that the bushes around Townsville should be eliminated as they restrict the view of CCTV cameras and are places of risk (see Figure 15.3). The young women were greatly offended and anxious about these spaces, as for them it portrayed a lack of social control and lack of ownership of public space.

Many of the young women attending the centre limited themselves to

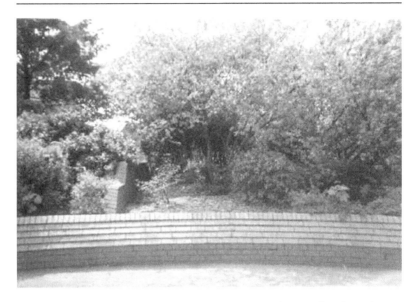

Figure 15.3 The bush is dangerous because someone will grab you, stalkers hang about here

indoor activities thereby reinforcing gender stereotypes and reducing their opportunity to develop their skills needed in the 'outside' world. As Pearce (1996) suggests, girls' access to specific spaces is limited, girls are often found to use 'inside' spaces and this can be of detriment to their psychological and social well-being, as they are often excluded from developing certain skills needed when accessing outside spaces.

When asked what they do and where they go in their leisure time, most of the girls said they 'stay in', listen to music, play board games, practise time-tables, clean up, baby-sit or dress up in each other's bedrooms. For these girls the increasing presence of overt methods of surveillance (CCTV) paradoxically is to them evidence that it is not safe for them to go out as they suggested that they felt safer indoors. This became evident in their photographs: for example Figure 15.1 showed the tunnel to the supermarket as unsafe, yet also the young women took photos of this space as having a CCTV camera present, which they viewed as a good point. However, the CCTV presence did not quell their anxieties about passing through the tunnel (see Figure 15.4).

Their distrust in the cameras and lack of information about how CCTV works limited its enabling capacity. There is also a tendency to blame women if they are attacked in places considered dangerous and where it is felt that they should not have been in the first place. Consequently women tend to

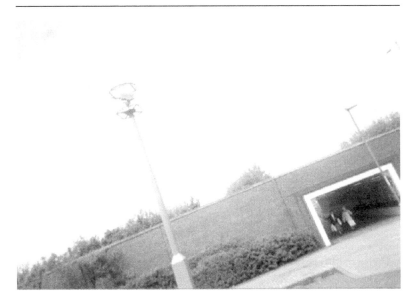

Figure 15.4 Good point because of security cameras – near tunnel

associate risk with places where attacks could occur rather than with the men who would attack them (Valentine 1989). Conventional crime-prevention literature reinforces these notions as it advises women to avoid certain places and therefore encourages their restricted movement through public space (Painter 1992, Stanko 1991, Yeandle and Morrell 1994, Valentine 1989). Women are advised to stay at home after dark, avoid certain places and be aware of their environment (Yeandle and Morrell 1994). In this way safety strategies are a double-edged sword in that advice aimed at preventing victimisation results in generating more fear and encouraging women's exclusion from public space (Stanko 1991). These centre-based young women played 'inside', identified as 'good respectable girls', attended baby-sitting courses, cooked, cleaned and generally prepared themselves for their future role that they referred to as a 'good mother'.

Sample two: girls 'hanging out'

The girls from sample two suggest that the CCTV cameras are intrusive and have developed strategies to deal with them. They argue that money and resources should be spent on catching the real perpetrators of crime and there should be facilities that recognise their own needs, desires and fears as young responsible women. For these young women who participated in the research, public space in the form of the street was a key arena for acting out of their daily routines and leisure experiences. In general, they were more confident than sample one and did not perceive the locality as dangerous. They considered being outside to be an everyday learning experience, which is more empowering than the centre-based club environment. They hung out in the evening and felt that knowledge gained through this experience enabled them to have greater spatial mobility than other young women.

> You learn where to go and where not to go . . . people make the danger their selves. (aged 16)

The street is traditionally envisaged as a space which presents more risk for women, especially in the evening. A lack of facilities and opportunities for leisure often led to some young women occupying the street as a meeting place. The street, however, can also become a site of conflict, as adults can feel that young people are threatening. Yet the young women also said that they perceive the street as a site imbued with intimidation and risk for themselves, especially when they are alone.

> Our presence annoys people not what we do. (aged 15)

> You can see them looking you up and down like . . . you know, like they expect you to go home like good girls. (aged 15)

> It's like the older people ain't it . . . like they're waiting for you to do sommat. (aged 16).

These conflicts therefore bring with them contradictions, as adults express a fear of gatherings of young people on the street, yet the young women themselves felt unsafe on the streets and seek to manage this through staying in groups.

They felt that they are often the target of the CCTV cameras, but do not see how this is justified and develop strategies to overcome what they see as a voyeuristic intrusion. They suggested that the technological surveillance or the way that it is put to use perpetuated the crimes.

> We're just outside having a laugh and that, it's the ones inside selling the drugs they [the police] want to get . . . they never do nothing. (aged 16)

> They just watch you [the CCTV cameras]. (aged 14)

> Yer, they watch you and nothing happens, 'cause. (aged 15)

> We were all drinking, weren't we. (aged 16)

We had about three cameras on us and everything like that, no there was about five in the end. (aged 15)

They were coming from the next town, weren't they. (aged 16)

Yer, but nothing happened, nothing at all. (aged 15)

When the police come, you know when they are gonna come, don't you, it's like when the lasers come on you know so long after they're gonna come so you move on. (aged 16)

So you just move along a bit more. (aged 15)

It's not surprising they get smashed and that like . . . yer like they're asking for trouble . (aged 16)

Discussion: CCTV and women's safety

Previous research indicates that women are likely to view CCTV more positively than men (Honess and Charman 1992, Bennet and Gelsthorpe 1996). Bennet and Gelsthorpe (1996) found strong support for CCTV amongst female respondents. Overall 64 per cent of the sample thought it was a good idea, but women were more likely than men to be in favour of it (Bennet and Gelsthorpe 1996). Women also expressed being more worried about interpersonal crimes such as assault and harassment, which it could be argued CCTV has little effect upon. However their research indicated a strong correlation between feeling vulnerable on the streets and being in favour of CCTV. A significant number of people also said that they would be more likely to use the town centre at night if CCTV was installed (22 per cent). Females were more likely to express this view (29 per cent of women compared to 15 per cent of men).

Interestingly within both our own research and the above research, when CCTV was rated against other measures it ranked lower than increased police patrols and better street lighting. This seems surprising when one considers the widespread support expressed for CCTV. One possible reason identified by the young women we researched with was a preference for an actual 'human' presence in the form of police patrols rather than the anonymous camera. It also appears that young women preferred to be able to see any potential attackers for themselves rather than have the cameras see for them; they therefore feel safer as a result of enhanced street lighting. Similarly our own research indicated strong support for CCTV with a strong correlation between high fear levels and being in favour of CCTV. Where women were more likely to be in favour of it, they demonstrated higher fear levels. Bennet and Gelsthorpe (1996) argue that CCTV should not be treated as the 'panacea' to women's fear of public space but as more of a 'welcome addition to their existing armoury of devices and tactics which they use for protection' (Bennet and Gelsthorpe 1996: 89). The study concludes with a strong statement of support for CCTV as a means of reviving urban centres:

> CCTV is potentially capable of providing a sense of protection. In the absence of any attempt to tackle people's fears of public places there is a danger that they will stay away from these areas and city centres will spiral into decline. The installation of CCTV cameras may be one way of encouraging continued use of these areas
>
> (Bennet and Gelsthorpe 1996: 89)

However, the above study views crime as a wholly public 'problem'. This does not reflect the true reality of women's experiences, where violence is more likely to occur within the private sphere (Hanmer and Saunders 1984, Stanko 1987, 1995).

CCTV may encourage women to feel safer within public space but, even where danger is presented primarily within this context, the effectiveness of CCTV is still questionable. Our own feminist approach to victimisation reveals a wider range of male behaviours which makes space uncomfortable for women but which are invisible to conventional 'malestream' criminological and crime-control discourses in what Kelly and Radford (1996) term the 'continuum of sexual violence'. This is not only as a result of their experience of victimisation and their fear of crime; it also encompasses a variety of other more subtle male behaviours as identified by the young women in our research. Consequently the value of CCTV in relation to women's safety must be reassessed as a separate issue from that of CCTV and crime-control more generally. There is a tendency to sound universalistic when one talks of women's fear of violence and public space. However, in relation to gendered violence and fear of crime, similarities between women are significant enough to risk the proposition that women 'as a group' fear violence in public spaces to differing degrees. The threat of men's violence, and more specifically, of sexual violence, acts as a frequent constraint on women's lives. Of course it must be acknowledged that men fear and are victims of violence also; however, the prevalence of women as victims of men means that it is a gendered phenomenon.

Although women are 'encouraged' to fear public spaces and the strangers who inhabit them, numerous studies have revealed that the domain where women face more physical and sexual danger is within the private sphere of the home amongst known others (Hanmer and Saunders 1984, Stanko 1987, Stanko 1991). This leads us to question the effectiveness and use of CCTV to ensure women's safety on the streets. We do not want to downplay incidents of physical and sexual violence which occur against women in public space, but these are isolated acts which are exaggerated. In public settings such as the street, women are more likely to experience routine harassment such as staring and name-calling – the type of behaviour which in all likelihood would be rendered invisible to CCTV cameras but which still violates women's occupation of public space.

Now I see you now I don't

According to Coleman and Sim (1998), the approach to crime-control of which CCTV is part emphasises the risks associated with public space, ignoring the less obvious private dangers as well as more 'subtle' forms of harassment which take place within public spaces. This originates from the ability of the dominant masculine crime-control discourses to define what counts as risk and danger and to define the social settings which represent potential risks to the safety of individuals. However, research has found that, even where behaviour transgresses 'subtler' forms of harassment and it is obvious to CCTV operators that a woman has been attacked or suffered physical abuse, male operators do not take incidents seriously. According to Norris and Armstrong (1999) public incidents of domestic violence were treated with amusement rather than concern and CCTV operators demonstrated attitudes towards domestic violence similar to those within police occupational culture. The authors found that the 'protectional gaze' of the camera in relation to women was virtually non-existent. Lesser acts of violence perpetrated between men appeared to arouse more action from operators; women stimulated more interest as sexualised objects of the voyeuristic 'male gaze'.

> CCTV also fosters a male gaze in the more conventional and voyeuristic sense, with it's pan-tilt and zoom facilities the thighs and cleavages of the scantily clad are an easy target for those male operators so motivated. Indeed, 10 per cent of all targeted surveillances on women, and 15 per cent of operator initiated surveillance were for apparently voyeuristic reasons outnumbering protective surveillance by 5 to 1.
>
> (Norris and Armstrong 1998: 129)

Our own experience of the CCTV centre we visited reinforced the above findings. A distinct lack of protective concerns and voyeuristic tendencies towards women amongst male CCTV operators was also apparent within our own research. Our findings demonstrate that, although female operators displayed an acknowledgement of the subject's right to privacy and were unwilling to 'zoom in' on individuals for no apparent reason, male operators were more than willing to do so. The two male operators, when asked to put the camera on the street where one young woman lived, zoomed in as close as the camera eye could get following the young girl's mother down the street. The mother was followed at close range from just inside the front door step of her home and out of her garden into the street. The camera viewed her up and down whilst cajoling with youngsters as she walked to the local shop and back to buy a pint of milk. The male operators showed off their skill further on other unlikely suspects as the session went on. The following session we arrived at the centre to find there were two female operators: when asked if they would zoom in on someone a young woman recognised, they refused blankly as it would break privacy laws. Also female operators expressed a much more protective concern for the well-being of young women on the streets at night where they recalled how they would 'follow' at a distance women late at night after nightclub closing time to make sure they were safe. They suggested that male operators also followed women but insinuated that this was for different reasons. Again this is consistent with Norris and Armstrong's (1999) research where female operators appeared to take more of an active interest in women.

According to Brown (1998), it is necessary to assess CCTV from a gendered perspective which questions its value as a community-safety initiative and its relevance for women's safety. She correctly asserts that the installation of cameras in town-centre consumer spaces was fuelled by commercial interests and private enterprise rather than a concern 'to improve public safety, or more specifically women's safety' (*ibid.*: 217). In addition the potentially voyeuristic gaze of the 'electronic eye' could supplant any use CCTV may have in relation to women's safety and merely serve to reiterate the surveillance of women in general.

> Our studies of the gendering of town centre spaces suggest that CCTV, which is essentially a tool of *surveillance*, is likely to be of limited benefit to women. They are already subjected to policing by male attitudes and behaviour; they already police themselves by avoidance behaviour . . . It is not so much a question of whether CCTV can improve women's safety, as one of whether CCTV relates to the ways in which women are made to feel insecure.
>
> (Brown 1998: 217)

Concluding remarks

We would argue that CCTV represents a heightened manifestation of the male gaze with technological advancements allowing men to put women under surveillance yet again as the sexualised 'other'. Indeed, the additional mechanisms of CCTV allow the voyeuristic and sexual nature of the gaze to be further intensified. CCTV may promise to reduce crime and provide enhanced feelings of safety: however, when one deconstructs the nature of public crime using gender, it becomes apparent that CCTV is of little use in relation to women's personal safety and sense of well-being in public space. As argued by Burgess (1998), the argument is based on the premise that what is perceived to be risky or dangerous is real in its consequences. The young women's own perceptions of public space are not just upon on the structural design of spaces. Importantly, their perceptions are premised upon real feelings, fears and anxieties, depending upon where they are situated in the locality. It is our belief that an understanding of the subjective nature in which young women come to negotiate their use of public space is crucial for policy-makers, planners and CCTV operators. Those in authority might seek to impose their own definitions and understandings of female life space upon them which is situated in gendered discourses of power/knowledge and desire. Their understanding of where for example, is dangerous, where cameras should be situated, what constitutes suspicious behaviour and who should be watched may be invalidated by subjective knowledges and assumptions about an area. As Fiske (1998: 156) suggests, 'technology does not, of itself determine that it *will* be used or *how* it will. Similarly, technology may limit what can or cannot be seen but it does not dictate the way it is watched. Technology may determine what is shown but the social determines what is seen.' In short, the camera may or may not show difference, but who sees it is a function of social and cultural factors and, while the operators may control the tele-scene or real-time images, everyday life continues without them.

Notes

1 *Home Office Anxieties About Crime: Findings from the 1994 British Crime Survey*, Research Study No. 147, Home Office, London, 1995, cited in Coleman and Sim 1998.
2 For a detailed coverage of the 'rise of CCTV' see Norris and Armstrong (1999), chapter two.

Part IV

Policy implications of community informatics

Community informatics, community networks and strategies for flexible networking

Michael Gurstein

Introduction

The 'grand conflict' of our time, it is becoming increasingly evident, is that between the global and the local – between those forces and agencies which are promoting the free-floating rootlessness of capital and trade and those looking to resist this through the strengthening of local culture and local communities.[1]

Opposition to 'globalisation' of markets, of capital and of the rules governing trade emerged into public consciousness in Seattle amid the conflicts around the activities of the World Trade Organisation. But it also includes the strictures of the IMF as an enforcer of open trade and (tariffless) borders; and the actions of globally distributed megacorporations increasingly concentrating wealth and power in fewer and fewer corporate hands. In all of this it has become evident to many that the 'tool' of choice, the 'Force' which is empowering this globalisation, is the invisible flows of digital messages through communications channels and from computer to computer.

Certainly, the history of computing and of computers is intertwined with the development of military communications and with the rise of global systems of management and control. Not for nothing is the primary stream of applied technology known as 'Management Information Systems'. The central design objective of most traditional applied information-technology research has been to extend the power and reach of management to co-ordinate production and distribution organisation-wide, then nationally and now globally.

There were early attempts, as we will note below, to provide computing opportunities (and thus access to management and control capacity that might follow) to other groups in society. However, it remained for the development first of low cost 'personal' computers (that is, computers that could be used and afforded by the general public) and then the Internet (which wedded the information management power of low cost computing with low cost communications capabilities) to make available widely and 'locally' opportunities which previously had been accessible only to the wealthy and powerful.

Globalisation and local communities

Globalisation 'hollows out' local communities. More highly valued, more knowledge-intensive activities are centralised. An artificial specialisation is forced on to the local economy. Local production has to compete globally on the basis of wage rates, benefits and taxes. Communities become ever more subject to external forces over which they have little or no control.

As the globalised economy shifts into higher levels of technology, the need for capital increases, while the supply of capital available for local investment is stagnant or in decline. The life or death of local economies becomes simply a by-product of what many are terming the 'casino economy', where a few are big winners but most are losers. The result is local decline through the centralisation of financial and public servicing, the introduction of very large stores in retailing, the increasing emphasis on research (capital) intensive processing and production and similar processes. Whole regions, including their communities and residents, become expendable in relation to these overwhelming global forces.

The 'local' by contrast with the 'globalised' is where enterprises and activities respond to the issues, conditions and future needs of the local community. Local enterprises, which share the fate and future of the local community, are likely for the most part to be more sensitive to local requirements and conditions than a branch plant or subsidiary of a transnational with its headquarters in some distant city or even distant country.

ICTs may support local communities as they attempt remote or distributed self-management. Decentralised computing capacity linked to a communications capacity allows for work to be done from any networked remote location. There is an opportunity for remote access to skills and training. The playing field for technology-oriented education and training is being levelled. One intriguing possibility is that, in the future, information-intensive public-sector activities could be decentralised in order to equalise employment opportunities between rural and urban areas (Dienes and Gurstein 1998).

The character of the functionalities supported by ICTs presents significant opportunities and even advantages to local communities. At the least, these functionalities reduce barriers of distance and location, giving argument to the inevitability of metropolitanisation as a necessary accompaniment of the widespread introduction of ICTs. But these characteristics also include distance-insensitivity: that is, information distributed by ICTs does not for the most part reflect the condition of its physical location.

In this context, local information can have the same status and sophistication in its treatment when managed and controlled locally as part of a network, as when it is centrally managed and controlled. This presents the opportunity for local ownership and management of local information; the opportunity to work or act on or to participate in information-intensive activities at a distance; the capacity to take advantage of local nuance, accent or timbre in the processing of information and of products; and the means to take advantage of economies of disaggregation, the synergies of distributed production networks and the flexibility of small-scale distributed management and control. For small communities, this can mean access to markets and suppliers, to information providers and to others for mutual support and the possibility of competing effectively if remotely with globalised producers (Gurstein 1998).

The very rapid growth in Internet-enabled activism and local organising, particularly around such areas as the anti-WTO protests and with the Indymedia (Independent Media) developments,[2] suggests some of the other directions in which distributed opportunities for information-management and information control may develop. Local groups can emerge, inspired by the activities of others in distant places but with common concerns and common goals. Information can be shared seamlessly back and forth and in individual locales. Local concerns and local resources can supplement and complement the broader frameworks and add strength both through numbers and through technical and other speciality contributions to the overall project.

Indymedia for example, relies on software developed jointly by an Australian and a US software developer each working in electronic collaboration but physically separated from each other. The software, which is available for free download from the Net, is now being used in some thirty independent sites in ten or so countries (at last count), and all of this developed in less than one year. In this way individual 'nodes' (local sites) can work independently while levering the entire network of interdependent local information-processing centres and inter-communicating hubs. The network is open to everyone, but participation is through the individual nodes where local rules of participation are developed and enforced.

Community informatics and community networks: enabling communities with information and communications technologies

Community networks or community networking are ways to develop and control locally based information systems to support local development. Community informatics (CI) is the 'science' or methodology by which such processes may be implemented and can provide direction and support for achieving such effects as local empowerment through the management and use of local systems.[3]

CI is concerned with the design and development of 'community' information systems and community networks which, in parallel to 'management' information systems (MIS), look to provide the tools to realise local interests, objectives and responsibilities. CI provides methodologies for those in communities looking to use the technology to manage local processes and to participate in global processes. Not infrequently of late, those local processes are in opposition to or even in direct conflict with globalised and remotely managed technology and economic activities.

The methods of CI draw from a range of sources and inspirations. On the one hand they draw on long traditions within applied technology and technology theory; on the other hand they draw on insights from community research from anthropology, sociology or other social sciences. But CI also draws on ethical traditions of equity and inclusion, of community efficacy and of distributed control. The ultimate tests of its theories of course, are in their practice not their elegance, and methods are pragmatic and syncretic, concerned with understanding input means and output measures.

Where MIS empowers and enables managers and particularly corporate managers to extend the power and practice of increasingly globalised corporate structures, community networking and CI are looking to enable local communities. They are developing the means and the capacity to counter the typically hierarchical processes of large-scale organisations. In this they are using technology systems and particularly networking capacity to support the management of local activities and to create mutually supportive networks of efforts whose functioning acts to distribute control rather than centralise it (Gurstein 1999).

Manuel Castells[4] sees this approach to community networking as being a basis of opposition to globalisation. CI, determining the means for enabling community processes with ICTs, is thus developing the pragmatics and the theories to extend and to realise this while providing the methodological underpinning to the variety of community processes made possible – community development, e-health, e-culture, e-government and e-politics and not least e-exchange and e-commerce.[5]

Community networking is a common organisational strategy for grounding a local framework of computing within a local community.[6] Included within these strategies and mirroring the directions taken by MIS but using lower-cost technology, and freeware or shareware are such applications as computer-supported community work, that is, managing locally based computing as a support to collaborative community-based activities.

In many cases the Internet has come to be a central element in areas of social development and particularly in social advocacy. Those involved with this are developing innovative Internet-based approaches and even applications, which are resulting in lower costs and increased scope. Also there is activity at the community level to develop and implement strategies for bridging the 'digital divide' (Gurstein 2000b). It is the extension of individual empowerment through computing access which develops the real power of local computing by integrating individuals into local structures of computing and community (and of community computing).

There are multiple and parallel applications which arise in the community as computing facilities are made available. These include the opportunity for the community to take possession (and ownership) of its own 'memories' and particularly the outputs of its own culture and language. Thus, as the larger forces of globalisation are increasingly looking to capture broader and broader swathes of culture and knowledge as intellectual property protected by rules of copyright and patent, communities in turn can use the technologies to preserve, capture and exert ownership over the results of local cultural development, production, history and knowledge (Turk and Trees 2000).

Also of critical importance is local and community empowerment in the area of health and well-being, community tele-health and tele-medicine. Having access to Internet-based information and remotely based but Internet-delivered medical or health services will significantly enhance the health care available locally in remote or underserved areas and support the development of local processes of health-care management. Through the combination of remote service and support and local management and delivery, local health care can be improved and individuals can develop increased responsibility for managing their and their communities' health (Dienes and Gurstein 1999).

User-friendly interfaces and ever more sophisticated database management software are allowing geographic information systems to have a significant role in supporting communities to exert democratic control over local physical and socio-economic resources. By displaying and processing data in graphic and map-based forms, even the least literate of citizens can understand and begin to act upon patterns of resource distribution (and mal-distribution), environmental issues, matters of health epidemiology and so on (Krouk *et al.* 2000).

Finally, those with highly developed technical skills and a social-activist perspective have been involved in the free software movement and open source developments such as Linux. The significance of free software, shareware or open source software for community-technology initiatives is in part that many community initiatives use these software platforms and products because of cost and to a degree because of a belief that there is a shared set of broader social values.[7]

Background: history

The ancestors

Of course, community or citizen technology has a history and even a pre-history. Among the earliest ancestors was what became known as community memory. Lee Felsenstein, one of the founders of community memory, discussed this in an interview as follows:

> by 1970 I knew that broadcast media were never going to serve the cause of decentralisation of power within society . . . In August of 1973 we were able to try an idea proposed by Efrem Lipkin and placed terminals in

public places (a record store in Berkeley, followed by a branch of the SF Public Library) which people could use as a bulletin board. We called it 'Community Memory'.

What happened was that an agora[8] appeared, with an unknowable number of different needs, desires, suggestions, proposals, offers, statements, poems and declarations cropping up. The researchers, who had expected only a few categories of classified-ad items, were amazed at the discovery. It became clear that the crucial element was the fact that people could walk up to the terminals and use them hands-on, with no one else interposing their judgement. The computer system was not interposing itself between the individuals who used it, either.

Many a well-financed 'videotex' system has foundered and sunk because the operators would not consider opening the system on a person-to-person basis. People do *not* want to be subjected to centralised information. They *do* want to be able to explore the social space of their surroundings and to ask the question: 'Who's out there?'

It was some of this same spirit of looking to the power of computing as a tool for creating community and distributing access to empowering information which infused the early work in the US Defense Advanced Research Program Administration, although of course, in this case the desire was to distribute the information not to the larger community but rather to a more closed community of researchers and scholars. However, the power of the opportunities which this technology afforded was too great to be kept for use only by a small circle. The community of users of the distributed communications and information management system originally known as DARPANET and eventually the Internet, became available first to universities additional to the initial two or three, and then to additional students and faculty within those institutions. Eventually, as some of these moved on to other places, the facilities became more widely available among the technologically literate population in a number of cities within North America.

It was however, with the development of low-cost personal computers at the beginning of the 1980s that these opportunities began to take off. As computers and computer-to-computer communication became more widely understood and technology for sending and receiving messages from individual personal computers became available, store and forward (bulletin board systems) were established.

At the same time as personal computing was being created by Apple Computers, parallel initiatives allowing for widely decentralised telephone-based text messaging were being developed in Canada with Telidon/Videotex, in the UK with Prestel and in France with Minitel. Each of these technologies in its own way was looking to provide parallel solutions to the problem of linking computer-based text-management with telephone-based switched communications and thus to give widely distributed access to computer messaging and remote information processing. All of these technologies were attempting to provide a new type of computing which was decentralised, requiring much lower skill levels for use and designed for widespread and popular application. Only Minitel, with its backing from the French government and its application as a substitute for the French telephone directories, survived the initial period of launch in anything like a commercial form.

First generation: personal computing leads to community computing

The first generation of community networking grew directly out of the development of personal computing and the desire to provide the opportunities presented by Internet communications to a broader audience beyond universities and commercial organisations or governments. In many cases these grew out of the bulletin boards which had been established by early computer hobbyists as ways of providing messaging services for themselves and their friends. Many of the initial establishments were based on an idealism and principles similar to those already quoted from Lee Felsenstein. This, combined with early 'hacker' ethics of information-sharing and code-sharing and notions that 'information wants to be free', led to the development of freenets where access to Internet facilities was provided to the community by volunteers without charge (Schuler 1996).

Parallel to these operations and particularly in the US, again with the availability of low-cost personal computers, community technology centres were established, which, while not linked to the Internet, were designed to provide upgrading and skills training for low-income and minority populations in US urban areas (Miller 2000).

Second generation: community computing matures

The first and pioneering generation of popular computing led to the establishment of a network of freenets and then community nets throughout North America and in western Europe. With the advent of the widespread recognition of the functionality and power of the Internet, governments throughout the developed world began to look at ways of ensuring the broadest base of access to the technology as a way of ensuring a 'wired' citizenry and an educated labour force and as a market for electronic-based commercial and governmental services. These programmes – in Canada the Community Access Program,[9] in the US statewide programmes such as Missouri Express[10] and others – brought low-cost connectivity to relatively rural and remote areas and, in Canada at least, provided a basis for a national 'connectivity' strategy.

At the same time, however, the cost of Internet access was declining dramatically and the role of the community nets as local Internet service providers was being undercut. Parallel with this, commercial community networks (really commercial World Wide Web portals with some local news facilities) were developing. Often developed as franchises (Microsoft was one such franchisee) and frequently linked to local news outlets (for which the local news was re-purposed), these 'community portals' flourished as stock-market-driven 'dotcoms' for a period, but most have now disappeared or become simply another in a huge volume of local portals competing for a limited 'clickthrough' local e-commerce traffic.[11]

In Europe public authorities at the same time were in the process of sponsoring 'civic networks' which had partially overlapping objectives to the North American community nets but were very much more enmeshed in formal local government and political discourse (de Cindio 2000). These civic networks (the best-known of which was the DigitalStaat or digital city in Amsterdam) have been having their own difficulties as the civic authorities, who were in most cases the sponsors, have decided, now that the Internet has become so successful, to take direct responsibility for the civic Internet presence. This has meant that the funding for a number of these civic networks has been curtailed, and some, such as the Amsterdam network, having first attempted to become private corporations but not having found this to be financially feasible, have now closed.

Third generation: getting down to business

While the immediate and most visible of the community-based technology initiatives with community networks and freenets now find themselves in financial trouble as their revenue base in providing Internet services has disappeared, the base of alternative community-based technology initiatives has expanded and broadened. These initiatives cover a very wide range, including local e-commerce, community-learning networks, local e-health, local electronically enabled social development (digital divide), local advocacy or e-democracy, local e-government and local e-culture initiatives.

Developments in each of these areas and the prospect of in effect unlimited and virtually free local bandwidth, with broad-band communication in developed countries and through satellites in developing countries, present enormous potential for local initiatives and empowerment through the use of the technology. How and whether these opportunities will be developed still very much remain to be determined, but the opportunity locally to create, manage and distribute information in a context where information is becoming the most valuable economic resource is rapidly becoming available.

In addition, the means for peer-to-peer communication and exchange and, not incidentally, commercial exchange – as, for example, between communities but bypassing middle persons and circumventing the inter-mediary and frequently coercive powers of the state – is equally coming available. Of course, with these opportunities go commensurate risks: the loss by the state of tax revenue (and thus its capacity to support public and social services), and of its ability to ensure fair rules of transaction, for example.

Using new technology to build a new community: strategies for local development

In addition to theorists who have extrapolated the positive and negative visions of technological change, there is a growing community of individuals and organisations who are actively working to create workable applications for local users. Community networks, community technology centres, community learning networks and a wide range of supporting institutions make up what has been called the community technology sector. These groups aim to create communities with fiscal sustainability and reduced poverty, or opportunities for young people to find satisfying work while staying in rural homes, or finding ways of assisting small local businesses to compete effectively with global enterprises. They value principles of community economic development, looking for opportunities where there is a significant degree of local control of the economy, of development and of growth (Gurstein 1996, Gurstein and Dienes 1998).

Organisations are using the new technologies to support local economic development in the following ways:

- ICT *enables* local residents to do the activities they have always done better, faster, more cheaply or more efficiently, thus maintaining their competitive position in the larger economic context.
- ICT is a *resource* for new social and commercial enterprises, new styles of development and new initiatives, doing things at the local level which have not been done before as a base for local economic advance.
- ICT is a means to link into larger *networks* where the local economic activity might not be sustainable and effective when undertaken in a fragmented or piecemeal way.

ICT as an enabler of local development

The Net also has immediate use in equalising access to information and external resources. Individuals living in remote locations now have an easier time accessing government and other information. Development agencies that work directly with communities can assist clients to conduct more complete job searches online, or access education and training materials. For the most part, however, these applications are simply replacing an old medium (telephone or print) with a new one that's a bit faster or less expensive. The basic strategy for development remains the same.

ICT as a resource for new kinds of development

Many organisations have emerged to translate new opportunities presented by
ICTs into significant local development. Some are existing community
resource centres often linked to universities, colleges and economic development agencies. But a major new influence in this area has come from the
community-technology 'movement' – specifically, community networks and
community access technology centres which have developed out of the
volunteer sector. Of the latter, while each is locally based and community-
driven, community-technology organisations have nevertheless built a
significant 'grid' of dial-up and walk-in Internet resources across North
America.

While many community networks and access sites have worked on
development in the broad cultural and educational sense, a growing number
are looking at development in a new light. They have built on the provision of
raw 'access' to technology by translating this access into opportunity for
enterprise growth or development. Community enterprise centres have
emerged to address the specific technology needs of very small businesses,
and to facilitate development by acting as a training resource or a business
incubation facility for new, high-tech enterprises.[12]

Perhaps the most interesting developments are those where the technology
is being used directly in service delivery, as for example in providing online
support for medical and psychological conditions; the development of
electronically enabled 'communities of practice' (as supplements to or
alternative support communities for professional activities); or the use of
web strategies as hubs for consolidating and redistributing information and
resources to the voluntary sector (also of course, within the private sector).
The role that ICTs are playing and can play in transforming the base of
opportunities for those who had previously been marginalised because of
location or income differentials is now being actively explored (Schon *et al.*
1998, Gurstein 2000).

Networking as a strategy for ICT-based development

Whether traditional development organisations or newly established
community-technology centres, the most successful strategies for ICT-based
development involve networks. This meaning of the word 'networks' doesn't
simply refer to a network of computers but rather to the process of linking
people to people with the aid of computers – combining the technology
resources with local capabilities in flexible, creative structures.

New types of networked small enterprises, both public and private, are able
to take advantage of the synergies of scale and of intra-organisational
linkages (ease of communications, common administrative systems, creation
of common organisational cultures) which had previously been available only

within larger corporations or other organisational forms. Some examples include the creation of 'virtual cities' or 'smart regions' which are networks of linked enterprises, both public- and private-sector, working together towards common objectives and, for some purposes at least, presenting a common face to the outside world. In the private sector this leads for example, to targeting new markets for local products, and creating highly resilient small-run production or small-scale information-industry companies among others. This in turn can lead to the realisation of what are emerging as economies of 'disaggregation', in contrast to economies of scale, where enterprises can have the best of both worlds – the advantages of the scale of larger firms while still maintaining the flexibility and independence of the smaller enterprise.

New types of networked organisations, structured for example as hubs and multiple self-sufficient nodes, may be created to strengthen each of the members collectively. Collaborative specialisation, information-dispersal and multiple or distributed ownership, decentralised and horizontal support structures, and a high degree of local self-sufficiency (and thus structural redundancy or survivability) characterises these new organisations. These structures allow for a speed of adaptation, highly efficient (low-friction) horizontal rather than vertical information flow, and the economies of mutual rather than functional support. Client or end-user needs can be met more directly, both geographically and culturally, creating powerful and globally competitive marketing opportunities (Gurstein 1999, 1999a).

This in turn would map on to the strengths and competitive advantages of local enterprise and development efforts. Highly adaptive responses to external economic, social and political conditions would help those locally to evolve towards information intensity, increasing complexity and functional elaboration while integrating clients or users directly into dispersed supplier and producer chains. The resulting disintermediation between user and supplier is precisely what many are predicting as the organisational model of the future marketplace.[13]

Towards flexible networking and local development

The concepts described above aren't unique to technology-based development. In fact, the idea of 'flexible business networks', current in small-business management circles, is very relevant. Flexible networks are groups of firms (or, in this case, community organisations) which work together to achieve something any one member of the network couldn't achieve alone.

The most easily understood form of this type of arrangement is the flexible *manufacturing* network, in which small firms collaborate to make a single finished product. A maker of chairs agrees to buy lumber from a small woodcut owner, for instance. Between the two of them, each may have more secure markets and supplies, giving the small business the benefits of a vertically integrated firm.[14]

It is harder to explain how flexible business networks (as opposed to flexible manufacturing networks) are of benefit. Flexible business networks are informal groupings of enterprises that share information, contacts and resources. Sometimes, two or more members of the network may collaborate on a project. But often the formal relationship ends at the completion of the contract, and the two enterprises return to being colleagues but not business partners.

The famous example of the value of flexible business networks is in northern Italy. In the Emilia-Romagna region, a number of very small furniture, ceramic, textile and metalworking firms have organised as flexible networks. During the 1980s, after implementing the flexible-business-network idea formally, these firms grew rapidly. The region changed from one of the most stagnant to one of the most prosperous economies in Italy.[15]

In applying the lessons of flexible business and manufacturing networks to local economic development, one observation stands out. The success of small enterprises may have less to do with the availability of capital (as is often the implicit assumption in economic development strategies) and more to do with access to the right kinds of information, training and marketing support for their products.

A virtual (electronic) network could be established in this way, which for practical purposes would function as a 'virtual enterprise' and take advantage of the very real changes in operational functionalities which the technology affords. A virtual firm could optimise the advantages of ICTs: distance-insensitivity, local ownership of local information and the lower-cost structure of distributed rural or small-centre locations. New types of networked enterprises could take advantage of network synergies.

From flexible networking to community power: ICT and distributed networking

A significant new opportunity is presented by ICT through the formation of online networks for distributed social, economic and political organisation and development. The capacity of the technology to allow for continuous communication, work-sharing, remote administration and management, seamless presentation and co-ordination of multiple centres as a single presence to the world is only beginning to be explored as a basis for community action.

The notion of 'flexible networking' is one which has been widely researched in the context of regional economics and particularly the phenomenon known as 'Third Italy', but has been only implicitly applied to broader issues of local or community 'networking'.

This approach emphasises co-ordination of production based on optimis-ation of selective advantages within the network, and the use of the larger-scale capacities of the network to undertake more elaborate activities. Both of these lend themselves to application in the variety of areas of community enablement through ICT including e-health and e-culture.

This could be a major source of opportunity and strength for local communities which previously had been restricted in the range of their activities by limitations in scale, access to skills and the advantages which arise from specialisation. Thus, a flexible network can draw advantages both from the specifics of particular geographic locales and from the economies and efficiencies of scale as a component of a larger network of local and independent actors.

It would in principle be possible to establish or to extend a virtual (electronic) network that could for practical purposes function as a virtual enterprise or an extended networked virtual city including a number of smaller localities interacting and co-ordinating with each other through horizontal electronic communications. Such extended electronic 'localities' could take advantage of the very real changes in the operational function-alities that the technology affords. These include allowing for the locale to function so as to optimise the advantages of ICTs including the lower-cost structure and flexibility of response of distributed locations.

The successful projects in this case share a common strategy. They expand the resources and information available by collaborating with related efforts at the local, regional or international level. They participate in 'flexible networks' of one form or another.

The idea that business or non-profit organisations would collaborate on issues of mutual interest is not new. The concept of flexible networks, however, is more than a simple joint venture. In the community technology sector, effective participation in a network often means the ability to identify and join the networks that are likely to be useful, in advance of the need. This is different from joining a networked 'coalition' which responds to a crisis.

These new types of networked organisations are structured as hubs and multiple self-sufficient nodes with collaborative specialisations, information dispersal and multiple or distributed creation and ownership of information. They have decentralised and horizontal support structures, and a high degree of local self-sufficiency. With this, of course, goes a speed of adaptation and of information-flow horizontally rather than vertically, and economies of mutual rather than functional support. Add to this the opportunity to adapt responses closer to the precipitating events both geographically and culturally and this can be highly 'competitive' in larger, even global contexts (responses to the actions of global corporations or multilateral institutions such as the WTO are examples of this).

The opportunity to develop locally based structures and organisations which can act as a counter-force to the centralising and globalising forces of neo-liberalism is significant. It should be noted that we are talking of new and local foci of power, which are not necessarily structured in relation to centralised systems of power. This is leading to 'networked' power, where power is available in distributed nodes, linked electronically and capable of working in concentrated, cohesive and co-ordinated fashion where necessary (as for example when dealing with larger-scale issues) but where there need not be such cohesion or co-ordination when it is no longer necessary (as for example when responding to issues of local concern).

All of this, of course, would be mapping on to the strengths and competitive advantages of the existing communities in local areas and providing highly adaptive responses to external economic conditions while helping local communities to evolve towards increasing information-intensity, increasing sophistication of existing markets, increasing complexity and elaboration and being able to integrate directly into dispersed decision-making structures. The resulting disintermediation between 'user' and 'supplier', citizen and the 'state', is precisely what many are predicting as being the organisational model responding to the Internet-enabled polity of the immediate future.

The model: using ICT for local development through flexible networking

In examining the possible application of the concept and techniques of 'flexible networks' to the linking of community sites as virtual IT action networks, it is necessary to make a number of assumptions about the opportunities which flexible networks present.

Assumptions

First, in synergy there is strength. It is evident that, for example, there is neither the skill nor the population base for the development of a 'home-grown' IT-based activity centre in a single centre in rural Nova Scotia. The population base is too scattered and the density both of residents and of resources is too low for there to be the base for such a development. On the other hand, if one is looking not simply at the catchment for a single community site but rather at the network of these sites either regionally or for some purposes even nationally, then both the skill and capacity base would be sufficient to support significant actions and organisations in a 'virtual' format. Thus, where the unit of development of organisational structuring is the network rather than the individual sites or nodes, there is the potential for significant synergies as between the sites and within the network – including being able to optimise the skills and information of the various parts of the network in support of the response to the needs in a specific situation.

Second, the local node is a focal point of the action or activity – even while the 'network' is the basis for the virtual structuring and presentation of the virtual 'enterprise'. It is at the local node or individual site that an activity is likely to take place. The local node will be a place where experimentation and innovation may happen.

Third, ICT is the enabler of the model: without ICT the type of co-ordinated action which is envisaged for the network would hardly be feasible. In fact it is the availability of low-cost communication, of widely distributed electronic access to information, of widely distributed electronic access to training and support, the capacity for action at a distance and ICT-enabled remote management and administration which supports the possibility of a distributed or flexible network of community sites working together to become a 'distributed' but co-ordinated IT enterprise or activity centre.

Fourth, the model may work at multiple levels of network aggregation, that is locally, sub-regionally, regionally, nationally and globally. That is, a very local network can be aggregated electronically into a region. The individual nodes can be linked electronically into other nodes externally for specific actions or activities; or the regions can function as individual nodes for some purposes and have their activities linked into and co-ordinated with other 'regions' and so on up to national or global and globally co-ordinated networking.

The multiple nodes of public access

In the communities network there will of course be multiple nodes. These nodes will provide access to opportunities for participation by those without linkages to external resources and in this way be the means for many to enter into the broad range of political action and participation. There will, however, in the model presented continue to be local 'ownership' and direction of the node based on the notion of local control over the individual community site or node. The effect of this will be quite intense com-munication within each node and between nodes, since they will be linked laterally rather than vertically, the notion being that there will be the development of plans and strategies locally along with local management and administration of local resources and local marketing and local entrepreneurship.

Mediation and support of public access

Even (or especially) with the local control of local nodes there will be the need for trained mediators between the technology (information) and the end-user. These will act as guides or interpreters of the use of the technology for the specialised purpose to which it is being applied as well as providing technical support, training, information 'brokerage' and selection or interpretation.

The generative core (multiple cores or hubs)

There will also be the need for a 'generative core' or hub to handle a number of specialised and skill- or resource-intensive functions. Only by chance might there be a local capacity to undertake effective action at the level of the individual node. In some instances, with planning and over time it may be possible to develop certain of these functions in one or another of the individual nodes but it will be necessary to proceed with the network based on the hub and nodes model in advance of this arising. The hub then would provide specialised skills, a support or leadership role to nodes or network, standard setting and quality control, network maintenance and support, network resource management and administration; innovation support and research and development; network marketing; network-wide entre-preneurship; and external relations with extra-regional, national and international linkages.[16]

The overall impact of this could be quite dramatic in supporting the revitalisation of local communities and resistance to the various local incursions from corporate globalisation. It could also provide a means for generating locally skill-intensive employment opportunities, a resource and skill base for local ICT development and support for the upgrading of the quality of local public and other services.

Some thoughts on outstanding 'research' issues

What then are the outstanding issues in the area of community informatics, which in turn will support the position of local communities in their attempts to resist and develop local power and citizenship in the face of the almost overwhelming forces of globalisation?

Access, inclusion and the digital divide

There have in recent times been a very large number of discussions concerning access and particularly what is perceived as the 'digital divide', that is the gap between those with the means to use the technology (physical access, training, infrastructure and so on) and those who lack this. However, issues as to why a 'digital divide' might be of concern – and particularly what the access to the technology, once achieved, would be used for – are much less frequently addressed.

In the context of the discussion above, it should be clear that the issue of access and of the digital divide might more properly be seen as one of having access to the means to the personal empowerment which the technology affords and particularly access to these as means for participating in local and community empowerment. Thus access is not simply about having the means to use a computer or the Internet; rather it is about having the means to use a computer or the Internet to participate in the processes of local empowerment and citizenship.

Access then becomes not a process of enabling one-way access to the means of consumption but in furnishing the skills and opportunities for two-way communications as the basis for effective local (and global) citizenship.

Sustainability

The major challenge confronting local community-technology installations worldwide, whether they are community networks, telecentres, community-based health initiatives and so on, is the question of how they can survive financially, that is be 'sustainable' in the longer term.

This question should be seen in a larger context. First, of course, there is the issue of what precisely might be meant by 'sustainability'. The use of ICTs involves an ongoing cost whether to a corporation, a community or an individual. There is the cost of the equipment and amortising the ongoing maintenance and replacement of the equipment, both what is directly used and the infrastructure which supports the communications capability. This means that there is a recurrent cost for technical usage, and in the case of community applications or access points there is also likely to be the cost for employees, trainers or support workers, for a physical site to support the access point and for management.

The issue of sustainability to a community is how it can generate the funds to pay for these ongoing charges or, alternatively, how the facility can generate enough funds to maintain itself. Notice of course, that the two previous formulations differ in quite significant ways and have quite significantly different implications with respect to the issue of 'sustainability'. If the facility is seen as providing community service then the ongoing sustainability can be understood within the context of the ongoing sustainability of other community services such as schools, health facilities and so on and can be drawn from whatever sources (taxes, grants in aid and so on) are supporting those services.

However, if the facility is seen as only providing a service to specific individual users, then the model of sustainability must necessarily be one of identifying individual revenue sources (fees for service) and immediately puts the facility into the context of a market-driven mechanism.

If, as we have been arguing, this facility is a necessary component of capacity development for local citizenship, that is of maintaining a local empowerment, then clearly we must look at the issue of sustainability in the first context. The aim of the research then becomes identifying the manner in which the facility can become sufficiently and visibly embedded in the community so that it is recognised for what it is, a necessary component for community survival. Doing this, of course, requires the development of strategies and applications which link the facility directly into other and necessary community processes and involves determining how to use the technology as the basis for more effective and efficient organisational management.

Training and diffusion

Key to the broad use of the technology is the availability of training and strategies for technology-diffusion. Much of the attention to date, perhaps because of the links to the 'digital divide', has been on providing 'sensitisation' or training on how to use the Internet. This, of course, provides only the most basic of skills and knowledge.

If, however, one looks on use of ICTs within communities as a basic prerequisite for contemporary citizenship, then the question should be how to train effectively for digital 'citizenship' rather than simply for access or use, that is as a digital consumer. In this context there is the need to identify what the elements of 'digital citizenship' might be, that is the minimum requirements for the citizen to be able to participate effectively in the digital sphere as a user or creator. This approach suggests that training and diffusion of ICTs within communities should be towards facilitating active participation in specific application areas rather than simply opening up the opportunity for passive use.

The future

The obvious and profound changes in ICTs have transformed the nature of public affairs. Technology change has made globalisation possible. However, the technology also provides the means for very low-cost information distribution, remote accessing and information-processing, distributed goods production, direct delivery of the variety of information-intensive services and universally accessible and globally distributed electronic commerce. These resources are increasingly available through non-fixed-link networks, such as satellite or cellular communication. All of these could support localised development as easily as 'globalised' concentration: this presents the intriguing possibility that people in rural and remote areas could have access and information control capabilities equal to those in a large metropolis. (In theory, it matters little if the electronic 'storefront' is physically in a city or in a very remote place.)

However, ICT should not be seen as inevitably leading to local development, or even that it is a necessary 'ally' of such efforts. Rather, ICTs can be seen as a two-edged sword. On the one hand, it slices away the barriers to the free flow of jobs and capital and locally anchored economic well-being. On the other hand, it provides a resource for the local, the individual seeking a local livelihood in a home town or a community looking for a new means of survival as its traditional economic base declines.

The vision of the 'information society' has largely been a dream of the 'winners': wired condos in the sky, high-tech communications between the suburban semi-castle and the Caribbean island time-share, wired cities speeding the commerce of the rich and bringing enlightenment and education to everyone else. The real applications of the technology – how it would actually work in the 'local' economy, what the new 'wired world' might look like for those who will not necessarily be its beneficiaries – has been left largely unexplored.

The promise of the microcomputer, however, is the promise of decentralisation. A concentration of computing power and the supporting technical resources characterised the mainframe era. Personal computers allow for enormously powerful yet decentralised computing not only for those who can afford specialised technical support but also for local and rural users. Commentators have repeatedly noted the potential for local (and individual) empowerment arising from the personal computer revolution.

And, of course, the torrent of technologies is not stopping. We have the prospect of effectively unlimited communications capacity with broadband and of completely mobile communications with wireless. We have the prospects of 'ubiquitous' computing, that is computing anywhere and everywhere and we have the convergence of media – text, sound, image, motion and eventually smell and touch all available for distribution and manipulation. But even within this cornucopia, there remains the prospect, even the requirement, for physical locale and localisation. There is the need to communicate from and to place, to connect with our physical selves which will always be in 'place' or 'locale' – we need to eat and sleep, to procreate and manage our wastes – and virtuality will have little effect on this. And for each of these to be accomplished effectively and efficiently and even pleasurably we need not only the individual but also the family and the linkages to other families and to the networks within our locale functioning as communities.

Even as the technology rushes forward, it does so by presenting greater and greater opportunities and powers to individuals and to the collectivity that they choose to create. That one of the most fundamental and long-lasting of these collectivities is the community suggests that at least some and perhaps much of the power presented to individuals will in fact become the power of 'citizens' acting within institutions. They have willed these into existence and now they are expected and enabled to reflect what the technologies can ensure – transparency, flexibility, the summative power of networks and networking, and where 'open source' refers to how the major institutions of community operate in their governance superstructures as well as in their technical infrastructure.

In fact, as a prediction, it is likely to be in the zone of interaction between the virtual and the real in communities that the future nexus of power and the recreation of citizenship are likely to reside. Where physical communities are empowered by the global reach of the virtual and where the virtual is empowered by the physical force of the real is the point where the true resistance to the global and the globalising will develop and prevail.

As a further prediction, the attempt to commercialise communities, whether virtual or real, will fail because most of the values and valuable activities within communities are those which are closer to the ethic of the 'gift' and the 'hacker' culture than they are to the commodity cultures of the e-commerce juggernauts. Communities are for the most part about taking collective responsibility for one's environment – whether the physical environment of the land and the sea, the cultural environment of the education of children, the reproduction of ethical systems, the invention and play of art or the virtual environments of communications and vital usable information. Communities are also about exchange and commerce but as an element of re-creation not as the sole objective of the 'enterprise'.

The power in this will come when the force of the virtual empowers the physical and where the 'hi touch' of the physical is reinforced by the 'hi tech' of the virtual.

Notes

1 This characterisation is of course, a gross generalisation. Also, while the forces of 'globalisation' may be evident, those who oppose it are certainly not all 'localists' and while an ideology of globalisation (neo-liberalism) is widely articulated, not least by the spokespersons for such agencies as the World Trade Organization, the International Monetary Fund and the World Economic Forum (Davos), no clear positive alternative position has yet emerged around which there is a consensus among globalisation's critics.
2 Cf. http://www.indymedia.org.
3 For an introduction and overview of Community Informatics see Gurstein (2000b) and Loader *et al.* (2000).
4 In a verbal presentation to the First Global Community Networking Congress, Barcelona Spain, 30 October 2000.
5 Gurstein (2000c).
6 See, for example, Schuler (1996).
7 Much of the discussion on these issues takes place in the context of specialised e-lists such as 'Linux Without Borders' or on websites such as http://www. slashdot.org.
8 The term 'agora' is often used in discussions of electronic democracy as a way of designating public (electronic) discussion space. It is even one of Excite's analytical web categories. Cf. http://www.mckinley.com/lifestyle/cultures_and_ groups/citizenship/electronic_agora/; or http://www.valdosta.edu/~rbarnett/phi/ phicyber/; or http://www.cci.wmin.ac.uk/HRC/manifesto/hmm.18.html.
9 http://cnet.unb.ca/cap/.
10 http://extension.missouri.edu/moexpress/.
11 Gurstein (2000c).
12 For a description of one such centre see Gurstein (2000a).
13 This seems to be what Castells was referring to when he talked of local information producers such as Community Networks or the Zapatistas as providing the new and networked base of resistance to globalisation; cf. Castells (1997).

14 Adapted from Gurstein (1999b).
15 See Piore and Sable (1984) on the highly successful flexible networking approaches to production as found in Emilia Romagna in northern Italy.
16 An example of what is being referred to here can be seen at Gurstein (2000a).

Chapter 17

Cultivating society's civic intelligence

Patterns for a new 'world brain'

Doug Schuler

Societies are, and will always be, shaped among by social actors, mobilised around interests, ideas, and values, in an open conflictive process.

Manuel Castells (1998)

Technological ambush?

In a recent issue of *Wired Magazine*, consummate computing pioneer Bill Joy (2000) unveiled a trio of apocalyptic scenarios that he believes could be unleashed in the not-too-distant future. These unpleasantries, resulting from unrestrained, unprincipled and unregulated genetic engineering, nano-technology and robotics (GNR), can be added to the list of big nightmares of the twentieth century, such as environmental disasters and nuclear and bacteriological warfare, which may yet plague us. Each of these technologies, according to Joy, could abruptly unleash problems on so vast and unprecedented a scale that any of humankind's responses would be completely overwhelmed. That such a notable 'priest' had so seriously challenged the central teachings of the technological (and economic) church was not missed by the US media, where the story was featured on the front page of the *New York Times* and other prominent newspapers.

Ironically, computers are at the forefront of the problems Joy describes; without them those catastrophes would be inconceivable. Computers, in fact, are the only indispensable element in each of the three problems. Joy's scenarios centre on technological development outstripping humankind's ability to control it. Our 'fail-safe point' may have been passed according to Joy. A variant on Malthusian predictions (much disparaged but impossible to disprove) may be finally bearing the bitter fruit that Malthus foresaw. The planet's burgeoning population and its deteriorating environmental condition, coupled with humankind's propensity towards disagreement and strife, its disregard for nature and its penchant for exploiting its innermost secrets, may provide an ideal set of preconditions for a sudden and profound technological ambush.

Joy, of course, is not alone in his warnings. Indeed, our era could be characterised as the age of such warnings. Many scientists have documented the monumental changes that humankind is currently loosing upon the natural environment. In another recent article scientists concluded that the human-originated changes currently being wrought on the planet have attained the magnitude of a geological force (Karl and Trenberth 1999). Nobody knows the consequences of ignoring these changes. Yet it is a matter of obvious importance to the inhabitants – human and otherwise – of the earth. A cavalier disregard may be catastrophic.

Anticipating and possibly averting ecological and other nightmares would likely require changes to our ways of thinking and acting; changes which, depending on their scope and severity, are likely to be extremely difficult to enact. People are loath to change habits developed, cultivated, and rationalised over a lifetime. Humankind, similarly, is unlikely to modify cherished habits to avert problems of the future based on contested evidence of new circumstances, especially ones that may not seem to appropriate to their lives.

Joy's predictions border on the apocalyptic; in his mind human extinction within a generation is possible. Assuming that his predictions have even a germ of possibility, the obvious question is what can be done to understand the situation, avert potential disasters and develop a more sustainable relationship with our social and natural environments. The equally important but less obvious issue is identifying the underlying conditions that would help make even a partial resolution of the problems become conceivable. This chapter is an attempt at describing these conditions and how the idea of a 'civic intelligence' might play a useful role.

The world brain and other utopian visions

Joy's concerns, and others like his, were formerly found only in science fiction, for it is in that genre that technological and social possibilities are most creatively explored. For that reason I would like to invoke the memory of H. G. Wells, the English science-fiction writer, historian, generalist, and visionary, who did not live to see the Internet or other recent technological achievements. Wells was not just a science-fiction writer who integrated technological scenarios with social issues and outcomes; he was also a historian who searched for broad historical patterns: 'I dislike isolated events and disconnected details' (Wells 1971). Wells was also deeply concerned about the human condition and devoted considerable thought to the prospects of enlightened social amelioration. He discussed, for example, in the 1930s a number of collective problems that would become increasingly apparent in the following seventy or so years (including environmental problems and weapons of mass destruction).

Wells believed that there was a 'conspicuous ineffectiveness of modern knowledge and . . . trained and studied thought in contemporary affairs'. As a collective body, we are failing to address collective problems in spite of immense individual talent and specialised knowledge. In his quest for possible antidotes, he dismisses all types of ideologies and religions as unsuitable. He also rejected rule by 'some sort of *élite*, in which the man of science and the technician will play a dominating part'. Bill Joy, of course, would be a member of such a group, even though that group is responsible to some degree as the perpetrator of the challenges that Joy warns about. Wells places his faith in '*science*' and not '*men of science*'. Science in his view should 'enlighten and animate our politics and determine the course of the world'. To this end he asks, 'Is there any way of implementing knowledge for ready and universal effect?' His answer is a *world encyclopaedia* which would provide an intellectual backbone for the human race, a 'world brain' which 'would do just what our scattered and disoriented intellectual organisations of today fall short of doing. It would hold the world together mentally.'

Wells placed his faith in the establishment of a world encyclopaedia, a single artefact packaged as a series of bound volumes which would apparently be so *accurate*, that people would have little choice but to make the right collective decisions based on diligent study. Unfortunately very few people could afford to purchase this set of volumes and fewer still would read them in their entirety and absorb the knowledge therein. Nor are the existence of facts tantamount to the existence of 'objective' interpretations of the facts or obvious policies or courses of *action* based on those facts. 'Facts' have meaning only when *interpreted* and they have power only when they have consequences. Without saying so directly, Wells suggests that society becomes more 'intelligent' by making its citizenry more mindful of the facts.

Perhaps the most ambitious project along these lines was the one proposed by the German philosopher Leibniz. Leibniz was an advocate for artificial intelligence some three hundred years before its inception. Leibniz conceived of an invention that would be a type of artificial patriarch, almost a god. He immodestly proclaimed in 1679 that his

> invention uses reason in its entirety and is, in addition, a judge of controversies, an interpreter of notions, a balance of probabilities, a compass which will guide us over the ocean of experiences, an inventory of all things, a table of thoughts, a microscope for scrutinising present things, a telescope for predicting distant things, a general calculus, and innocent magic, a non-chimerical Cabal, a script which all will read in their own language; and even a language which one will be able to learn in a few weeks, and which will soon be accepted amidst the world.

The system had two extremely powerful components: a universal representation system, and a universal calculus for ratiocinating over the facts in the system's vast information stores. Leibniz anticipates Joy's concerns but, unlike Joy, appears to be an uncritical promoter of at least the particular manifestation that he envisions. He presupposes that some type of ultra-rational system could actually be constructed and that it could – and would – be used for decision-making that was best for all; the idea that the system could be somehow subverted or *misused* was not considered.

History indeed has furnished us with a host of projects that would enlighten us in some near-mechanical fashion. These include Bacon's House of Solomon and Otlet's Office of Documentation and Palais Mondial. Some years earlier, in 1888, the prominent American pragmatist John Dewey also believed that what was wrong with society was a failure of intelligence and information. Dewey, along with support from Franklin Ford, a financial journalist planned to offer his own version of a 'world brain' in the form of a weekly newspaper entitled *Thought News*. This ill-fated idea was universally panned and Dewey and Franklin failed to produce a single issue.

The projects unravel before they begin

Schemes such as those advanced by the visionaries above always fall short of their utopian objectives; they usually fail to recognise one or more funda-mental barriers that stand in the way. Their projects are often disconnected from social realities. Some of the projects, Wells's world encyclopaedia, for example, would depend on the ability to mobilise large numbers of people in the development of some single artefact. On top of that, there is little or no social or cultural desire demonstrated for the product, or evidence that it would be used at all, much less with the utopian results envisioned by the encyclopaedia's prime advocate.

What many visionaries fail to notice is that a grand idea, however obvious to the perpetrator as a 'solution', must be coherently embedded in a system of *existing* social forces, institutions and conceptualisations. While we will later discuss some ideas for a 'world brain' that avoids the undoings of the other utopian projects, we will first examine two additional arguments why establishing a 'world brain' or other utopian scheme is difficult.

The 'impossibility' of democracy

The co-operation of the people is likely to be necessary for any required changes in our techniques for addressing the problems that Joy and others have presented. Co-operation that is willingly embraced through non-coercive means is more reliable and more easily sustained. For those reasons, it appears that *democracy* in one form or another may be necessary. In addition, the potential reach and malleability of the Internet and other new communication technologies further suggest that it may be possible to devise applications, services and institutions within the evolving world-communication network that would support and strengthen these democratic approaches. Communi-cation, certainly, is key to any effective democratic system. Projects along these, while reminiscent of Wells's world-brain visions, would need to be more aligned with the preconditions that support conceptual and technological innovation if they are to be used and useful.

Democracy, as nearly everybody knows, is highly flawed in practice: the wrong people can become elected for the wrong reasons and do the wrong things once in office. Candidates can be favoured for their tousled hair, their dimpled smile, their lineage and the slogan *du jour*. Once in power, elected officials may acquiesce to special interests (Greider 1993) or be undermined through media-induced scandal (Castells 1998). Running for office (in the US) is so costly that only the very rich have any chance of getting elected. (The New York State Senate race will probably cost over one hundred million dollars.) The role of the media, lobbyists, rich patrons, professional public relations campaigns and dirty tricks further frustrate any attempt to understand or to participate meaningfully in the 'democratic process'.

The task of collective self-rule – democracy – has been called an impossible task. Indeed, its impossibility can even be 'proved', in much the same way that engineers had 'proved' that bee flight is impossible. The task of democracy – if it's done remotely well (so the story goes) – is so exacting, so all-encompassing, yet so frustrating and ultimately unpredictable, that it's been called an 'impossible' enterprise. Walter Lippman (1925) in particular, was sceptical of the idea of an 'omnicompetent' citizen who possesses sufficient knowledge to participate effectively in the political process. Lippman notes that, even though civic affairs was his professional avocation, he was unable to monitor the relevant data, initiatives and ideas that he believed would minimally be necessary for him to sustain competence in this area. To be minimally competent in the area that this chapter addresses, for example, a person should be well acquainted with democratic theory, world systems, communication technology, political economy, public policy, environmentalism and the state of the world and many other topics. Each of these areas is characterised by shifting opinions, initiatives and discourses, in addition to an overabundance of empirical, verifiable data (whose interpretations are then disputed). (Interestingly, as Wells points out, our elected leaders themselves are far from omnicompetent. Their chief skills, campaigning and political manoeuvring, are, in large part, responsible for their success, while their competency in other matters may be under-developed.)

A similar criticism can, of course, be directed towards any elite body, however humanely and well disposed it is towards *governing* the rest of the citizenry. But does Lippman's critique render democracy 'impossible' or merely the idea of 'omnicompetence' and its purported indispensability? I would claim the latter. Reality is unfathomly complex and we are each incapable of 'knowing' even one aspect in its totality. But, impossible or not, democracy or some approximation of democracy is not optional. Decisions have to be made. We have no choice but to cultivate systems of governance that can help us constructively engage with our collective concerns. Lippman's critique is valuable, but not to support the conclusions for which it was originally marshalled. Lippman demonstrates the fallibility of basing a system of governance on the idea of omnicompetency. Indeed, any system of governance should *assume* the impossibility of omnicompetence and the inescapable reality of imperfect competence, while not allowing ourselves to be defeated by it. This means, in software parlance, turning a 'bug' into a 'feature'. It may be, in fact, the impossibility of omnicompetence that makes democracy the *only* viable choice for a system of governance.

Dumbing down the citizen

In the early 1970s Harry Braverman's *Labor and Monopoly Capital* (1974) demonstrated how the process of 'dumbing-down' workers, primarily through severely reducing their on-the-job responsibility, flexibility, and autonomy (often called 'de-skilling'), increases management control and, hence, profits to the advantage of capital. Since we will be soon discussing the idea of civic intelligence we may hypothesise briefly about whether these ideas may also have some applicability outside the workplace. Is it possible that the citizenry is being 'dumbed-down' in similar ways? And, if so, can we 'run the processes in reverse' to undo the damage?

The key to Braverman's analysis is the decomposition of broad workplace responsibilities by management into discrete constituent parts, which are then used to force workers to perform within circumscribed ranges. This process, often in the name of 'efficiency', dramatically lessens the scope and directionality of worker power. How could this process be replicated in realms outside of the workplace? The first responsibility to be jettisoned (as 'outside' their primary work responsibility) in the civic sphere under such a redefinition would be the consideration of issues relating to general social implications. Thus workers and labour unions should focus exclusively on jobs and job security (and not, for instance, the social consequences of the jobs); artists should explore and express their *individual* feelings; scientists and researchers should pursue what is fundable within a narrow, specialised niche – computer science, physics; and other 'technical' disciplines would expel implications of their subject matters from the curriculum, while measuring success purely in terms of monetary return on investment. Citizens of course would spend much of their non-working life shopping, buying items that would maximise their individual comfort and status while keeping the economic machine running at maximum capacity.

This general process removes the 'politics' of labour, leisure, and learning; indeed it naturally results in the 'de-skilling' of the citizen. Economists are the pioneers in this process by adapting and advocating the use of an economic calculus as the sole determinant for all of our decisions. This is the ultimate dumbing-down; it reduces human aspirations and agency to that of a greedy and unthinking automaton. The media 'de-skills' the citizenry in several ways as well, according to a variety of scholars. Castells (1997), for example, shows how the media's fixation with political scandal encourages cynicism and political disengagement on the part of the citizenry. The media often promote 'the spectacle' (Garber, Matlock and Walkowitz 1993) at the expense of the intellectually taxing. The ill-effects of money on the media, politics and elections also further increase the distance between citizens and public affairs (Schuler 2001). Furthermore, Robert Putnam shows convincingly that, at least in the US, the virtually overnight spread of commercial broadcast television has been a primary culprit in the steady degradation of American civic life over the last several decades (1996). One can only wonder what effects this new electronic 'opiate of the masses' will have as it continues its spread on cultures outside the US.

The questions as to whether and to what extent citizen 'de-skilling' has been orchestrated, and by whom, will not be discussed in depth in this chapter (although the transformation of the US from a country of citizens to a country of consumers is certainly an appropriate and provocative topic to contemplate in this regard). It is sufficient to say that civic de-skilling is likely to dampen civic intelligence by influencing the content of issues, and the conditions under which they are placed on the public agenda, and by trivial-ising and polarising discussion and deliberation on important public matters. Certainly each de-skilling step introduces changes in both institutionalisation, the prescribed processes through which actions are advanced and validated, and in conceptualisation of what everyday life entails; each step helps erect ordinary and the extraordinary barriers to civic intelligence.

Who – or *what* – will govern?

If the dire scenarios that Bill Joy describes (or even the less dramatic but no less worrisome, environmental catastrophes that atmospheric and other scientists warn us about) have even a minuscule chance of occurring, an urgent need to consider ways to avert them arises. Since 'solutions' to these problems are likely to be protracted and multi-pronged, and involve large segments of the citizenry, a correspondingly urgent need to analyse the preconditions underlying the development and successful implementation of these 'solutions' also arises. What 'environments' – social and technological – would be hospitable to the satisfactory resolving of these problems? If we could imagine humankind finding better responses to our myriad problems old and new, what circumstances and resources need to be in place and what steps could be taken that would support these new responses? These preconditions and steps we can call 'civic intelligence' or perhaps a 'world brain'.

What choices face us in the design of this 'civic intelligence'? What attributes could it have? One hypothetical expression of 'civic intelligence' would be a massively complex computer system, which would make intelligent decisions on society's behalf. This option would be a twenty-first-century manifestation of Leibniz's dream, a terrifying cybernetic Frankenstein-on-a-chip from the same cupboard of nightmares that Joy opened in his *Wired* article. The limitations of this approach are manifold but are worth briefly mentioning; the impossibility of accurately, adequately and comprehensively representing infinitely complex situations with discrete computer logic comes to mind, as do the problems surrounding the implementation of the decisions. Would police or other armed organisations receive their instructions from such an 'intelligent' system? The problem of the biases and assumptions of the system's creators becoming embodied – for ever? – in such a system is also a sobering and disturbing thought. Imagine an International Monetary Fund (IMF) 'expert system' free to impose economic 'restructuring' on hapless regions according to the arcane theorems of economists!

Other approaches which rely more heavily on intelligence of the non-artificial variety include having a small elite group making the decisions, nobody making decisions (let the 'free market' reign, for example) or a system in which citizens play a strong role. Political scientist, Robert Dahl (1989), suggests that these three systems – dictatorship, anarchy, and democracy as well as 'polyarchy', a hybrid of the others – constitute the entire list of possibilities.

Wells suggested that scientists (at least in his day) would sometimes yearn for a society that would apply their (eminently reasonable) principles and clamour for their leadership, and Lippman believed that an elite group should govern because of the impossibility of omnicompetence. What Lippman didn't acknowledge was that omnicompetence is impossible for small groups as well as for individuals. America's 'best and brightest', for example, engineered America's tragic war with Vietnam. Regardless of the role of an elite, the non-elite citizenry will necessarily also have a strong role to play. If an elite group, for example, devised solutions or sets of solutions, they would then have the thankless and potentially impossible job of 'convincing' (through rational appeal, propaganda or force) the rest of us to accept their jeremiads and prescriptions. A democratic approach, on the other hand, would be to enlist the aid of the citizenry at the onset as part of the overall project. The population or at least a large majority may need to 'buy in' and adopt – without coercion or deception – ideas and actions which would be unacceptable without suitable participation in the process (Pateman 1970) which developed those ideas and actions. A more radically democratic view (and the one that might ultimately be seen as the obvious choice) is that the often neglected, sometimes 'dumbed-down' citizenry might provide the intelligence, creativity, energy and *leadership* that are needed to recognise, formulate and reconcile the problems that we are faced with.

As we have seen, governance shouldn't be entrusted to an omnicompetent elite or an infallible computer system: both are impossible to achieve. Nor should governance blind luck through the fantasy that the status quo and/or the 'free market' will miraculously solve current problems and avert future ones through benign and unanticipated side-effects. A democratic system of governance, then, is the only viable alternative, and civic intelligence that is strongly *democratic* – in spite of the problems previously discussed – shows the greatest promise for an effective and equitable system of governance. This approach increases distribution of creativity and attention while, at the same time, reducing concentration of power away from those people with vested interests in maximising their gain – often short-term – over the gain – often long-term – of the larger population. There is mounting evidence that this democratisation is occurring. As Bill McKibben (2000) points out, the vast majority of Seattle's anti-WTO protesters were demonstrating on behalf of *somebody else*, an impossibility according to *homo economicus*. Keck and Sikkink (1998) report out that 'advocacy networks' often involved individuals advocating policy changes that cannot be easily linked to a rationalist under-standing of their 'interests'.' An effective and equitable system of governance would help promote the creativity of the civic sector which is, as Castells (1997) and others remind us, responsible for launching the major social movements of the last century, including the environmental movement, civil rights movement and women's movement.

Civic intelligence: towards a 'world brain'

Civic intelligence as I propose it, is relatively prosaic: it refers to the ability of humankind to use information and communication in order to engage in collective problem-solving. The term has nothing to do with the metaphysical musings on 'global consciousness', 'hyper-intelligence' and the like which are expected by some to emerge spontaneously at some time in the not too distant future ushered in by global communication networks. Like the 'intelligence' of an individual, civic intelligence is a relative form that can be less or more effective and creative. Thus it can be developed incrementally through human effort; not through sudden inexplicable revolution anticipated by faith or spiritual longing. Civic intelligence extends the notion of social capital (Putnam 2000) to include an agenda, an orientation towards action in addition to one of observation and study.

By transcending the individual, civic intelligence adds another level to the idea of 'intelligence'. Civic intelligence is a form of *collective* intelligence. It is a premise of this chapter that this type of intelligence, probably to a much higher degree than an individual's intelligence, can be improved and made more effective. And how people create, share, and act upon information is crucial to that.

Intelligence implies an orderly process for assessing situations, ranging over possible responses and determining and enacting appropriate actions. It also implies looking into the future in so far as that is possible, and making decisions in the present that will help make future situations advantageous at best, tractable at worst. Another important element of intelligence is the ability to acknowledge changing circumstances and to adapt appropriately. Plans and other templates for action are indispensable; unfortunately they're not infallible.

Intelligence is the latent capability to interpret, respond and survive. Its reference point is human and the seat of intelligence is the human brain. The human brain is, of course, a remarkable organ, one whose complexity is unmatched in natural or human-made products. The brain stores information in the form of memory and in reflexive and habitual patterns of responses. It takes in information about the environment in a variety of forms – from 'low-level' sensory data to highly symbolic and abstract conceptual information. It integrates all of this information, helps to regulate all the systems and functions in its body and is largely responsible for the body's thoughts and actions. Although the brain (and the nervous system) is the organ where thought and decision occurs in the human body, it is certainly not in charge of everything; it can't for example, *decide* to deprive the left foot of nutrients. This contrasts with social systems, which are more *reconfigurable*; at least in theory; the government, for example, can decide to stop funding health care programmes or subsidies to weapon developers. It is also important, for communication in the human body and for our analytic purposes, to realise that, although the collection of systems that constitute the human body (or, even, the brain) is an *integrated whole*, the relationships of its subsystems aren't wholly co-operative; there are conflicting needs and requests that can't all be met. Conflict – and the need to resolve conflict – is crucial in both individual and collective intelligences.

Most of these activities of intelligence are below the level of consciousness, and the decisions that the brain makes are generally habitual and definitely not optimum or *correct* in any sense. ('Correctness' by itself with no implied or explicit criteria is impossible to demonstrate. A 'bad' or 'incorrect' decision in the short run can arguably lead to a much better result in the longer term. But – similarly – better in terms of what? And *when* is the decision evaluated? And how much did a particular decision contribute to a situation?) There is simply too much (or too little) information, information that is misleading or inaccurate, inadequate time for processing information, and under-defined criteria for evaluating decisions to determine whether decisions are 'correct'. 'Muddling through' (Lindblom and Cohen 1979) is not merely an interesting side note but the defining characteristic of any 'intelligent' activity. For that reason, this is a core problem that 'civic intelligence' (or democracy) must contend with. This fact, however, does little to obviate the critical need to improve humankind's ability to evaluate and improve its collective decisions.

Since I am not a brain specialist (or omnicompetent) I am unable to go into great depths relating brain-oriented intelligence to civic or socially oriented intelligence. It would be interesting to see how far others would go with this analogy and where they believe it fails. Certainly there is a rich vein – too rich to be mined here – of work in this area. My assumption is that the metaphor goes only so far and that a too literal interpretation and 'force-fitting' of data into theory (and, perhaps ultimately, into people's consciousness and policy) would be counter-productive. Nevertheless, some additional exploration of issues raised would be useful. One of these issues is the relationships of the individual entities – people, to be less ambiguous – in a 'world brain' to each other. Are some of the individual people less important? What if a person's demise would lead to a better life for everybody else? Should the part be sacrificed for the whole? Also – what degree of autonomy should individuals be granted? Should people be treated as some type of functional unit whose freedom should be curtailed and behaviour routinised, for some greater good? The fact is that society has, in fact, embraced many of these decisions already, through innumerable mechanisms over the millennium. I will be arguing that relaxing some of these mechanisms, the current restrictions on behaviour and roles, and moving us away from both 'rationalised' and traditional constraints, will actually be more 'intelligent' and this reconsideration will help engender a collection of civic information, processes and attitudes that will help society *as a whole* to deal with its collective problems.

I am now prepared to present some preliminary considerations for a new 'world brain' or civic intelligence that is based on and addresses current social and technological realities. Similarly to the approach taken by Leibniz, Dewey and Wells, I am proposing an approach that relies to some degree upon the development and use of appropriate communication and information systems. Of course humankind's communication and information systems are currently undergoing massive changes at the global level. The civic intelligence challenge is to develop programmes, applications and policies that help shape this juggernaut into useful forms. We need to ask in what ways can connecting a huge and potentially unruly and fractious group of people from a multitude of cultures and life circumstances help society as a whole to deal more effectively and equitably with problems and other issues of shared concern.

Patterns for a new 'world brain'

Following the pioneering insights of Christopher Alexander and his colleagues (1977), I am proposing a creation of a set of *patterns* for the development of an improved civic intelligence. This discussion of patterns is tentative and incomplete as it is my first attempt at elaborating these ideas; it is not a 'general theory' of civic intelligence, but an assortment of ideas that, hopefully, can help underpin such a theory at a later date. There are six basic pattern categories in this proposal for increasing civic intelligence. *Orientation* describes the purpose, principles and perspectives that help energise an effective deployment of civic intelligence. *Organisation* refers to the structures, methods and roles by which people engage in civic intelligence. *Engagement* refers to the ways in which civic intelligence is an active force for thought, action and social change. *Intelligence* refers to the ways that civic intelligence lives up to its name. *Products and projects* refers to some of the outcomes, both long-term and incremental, that civic intelligence might produce. *Resources* refers to the types of support that people and institutions engaged in civic intelligence work need. We shall look at these separately.

Orientation

A thriving civic intelligence must stress values that support social and environmental ameliorism while acknowledging and respecting the pragmatic opportunities and challenges of specific circumstances. A central idea of a thriving civic intelligence is that an inclusive democratic mobilisation and strengthening of the civic sector are necessary for the purposes of addressing social inequities, human suffering, environmental devastation and other collective concerns including the social management of technology. Castells (1998) describes how the civic sector has been responsible for initiating the major social movements of our era including civic and human rights, environmentalism, peace and feminism. Margaret Keck and Kathryn Sikkink in their book *Activists Beyond Borders* (1998) state that networks of activists are 'distinguishable' from other players in international, national, regional and local politics 'largely by the centrality of principled ideas or values in motivating their formation'.

Unlike many previous 'utopian' projects that ignored social realities, a realistic approach to cultivating civic intelligence must be more pragmatic by recognising what factors promote innovation and by developing programmes with these in mind. It is also possible to help develop and promote the factors themselves. George Basalla writing in *The Evolution of Technology* (1988) suggests that three preconditions must be present in order for a technological innovation to succeed:

- existing models to extend and build on
- social environment that values the innovation
- intents, skills etc. of innovator.

To these three I would add a fourth: adequate resources for innovator. This fourth factor acknowledges the important role of resources for promoting innovation.

Although the innovations we're considering are primarily social and secondarily technological, Basalla's observations are pertinent. A civic intelligence would help promote social innovation by helping to ensure that these four preconditions were met. Each of these preconditions should be in place for civic intelligence innovations in all projects, large and small, and one of the objectives of any civic intelligence project should be improving the base of preconditions for future innovation. As a matter of fact, the entire civic-intelligence endeavour might be summed up as a way to ensure that these preconditions are continuously improved and strengthened and made to reflect abiding human values. In terms of Basalla's preconditions a civic intelligence orientation would help foster a social environment that values civic intelligence innovations, would motivate the creation and marketing of suitable models, inspire and educate potential innovators and identify and distribute resources.

Organisation

Since the purview and resources of this project are distributed throughout the world, a global 'civic intelligence' project is also distributed all around the world. It needs to be undertaken 'everywhere at once' to be successful. Also, since there is no central force or institution with the skills, resources or authority to direct the effort, the idea of a centrally controlled hierarchical organisation is irrelevant. The organisational structure of a critical intelligence becomes a medium of people and institutions that communicate with each other and share information. This network is necessarily composed of a wide variety of dissimilar institutions and individuals that co-operate with each other because of similar values and commitments to similar objectives. Neither authoritarian directives nor market transactions could provide the adhesive that would hold this evolving, shifting, growing network together.

This particular type of organisation has, of course, unique strengths and weaknesses. As Keck and Sikkink point out (1998) in their discussion of advocacy networks, a network's lack of 'power' in the traditional senses has made these networks largely invisible to the research community. Yet it is a result of these 'weaknesses' that the individuals and organisations consti-tuting the network must employ different strategies and organise themselves differently to get their jobs accomplished. Indeed 'intelligent' use of infor-mation and communication has evolved and become a significant feature. The number and effectiveness of what Keck and Sikkink call 'transnational advocacy networks' has exploded in recent years. In 1909 there were 176 international organisations according to the *Yearbook of International Organisations*. By 1996 the number had swelled to over twenty thousand (Runyan 1999). The success, also, of the open source or free software move-ment (GNU, Linux etc.) demonstrates the feasibility of large, distributed, loosely organised networks oriented towards the development of techno-logically sophisticated not-for-profit products. The preconditions that Basalla mentioned are doubtlessly contributing to this growth: motivated innovators, a somewhat receptive audience and the resources to develop and maintain the necessary information and communication capabilities all currently exist.

An effective network depends on many factors, and understanding these factors will be key to improving the existing civic intelligence and to anticipating and countering any threats to it. Probably the most important pattern to keep in mind is *consciousness* of the network itself. This means to a participating individual or organisation that they need to be an active, respectful and intelligent member of the network. They also must know that the network is in some sense *alive*; it must be sustained as well as used. Although some competition exists between members or nodes in the network(s) or civic intelligence, success in whatever endeavour will depend to some degree on others. This will vary according to the skill, interests and philosophical outlooks of the individual members. Providing ideas, contact information, references or other information that other members of the network can use is an important way to contribute to the network. Discussion among network participants helps identify critical issues and resolve internal divisions. The discussion of issues also lays the groundwork for the important transition from a discussion orientation to an action orientation. Projects provide an important focusing mechanism as an 'opportunity structure'. Finally, the networks should be accessible: important democratic interchanges take place at the 'margins of power' (Barker 1999) and these 'marginal' political settings should be encouraged to grow.

Engagement

Engagement is both a tactic and a philosophy. Engagement as a tactic means that the elements of the civic intelligence networks do not shy away from interactions with the organisations or institutions or ideas or traditions that are contrary to the objectives of the network. These organisations and the like may be promoting or perpetuating human-rights abuses or environmental damage. They may also be thwarting civic-intelligence efforts by their adherence to exclusion or other types of civic 'dumbing-down'. Engagement, of course, assumes many forms. A civic intelligence should, as we might expect, behave *intelligently*. This means that the nature of the engagement should be based on the precepts of this chapter – it should be principled, collective and pragmatic, for example. But at the same time, engagement is a philosophy and it represents an everyday and natural predisposition towards action; it represents a challenge and an acknowledgement that the status quo, although not likely to be good enough, can be improved. Engagement, ideally, is flexible and nimble and it is appropriate for the situation. Timing plays an important role in appropriate engagement. Research and study also have critical roles to play, but they must not be used as a substitute for action, postponing engagement while waiting for 'all the facts to come in'. [See Rafensperger (1997) for a good antidote to this malady.]

The experiences in Seattle of demonstrations against the World Trade Organisation in 1999 show that large numbers of people, even in a relatively prosperous city, share strong feelings – often vague and unarticulated – that many trends of today's society are heading in the wrong direction and that many of society's 'leaders', both individual and institutional, are not leading adequately; their objectives, modus operandi and integrity are compromised to dangerous levels. During the week of anti-WTO demonstrations, one representative from a protesting organisation stated in a radio interview that 'It shouldn't be necessary to break glass' to put issues on the public agenda. A functioning civic intelligence would, ideally, help put shape and meaning to citizens' unease with some of the directions of global capital and to bring these issues up for public discussion. This would, theoretically, help prevent some of the ruptures, riots, wars etc. that result from unresolved civic grievances. An effective and fully functioning civic intelligence would make it unnecessary for some people to 'break glass' to be heard. The 'space' in which these voices can be heard – and can confront the voices of power – is called, in a broad general sense, the 'public sphere' by Jürgen Habermas (1989).

Intelligence

A central conceptual ingredient to this chapter is, of course, that of *intelligence*. This may be the trickiest aspect of the concept, owing to the diversity of views on what 'intelligence' is. This section will attempt to elucidate in what ways our conceptualisation of a 'civic intelligence' could be labelled as intelligent and what people can do to develop this capability.

Intelligence implies that a reasonable view of the situation exists (or can be constructed) and that reasonable actions based on this view can be conceived and enacted on a timely basis. Clearly, the creation and dissemination of information and ideas among a large group of people is crucial. Learning is important because the situation changes and experimentation has shown itself to be an effective conceptual tool for *active learning*. Therefore, some of the key aspects include: (1) multi-directional communication and access to information; (2) discussion, deliberation and ideating; (3) monitoring; (4) learning; (5) experimenting; (6) adapting; and (7) regulating. As the concept of civic intelligence begins to be more fleshed out, these aspects would be turned into patterns in the sense that Alexander and his colleagues intended.

Let's briefly touch on one aspect of intelligence – monitoring – and some examples of new civic uses. Technology, it turns out, ushers in both challenges and opportunities. We find, for example, that at the same time as our technology and economic imperatives are creating vast problems, they are also introducing some provocative new possibilities for our civic-intelligence model. One recent innovation, a system employing seven earth-orbiting satellites, enables us to monitor Earth's vital signs from space (King and Herring 2000). While the system doesn't specify what we the Earth's inhabitants will do with the data, it's clear that we wouldn't have a good picture of the state of the Earth without it. This type of surveillance can expose other events to public scrutiny; it was the French 'Spot' satellite which first alerted the world to the Chernobyl disasters. Also, unlike previous enterprises, this project makes its data readily and cheaply available to people all over the world. The existence of 'emergency response networks' (Roeder 1999) provide excellent examples of provisional networks that can be erected in a relatively short time to meet specific threats to public health or welfare.

Projects and products

Projects – both campaign- and product-oriented – help to motivate and channel activity. A extremely large number of projects are important within the context of cultivating a civic intelligence. There is ample evidence that the 'project' is necessary to marshal sufficient force to accomplish the desired goals (Keck and Sikkink 1998). One such example is the manifesto or declaration that communication activists have been developing in recent years, often in conjunction with conferences. These collective statements offer a distillation and articulation of their beliefs and objectives, which they hope will then be used to help under-gird future projects and products. Recent examples include the People's Communication Charter, the Papallacta Declaration, the Bamako Declaration and the Seattle Statement. The People's Communication Charter is an initiative of the Third World Network (Penang, Malaysia) and the Centre for Communication and Human Rights (Amsterdam, the Netherlands) and was one of the first and most far-reaching of these statements. The Charter presents a holistic view of communication and covers a wide variety of important communication issues including respect and freedom, literacy, protection of journalists, cultural diversity, participation, justice and consumption. Key to their approach is the idea that people must be vigilant about defending their 'communication environment'. Besides seeking ratification from individuals and organisations, one idea has been to launch an 'international tribunal' to hear complaints and evidence related to issues in the Charter. The Seattle Statement was developed at CPSR's 'Shaping the Network Society' symposium, an explicit attempt to broaden the conversation on civic uses of new digital network technology. It was then promoted via email, and 'signatures' were harvested electronically and added, sorted by country of origin, to the electronic list on the Web. The impacts of these statements are hard to forecast and hard to identify. Inexpensive global communication via email is making this easier – at least to those with access; the Seattle Statement was reportedly used within Hungary to instigate discussion and help raise interest in public networking projects.

The Neighborhood Knowledge Los Angeles (NKLA) project as a broad partnership between academia and the community is a good example of a holistic approach to civic intelligence. One aspect of NKLA is its 'early warning system' in which housing conditions in Los Angeles are monitored. In 1995, for example, census figures showed that 107,900 apartments were infested with rats and 131,700 had no working toilets. (Of course we must multiply this figure by several orders of magnitude to get a realistic feel for the actual scope of this worldwide.) NKLA has been compiling 'early warning' information of this sort (including, for example, tax delinquencies, building code violations, unpaid utility bills etc.) on to their website, which is then used by community organisations to devise solutions – including policy work and engagement with government – to their problems. NKLA, along with countless other communities, is engaging in mapping community assets to help community members find out about useful resources – often unnoticed and under-utilised in their own midst.

Good projects combine many important ideas in a compelling way into a form that people can readily understand and become a part of, and that results in desired change. Two recent innovative projects from Seattle show promise for meeting those criteria. The first project, 'Sustainable Seattle', is a project that identifies and defines measures or 'indicators' that, reckoned over time, will reveal whether or not Seattle is becoming more or less 'sustainable'. The project was a citizen initiative, not instigated by the government or by business. Moreover, the civic sector set the agenda and the agenda was 'sustainability', not any number of other possible choices that business, government or, even, other civic sector organisations may have devised. The set of indicators, discussed and disseminated, now can be used as an ongoing foundation for civic intelligence, developing programmes and policies for promoting 'sustainability'. Noting how the values of the indicators are related to each other can also reveal hidden connections and suggest innovative programmes. Incidentally, the presence of the indicators on the Web has helped and will continue to help similar projects around the world. The 'Sustainable Penang' project, for example, was launched after activists in Penang saw Sustainable Seattle's indicators on the Seattle Community Network.

Recently, another civic intelligence project, in a similar vein to the Sustainable Seattle project, has been launched. The 'Technology Healthy City' project with financial support from the city of Seattle is intended to take a series of information and communication technology (ICT) 'snapshots' over time to assess the impacts of technology on the region. The project thus far has been citizen-led. One of the explicit caveats was to devise indicators that were designed for *civic-sector* – not government or business – benefit. As ICT is widely acknowledged to be having major effects on the psychic as well as the physical aspects of the region, it will be interesting to see what role, if any, this project can assume in ongoing assessment and actions related to the use and effects of ICT in the region.

There is no shortage of potential projects: a search engine for non-profits, for example, or, even, a classification scheme for civic-oriented web pages, would be very useful. A number of projects that we might call critical information systems are also possible. These systems could provide access to information and to organisations and initiatives. TAO in Canada (http://www.tao.org), One World (http://www.oneworld.org) in Britain and Kabissa ('Space for change in Africa', http://www.kabissa.org) provide good examples of this. Tele-centres (or, in the US, 'community technology centres') provide physical places for people to access and engage with new communication technology while community networks such as the Seattle Community Network (Schuler 1996) can provide a wide variety of technological and other support service for communities. The many faces of 'globalism' remind us that new social, economic and political realities don't stop at the borders of geographic communities.

Resources

Adequate resources, including time, money, physical facilities, communication capabilities and focused initiatives for people and institutions are necessary but not sufficient for effective civic intelligence. Although it would be difficult to measure the magnitude of the need for these resources, the overall project can't wait until all the 'necessary' resources are at hand before starting. At the same time, helping to ensure that adequate resources do exist is critical for the project.

Challenges

Positive change is not impossible, although all major social and environmental changes, such as the abolishment of slavery in the US, probably appeared impossible at the onset of the struggle. It needs, also, to be pointed out that positive change is not inevitable either; there is no inexorable trend that we can rely upon to save us. Slavery is gone but new forms of quasi-legal servitude that would be considered slavery by another name are becoming increasingly common. Similarly the practice of torture, however antiquated it may seem, is also still pervasive throughout the developing – and developed – world (Pinter 2000, Conroy 2000). The propensity towards evil as a result of individual or institutional intent will always haunt us. History is ruled by ebbs and flows of immeasurable complexity. At the same time, people are the major architects of change – both good and bad.

The biggest challenge of course is to accomplish anything at all that leaves the social or environmental situation in a better state than it was before. Many efforts viewed from the advantage of hindsight seemed doomed at the onset; history, it was said, was 'against them'. Yet in some cases, history surprised us and the 'impossible' was accomplished. The campaign to abolish slavery in the US took over a century to accomplish its aim. Yet, even now, its tragic legacy persists, providing grounds for future social movements. When social or environmental ills exist, it is *society's* responsibility to address those problems despite bad odds. Unless the area of amelioration is uniquely immune, focusing on the task to be accomplished is more likely to obtain results than wishful thinking, the 'free market', historical 'inevitability' or just a run of good luck. We can move forward only by principled action based on what we expect and where we want to go from where we are. An effective civic intelligence links individual efforts with other individual events into networks that can accomplish greater goals than results generated through individual efforts. If these networks become powerful enough to help bring about broad-based positive changes in the world, then more effective civic intelligence can be said to exist.

As in the case of the movement to abolish American slavery, the 'advocacy networks' that Keck and Sikkink examined can emerge, accomplish (or not accomplish) their objective and then apparently wither away. In many cases the skills honed in one campaign are put to use in the next. For example, there is substantial evidence that the women's suffrage movement in the US was aided greatly by campaigners, ideas and techniques acquired during the anti-slavery campaign. While individual campaigns may still pass through these life-cycle phases, the spectacular rise in the number of transnational non-government organisations and advocacy networks suggests that a new era of heightened civic intelligence has arrived.

The question then arises in relation to responses of institutions outside the network. If this type of civic intelligence becomes more prevalent and powerful, it would likely become specifically targeted by those people and institutions that are threatened by it. If, at some point in the future, these new types of civic intelligence become sufficiently powerful (and it appears to be already happening in some cases), they will come into conflict with other existing institutions – network-based or not – that perceive themselves to be threatened. Indeed if they didn't come into conflict it would be either very peculiar or strong evidence that the networks themselves presented no threat to the status quo through either their impotence or their adoption of less threatening objectives. In any event, it is not the case that strong institutions are powerless in the face of heightened civic intelligence. There is no reason to presume that they are intrinsically incapable of counter-attack.

Although crystal-ball gazing is an inexact science, it seems clear that counter-tactics could be employed. Since information and communication are key to civic intelligence, the key to neutralising the effects of an active, engaged and effective civic intelligence would be found there. Many of these tactics have, of course, already been used. In the 1960s, for example, the US government developed the secret COINTELPRO programme based largely on disinformation and character-assassination to disrupt and discredit the Black liberation movement and the anti-war movement. US corporations sometimes create 'Astro-turf' front organisations based on economic incentives that mimic public interest organisations that have no economic stake in the issue. Thus the 'Farmers for Fairness' funded an extensive 'soft-money' media campaign against a politician working for environmental controls on hog-manure disposal in North Carolina. And *The Wall Street*

Journal reported that Microsoft and other companies have employed people to monitor Usenet news groups for unfavourable comments about their products and post (from a neutral, non-company address) comments to counter the negative claims. All of this 'info warfare' makes it much more difficult, of course, for the average citizen to obtain the information to participate meaningfully in addressing societal issues.

Too little, too late?

Unfortunately, humankind's problems may be so profound and our ability to respond so divided, unmotivated and feeble that attempts to deal with them are doomed to failure. 'Grand schemes' such as Wells's World Encyclopaedia, Dewey's Thought News, Kochen's WISE (1975), and Jungk's Everyman Project (1977) have periodically sprouted up, attracted a modest following, then faded away, apparently without a trace. The proponents are likely to be dismissed as cranks by the media and by the conventional wisdom of the era; their schemes are generally utopian, overly ambitious and, ultimately, unrealistic.

What can we do to ensure that our civic intelligence project is not dismissed as yet another crank scheme? There are two possible strategies. The first is to avoid risk by lowering the expectations, goals and rhetoric. We can dispense with the idea that we are historical actors who are capable of leaving a positive mark on the world. We can become thoughtful observers and theoreticians, for example. We can decide to forgo the idea of social and environmental amelioration – of civic intelligence – and retreat into academicism – or cynicism. The second approach is to ground our enterprise into the context and realities of our era and devise a programme that suits the demands of our lives and our livelihoods but is based upon values and social needs. It is probably possible to shape one's perspective incrementally to make one's work more consciously supportive of a civic intelligence if that transformation is prioritised. Research – be it academic study or 'street-level' information-gathering and assessment – can play a critical role, and a wide variety of academic disciplines have important roles to play (Schuler 1997). Research can and should be a tool that continually is brought to bear on the shifting, evolving realities of life.

Academics, stereotypically, are noted for their lack of emotional engagement. This is the purported product of rationalism; a cold, calculated, dispassionate assessment or mere reportage of data. But unless designed for entertainment alone (if *that* is even possible) any text, academic or non-academic, will have implications for *use*. Use, of course, may bring with it a challenge upon the world as it exists, a potential for altering the present course or shoring up the status quo. If the change is deemed important and the process through which the change could take place is plausible, hope is not unthinkable. Despair, on the other hand, exists when positive change is inconceivable; the future, presumably advancing towards a precipice, appears unalterable.

This project builds on the notions of networked groups of people and institutions that are working both within their own communities and outside across traditional boundaries using new communication and information technologies where necessary and appropriate. The novelty of this plan lies with the focus on the civic sector as a force capable of consciously and pragmatically constructing more intelligent capabilities. Beyond that I have identified some tentative 'patterns' that, if pursued, will help cultivate that intelligence. This chapter is not intended to provide a blueprint for the future. It is intended only to identify and attempt to pull together a number of reasonable suggestions based on the need for a renewed and stronger sense of civic intelligence. Critique may be easier to generate than action plans; it is also easier to digest as it asks for very little in the way of action, except, perhaps, for righteous indignation. Action plans, also, are necessarily based less on evidence and are inescapable proscriptive. Thus academics (whose written and spoken outputs have been circumscribed in various ways) are likely to eschew them. I hoped to integrate critique and activism in this chapter.

Most people, if they had their way, would prefer a social world that was just and offered opportunities to all people for a meaningful life. An environment that was safe and free of toxins and capable of providing sustenance and enjoyment now and for generations to come would likewise be among their preferences. Yet it is tacitly assumed that these goals are too 'utopian' and that they can never happen, or, paradoxically, that they're the natural consequence of capitalist, neo-liberalist development and all society has to do is 'stay the course'. It is acknowledged, of course, that arriving at this inevitable destination will take generations and that some people – *poor* people – will necessarily have to suffer as part of this 'natural' process. It is the central contention of this chapter that it is possible to harbour meliorist beliefs – and even to act on them – without being a crank. The opposite of this view would be difficult to embrace: That we are so 'dumbed-down' that we can't contemplate any improvements to our own 'civic intelligence'.

> When it becomes a program, hopelessness paralyses us, immobilises us. We succumb to fatalism, and then it becomes impossible to muster the strength we absolutely need for a fierce struggle that will re-create the world.
>
> Paulo Freire (1992)

An earlier version of this chapter appeared in *Information Communication and Society*, Vol. 4, No. 2, 2001 http://www.T&F.co.uk/journals/. Permission for publication given by Taylor & Francis Ltd. and the editors of Information Communication and Society.

Chapter 18

Participating in the information society

Community development and social inclusion

Peter Day

Introduction

Drawing from a longitudinal study of Scandinavian and UK community-ICT initiatives, this chapter contributes to the information-society policy discourse by examining tensions existing between policy and attempts to address social exclusion through community-ICT initiatives. It begins with an analysis of seminal information society policy documents at international and national levels and contests that the techno-economic determinism of many policy documents results in social tensions that can act as barriers to a more inclusive way of life. Attempts by the UK government to address social exclusion at community level are examined and a case is made for more participatory approaches to the design, implementation and development of community-ICT initiatives. Having contextualised the community informatics discourse within a participatory framework, the chapter concludes with a preliminary examination of the literature relating to the use of participatory tools and techniques at local level. This brief review of the literature forms an introduction to a research project currently being planned at the University of Brighton.

There is a view prevalent in policy-making circles today that society has entered a new social era known as the 'knowledge economy'. For many policy-makers, macroeconomic stability, technological development – especially in the field of information technology (IT) – and the utilisation of people as resources for this new economy are crucial components of the new age (Blair 2000). Such is the importance of the 'knowledge economy' to the policy discourse that the UK Prime Minister heralded it as 'the equivalent of the machine-driven economy of the industrial revolution'.

However, such views have been commonplace for some time. Over two decades ago, the sociologist Alvin Toffler posited that communication technologies would be utilised to create 'telecommunities' in the third-wave 'info-sphere' (1980) and prior to that, Daniel Bell forecast the post-industrial society as the third stage of human societal development (1973). More recently, Negroponte attested that social change resulting from digital technology was both irrevocable and unstoppable (1995). However, it was not only among theorists and social forecasters that such views held sway. Garnham (1994) signalled that social changes forecast by Bell and by Masuda (1981) started to form part of Western policy during the 1980s. So, despite an apparent new-found evangelism for information society issues, the notion that information and information communication technologies (ICTs) are driving revolutionary changes in an information or knowledge society or economy is not new, even in policy circles. The significance that the concept has taken on over the past five or six years is new, however.

Interestingly, this same period marked the emergence of a wide range of diverse community-based initiatives that utilise ICTs to underpin their activities. In spite of the techno-economic determinism often rooted in information society policy (Day 1996a), such initiatives attempt to make the information society more accessible to ordinary citizens but face significant implementation and development barriers (Shearman 1999). This view is supported by earlier research, which suggests that government and funding policies often create difficulties for community-ICT initiatives (Day 1996b, Day and Harris 1997).

An historical analysis of key information society documents: from macro to micro level

Much of the information society policy debate focuses on the development of what has become known as the information superhighway, or the information infrastructure (infostructure). Although somewhat clichéd, the metaphor provides a useful image of the structural impact of the communications network.

The National Information Infrastructure (NII)

The phrase 'information highway' is often attributed to US Vice President Al Gore, who used it in a speech to outline his views on the National Information Infrastructure (NII) (1993). However, the metaphor was actually used as early as the late 1960s in discussions of interactive cable-television systems (Dutton 1997). Despite this, Gore's speech was a public unveiling of the Clinton/Gore administration's vision of the societal role of ICTs. Its significance lay in the fact that it was a policy perspective of how ICTs could be exploited to change the way people work, learn and interact with each other.

A high-level information infrastructure task force (IITF) was established to co-ordinate federal government activities to turn the vision into reality. An advisory council was established to assist IITF in involving the private sector in the process of policy development (Kubicek and Dutton 1997). The resulting *Agenda for Action* document (IITF 1993) advocated the techno-economic use of ICTs to increase US economic competitiveness, reduce administration costs and make government more efficient and responsive (Kalil 1997).

A parallel development track

Although the Clinton/Gore administration is often cited as the catalyst for contemporary global information society developments, an analysis of policy documents reveals international parallels in ICT application, legislative, regulatory and policy development (Federal Trust 1995, Niebel 1997). The European Commission (EC), for example, in contrast to the NII vision, indicated a desire to express a comprehensive and integrated view of the new phenomenon (Niebel 1997).

Europe and the information society

Despite this apparent difference of approach, early EC policy varied little in actual content from the NII model. The 'Delors White Paper', for example, promoted a socio-economic framework for generating innovation and competitiveness through the utilisation of ICTs. The White Paper enthusiastically embraced the challenges and opportunities of a knowledge-based economy by promoting the economic case for the development of a trans-European information infrastructure or trans-European networks (TENs) (CEC 1994a).

A consequence of the 'Delors White Paper' was the constitution of a high-level group of experts (HLGE) on the information society, comprising mainly key industrialists and financiers. The group, headed by Martin Bangemann, recommended that market mechanisms should be the driving force behind the European information society whilst the public sector would foster critical mass by stimulating interest in and awareness of the infostructure's potential (CEC 1994b). The report promoted rapid deregulation and liberalisation of markets to facilitate private-sector development of the trans-European 'infostructure', applications and services. It emphasised entertainment services as the potential priority area, suggesting that existing satellite and telephone infrastructure would serve the consumer market, as pay-per-view and advertising revenues encouraged the private sector development of the information society.

At this stage of policy development, little serious consideration was given to addressing social exclusion (Day and Horner 1995). The same ethos of competitiveness and consumerism that underpinned the development of the NII was also to be found in EC policy (CEC 1994a). An unquestioning belief in market forces as the developer of this new form of human existence often accompanied an uncritical acceptance of the inevitability of the ICT revolution. 'The information society is on its way. A "digital revolution" is triggering structural change comparable to last century's industrial revolution with the corresponding high economic stakes. The process cannot be stopped and will lead eventually to a knowledge-based economy' (CEC 1994c).

National policies – the case of the UK

At the same time as information society policies were being developed in the US and EC, a similar process was under way in the UK, and again market forces were seen as the motivating force (Taylor 1995). A Department of Trade and Industry (DTI) White Paper set out the Government's vision for developing superhighways in the UK (DTI 1994) and a subsequent DTI report summarised the need to improve the standard of government services (1995). The Computer and Communications Technology Agency (CCTA) also adopted this theme (CCTA 1994 and 1995) and in 1996 the government published a Green Paper, Government.direct, with this in mind (1996). Whilst the Green Paper acknowledged the importance of access and ease of use, its focus was on one-way delivery of government services.

However, by 1996, pressure within Parliament for a socially broader approach to policy-development emerged. The House of Lords Select Committee on Science and Technology argued a case for subsidies and assistance for *wiring* schools and public places (House of Lords 1996). Significantly it also suggested that, by facilitating the electorate with direct online access to the political process, the government would show leadership in the provision of public information (Tang 1998).

In the same year, the DTI launched the Information Society Initiative (ISI), a four-year programme to promote the use and development of ICTs in the UK (DTI 1996a). The venture, which made £35 million available, was aimed at the business sector (ETHOS 1998). However, conscious of criticism that ISI was not aimed at a broader social agenda, the government announced the 'IT for All' programme as part of a revamped ISI in December 1996 (DTI 1996b). This aimed to:

- raise public awareness of and access to ICTs,
- demonstrate the benefits of different technologies to people in everyday life,
- break down barriers for people in the information society, and
- expand the UK market for companies through greater public use of ICTs.

The four-year programme was a one-off awareness-raising initiative, which sought to facilitate partnership projects between central and local government, business and the voluntary sector. However, although the inclusion of the voluntary sector appeared to signal a more inclusive approach to policy, the concern remained that little was being done at grassroots level.

The plethora of 'electronic' attempts and initiatives by government are less than cosmetic, but it is troubling to note that these measures, as they are, are still largely aimed at business, the educated and affluent groups of the population. Much less effort has been addressed at reducing the gap between access to these information services by the 'computerised' and the 'less computerised' communities.

(Tang 1998: 192–3)

The year 1997 heralded a change of government and hopes that more inclusive information society policies would be effected. These hopes were based largely on the stated aim that a Labour government would ensure that everyone could participate in the information revolution (Labour Party 1995). The new government's vision of the future was set out in *Our Information Age* (Central Office of Information 1998) and, although it emphasised social uses of ICTs, the focus was still on competitiveness. The sense of altruism found in *Communicating Britain's Future* had given way to a consideration of the effects of exclusion on UK plc, and references to democracy had disappeared (Marshall 2000).

However, the White Paper *Modern Local Government: In Touch with the People* put forward a number of proposals for improving representative democracy whilst emphasising the importance of innovations in participative-democracy innovations (DETR 1998). The Paper stressed the government's wishes for consultation and participation to become embedded in local-authority cultures. To this end, consultation was linked to Best Value proposals, where failure by local authorities to respond to consultation exercises would be grounds for transferring services to other agencies. Although specific mechanisms of consultation were not made clear, the need for public participation was. Here, the emphasis on targeting the socially excluded was seen as central to the government's agenda of enhancing democracy (Wilson 1999).

In 1999, the term *joined-up government* took centre stage, and plans for reforming the organisational management of government and the delivery of public services using ICTs were published (Cabinet Office 1999). *Modernising Government* differed from the previous government's approach in the commitment it made to involve 'people' in the decision-making process. The People's Panel, a 'nationally representative' group of five thousand – set up by MORI – was referred to, and citizens' juries, community forums and focus groups were also cited as examples of consultation. However, the fact that these consultation processes would be administered by senior civil servants acting as champions of the information age suggests a top-down approach to consultation (Marshall 2000). Despite this limitation, the undertaking that all groups would 'have proper access to information age government' was a significant policy pledge.

Access to the UK information society

Until this point, the government's focus on public access to ICTs had almost exclusively centred on the networking of public libraries (LIC 1998). Although commissioned by the previous administration, the government supported *New Library: The People's Network* findings by making £270 million available from the New Opportunities Fund to create an electronic network of public libraries (Blair 1999). However, a government-commissioned *Appraisal of Annual Library Plans* raised concerns about the capacity of some local authorities to grasp the potential of ICTs in addressing social exclusion, finding that the planning of technical infrastructure varied significantly between authorities. The appraisal also noted that public libraries appeared to lack a comprehensive review of social inclusion (Department of Culture, Media and Sport 1999).

Despite this, the government's investment in networking public libraries, positioning them as public-access points, should be viewed as an attempt, albeit limited in scope, to address exclusion. However, physical access to ICTs alone is not an adequate method of addressing exclusion, and the government announced its intention to make £252 million available to establish some seven hundred ICT learning centres in socially deprived rural and inner city areas in England (PAT 15 2000).

Based on a cross-sectoral partnership approach, the stated intention is that centres should be developed, organised and operated according to local need, with community involvement in the planning and use of the centres. It is clear from this that the government has taken on board the findings of past research (Day and Harris 1997, Shearman 1999). The understanding that learning centres should be flexible enough in their structure and organisation to meet local needs and reflect local culture, should enrich the lives of local communities and should stimulate a sense of community ownership, is pivotal to their sustained success. However, there are concerns that practice might reveal a different picture than that presented by the Department for Education and Employment.

This brief policy analysis reveals the underlying priorities of economic efficiency and competitiveness of many information society policies, and highlights their inherent techno-economic determinism. Indeed, the terminology used by governments, for example 'knowledge economy', 'information revolution' and 'we can expect information technologies to change the whole pattern of our lives', reinforces this point. However, the UK government has at last shown an awareness of the problems that social exclusion can cause, establishing the Social Exclusion Unit (SEU) in 1997 as part of its strategy to develop a more inclusive policy framework (SEU 2000).

Comprising eighteen policy action teams (PATs), the SEU reflects the government's cross-sectoral approach to consultation and is currently publishing a range of documents in key areas. In the context of the information society SEU established PAT 15 to address issues relating to the access and use of ICTs by people living in the poorest areas of the UK (PAT 15 2000). Underlining the importance of this remit, a recent report urges the government to take the lead in achieving universal Internet access in the UK. The alternative, the report warns, would be some twenty million people excluded from the 'knowledge economy', a situation that would have 'severe economic, educational and social implications' (Booz-Allen and Hamilton Associates 2000).

PAT 15's investigations raise a number of significant social issues and make some wide-ranging strategic and operational recommendations, as well as establishing a timetable for action (PAT 15 2000). It is too early to determine the effects of this document in terms of policy implementation and development, or for that matter to gauge its rhetorical value. Neither is it known whether the recommendations will or can be implemented at local level nationally. However, the concerns raised by the Department of Culture, Media and Sport in respect of the capacity of some local authorities to grasp the potential of ICTs in addressing social exclusion, together with the differences in local-level ICT infrastructure development (1999), give reason for caution.

Despite these concerns, PAT 15 is a signal that the government has recognised, theoretically at least, the social significance of community-ICT initiatives. For the community informatics movement, this is a huge step forward.

Reflections on information society policies

The early information society policy discourse points to overwhelming social changes in the lives of ordinary citizens. However, whether these changes herald a new age is open to conjecture (Webster 1995). Certainly the use of the word *revolution* to describe such changes should, as citizens, give us reason to consider the implications. Winner suggests we might want to study the fundamental goals of an IT revolution, that is its commitment to social justice and a system of democratic rule, before affording it support (1985).

In many policy documents citizens are viewed as consumers with little choice but to adapt their social conditions to meet ICT-driven changes. Bangemann, for example, defines the role of policy in the information society quite clearly. 'Preparing Europeans for the advent of the information society is a priority task. Education, training and promotion will necessarily play a central role' (CEC 1994b). The consumerist foundations of much of this information-society discourse have profoundly anti-democratic implications (Sanderson 1999). The choice of information services, especially in the entertainment field, is frequently presented as an end in itself. People are viewed as service consumers (public and private) rather than citizens of the information society. Politically negotiated ends for the provision of services, such as those provided by community-ICT initiatives, are often placed beyond debate, resulting in a depoliticisation of service provision.

This chapter does not advocate turning back the digital clock. It does, however, reject the techno-economic determinism found in many contemporary information society policies. The sense of inevitability, in terms of current socio-technical developments, inherent in these documents implies that no grounds for serious debate or inquiry into the design, implementation and development of the 'new' society exist. These are arguments based on the assumption which, to paraphrase Winner (1985), supposes that, as long as the economy is competitive, the human condition will take care of itself. Abundance and democracy are to be found in access to information and ICTs. Not only is such a value system wrong, it is also socially divisive and consequently dangerous.

It would, of course, be misleading to portray all policy attempts to shape the information society as lacking in social consideration beyond that of the economy. In fact, the EC's Information Society Project Office (ISPO) identifies health care, traffic management, education and democracy, among others, as areas where telematics could improve the lives of EU citizens (CEC 1995a) and proposes that ICTs should give people more control over their lives rather than becoming slaves to technology. ISPO also highlighted the need to prevent the emergence of a two-tier society (CEC 1995b) and charged a group of 'experts', in the form of the Information Society Forum (ISF), with assessing the social and cultural aspects of the information society (CEC 1995c). The Forum proposed open and easy access to information and the infostructure as a solution to the dangers of 'info-elitism' and social exclusion (CEC 1995d).

Whilst such sentiments are to be supported, it is in this culture of 'experts' that another aspect of the exclusionary nature of policy can be found. If and when policy-makers consider citizen participation in the information society, it usually takes the form of technical interaction, i.e. 'press this button' or 'touch the screen here': rarely do they consider participation in the policy-making process itself. Instead groups of 'experts' are appointed to consider crucial social issues such as the transformation of society (HLGE) and social exclusion (ISF).

This is not to suggest that there is no role for experts; on the contrary, expert knowledge is a crucial component of modern life but experts should not be seen as a source of unchallenged power and authority (Schuler and Namioka 1993). Instead they should be regarded as resources to be drawn on. In this way, policy development can become a partnership of responsibility between implementers and citizens (Day 1999).

Nowhere is this seen more graphically than with social exclusion. Social exclusion is not simply a rhetorical term or buzzword, it is a harsh fact of life that spells hardship and suffering for the excluded. It is a term that can be used to describe many states of the human condition and ranges from the unemployed or homeless to the disabled or the elderly. It can include single parents; those on low incomes; ethnic minorities; or members of other minority groups. It does not respect boundaries of culture, religion, gender, sexual orientation, geographical location etc. To address social exclusion, policies need to tackle its root causes. To understand these causes, policy-makers need to engage in dialogue with, and learn from, those who experience forms of exclusion. It is here that participation in partnerships of responsibility is of use.

Community ICT initiatives – vehicles for community development

The shift in focus from the international or national to the community-policy arena raises the often perplexing issue of what is meant by the word *community*. Rather than duplicating attempts for a hard and fast definition, Butcher's three interrelated senses of *community* (1993) can be utilised to provide a starting point for discussion.

* *Descriptive community*, often used by social scientists, draws on the word's etymological origins of having 'something in common'. This 'something in common' is usually referred to in a geographical or neigh-bourhood context but can also be applied to other social determinants such as ethnicity, religion, sexual orientation etc. and therefore relates to communities of interest as well as location.
* *Community values* in a society based on diversity are often contested, but Butcher asserts that solidarity, participation and coherence provide the value base that underpins community initiatives and policies in culturally diverse communities.
* *Active community* refers to collective action by community members embracing one or more of the communal values identified above. Such activities are purposively undertaken through the vehicle of groups, networks and organisations, where communication is paramount.

As the development of community policies is dependent on encouraging *active communities*, 'forms of practice and service delivery that embrace distinctive methods and techniques are required' (Glen 1993). What matters here is the recognition that communities are diverse social constructs. What works and is appropriate in one community may not work elsewhere. Community policy therefore should reflect a commitment to the objectives of community autonomy and responsibility for initiatives (Day and Harris 1997).

By developing an understanding of what *community* means, it is possible to develop policies that are meaningful and relevant to people in communities. One such example is based on an adaptation of Butcher's 'Key Elements of

Community Policy' model (1993), which provides an invaluable framework for the development of community-ICT policies. It also provides a useful context for the PAT 15's remit of reducing social exclusion by producing 'joined up solutions to joined up problems' (SEU 2000) (Figure 18.1).

Threats and barriers to 'bridging the digital divide' at community level

A central feature of the government's social inclusion strategy is the aim that each community should 'have at least one publicly accessible community-based facility' (PAT 15 2000). However, it is important that this target of seven hundred ICT learning centres should be seen as a first step toward addressing exclusion in the information society rather than an end in itself. Research shows that a range of policy lessons have yet to be learnt (Day and Harris 1997) and that the adoption of a 'job done' mentality risks stimulating disillusionment and resentment in local communities that will exacerbate exclusion in the long term.

Four areas of concern

The government's intention that ICT learning centres should benefit communities of both location and interest by addressing social exclusion is clear. What is not so evident is how government seeks to develop policy mechanisms that embrace community values and promote active communities.

The remainder of this chapter addresses four distinct but interrelated areas of concern raised by PAT 15 – provision, funding, partnerships and research – as a contribution to the social inclusion discourse.

Provision

In a review of existing local initiatives, PAT 15 suggests that local people often lack awareness of the potential of ICTs and do not appreciate their benefits. Whilst it is true that many community groups lack ICT awareness, there is a degree of the deterministic arrogance of the 'expert' in this statement. Community groups are often too involved in dealing with the day-to-day needs of communities to spend resources, financial or otherwise, on technologies that may be of little obvious benefit. That is not to suggest that ICTs are not potentially beneficial, merely that such benefits are not always clear to grassroots organisations with limited resources. Awareness-raising exercises and training workshops are identified by PAT 15 as tools useful for raising the profile of ICTs; however, they are only a partial solution in themselves.

Historically, significant numbers of community-based ICT initiatives have displayed similar signs of technological determinism to that identified above.

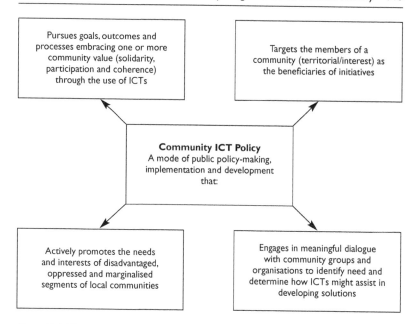

Figure 18.1 The key elements of community ICT policy

A number of 1980s and early 1990s community tele-cottages, or community teleservice centres were classic examples of this.

Usually driven by cross-sectoral partnerships with a predetermined community development agenda, these initiatives were often parachuted into a locality. The process normally involved some attempt to meet the community development or employment targets of statutory bodies and development agencies through IT training schemes. As a rule these initiatives were advised by IT advocates or 'experts' and often formed part of governmental research programmes. Little or no dialogue with local communities, to determine actual need, was entered into.

Such initiatives rarely solicited much in the way of public support and were sometimes met with outright hostility from the local community. One such example was that of Datariet, a teleservice centre established in Vestbyen, a working-class estate in the city of Vejle, Denmark (Day 1996b). Another was the Wiltshire Telecottage Network (WTN), where poor communication between and within agencies combined with failed expectations, disenchantment and hostility at grassroots level and led to the Network's ultimate demise (Day and Harris 1997).

Lessons from such experiences should not be wasted. If the sense of identity and community ownership referred to by the PAT 15 (2000) is to be established, communities need to be involved at all stages of an initiative's life-cycle: the design, implementation and ongoing development. The setting-up of neighbourhood plans, referred to in a number of PAT reports, should reflect this requirement by encouraging the active participation of citizens in the process.

Despite the paternalistic and top-down development approach of many controlling partnerships, many community initiatives have survived. Often overseen by management boards, comprising people with jobs and responsibilities elsewhere, the commitment and dedication of workers and volunteers, often of heroic proportions, have been decisive factors in this survival.

The job of the initiative manager is also very demanding, with responsibilities ranging from the broadest strategic planning to highly specific operational work. Managers have to draw from a variety of skills in areas as diverse as marketing, promotion, partnership-building, fund-management, building-management, proposal-writing, information service provision, administration and public relations (Day and Harris 1997). It is somewhat ironic and certainly worrying that cross-sectoral partnerships responsible for community initiatives, which possess a wealth of skills and expertise in these areas, have often failed to provide adequate levels of training and ongoing support.

Funding

One of the most sensitive and complex aspects of many community ICT initiatives is the question of funding. Case studies reveal a wide range of funding regimes, from the low-cost basic model in Herefordshire and Worcestershire to the substantial City Challenge and Lottery grants attracted in Barnsley and Grimethorpe (Day and Harris 1997). However, practitioners are often wary of being seen to criticise funding regimes through fear of threatening future funding. The reluctance of practitioners to engage openly in a dialogue of how such regimes could be improved is worrying. Those in the best position to suggest improvements to funding practices – community practitioners – are in effect being excluded from the debate.

Highlighting the confusing funding complexities within which initiatives have to operate, PAT 15 calls for the rationalisation of these funds through the National Strategy for Neighbourhood Renewal. Although such a call is both welcome and timely, exactly how the wide base of funders, which include a variety of central government and European Commission bodies, local authorities, TECs, businesses, charities and trusts, can be rationalised remains to be seen.

The report also recommends that public funding should be provided on a long-term basis but again fails to elaborate on what this means. Practitioners have in the past articulated that the gestation period for community-ICT initiatives is usually three years with sustainability sometimes being achievable in six (Day and Harris 1997). However, the usual period for 'project' funding is often between one and three years. This means that managers and staff spend enormous amounts of time and energy chasing sources of funding, time and energy that should be focused directly on addressing the needs of the local community.

In addition to this, initiatives are often forced to adapt existing services or develop new ones to meet the requirements and targets of funding bodies simply to survive. The bureaucratic demands of funders and the uncertainty of the funding climate frequently create problems that threaten the existence of community initiatives. PAT 15 correctly identifies the need to make the whole funding process more flexible. An apposite addendum to this would be that the funding process should be designed to meet the needs of local communities rather than the bureaucratic needs of agencies and public bureaucracies.

A related problem, apparently overlooked by PAT 15, is that of 'project culture' syndrome. If community-ICT initiatives are to address social exclusion then they must be regarded as long-term elements of the social infrastructure. The short-term and competitive nature of present funding sources, where socially excluded communities compete with one another for financial support, is wholly inappropriate for addressing social exclusion. Support for such a system, in which there are winners and losers, no matter how tacit, is support for a continuation of social exclusion. Initiatives require core public funding on an ongoing basis (INSINC 1997).

A small step towards addressing this issue would be to stop describing community-ICT initiatives as projects. The issue here is not one of semantics but one of perception and recognition of social status. The word 'project' has connotations of something temporary and/or of a short-term nature. However, it is not the use of the word that creates the problem so much as the perceptions it engenders. It is a failing of PAT 15 that the report consistently refers to 'projects' and appears not to have understood that 'the "project culture" is intrinsically inconsistent with sustainable public initiatives' (Day and Harris 1997).

Partnerships

As with many contemporary policy contributions, PAT 15 emphasises the role of cross-sectoral partnerships in achieving information society policy aims and objectives. Partnerships usually consist of formal or informal arrangements to work together to achieve a common objective. However, despite common objectives, a key issue with partnerships is that partners often have different agendas and consequently different interpretations of objectives.

The techno-economic focus of many information society policies advocating partnerships between public and private sectors has an inherent tendency to overlook the potentiality of social capital (Putnam 1993). Such partnerships are usually based on power. The private sector has economic power and the public sector has regulatory, administrative and legislative power. It is these powers that dictate and drive forward the development of policy. In this context, such partnerships have often stimulated social exclusion by failing to include representation from local communities and individual citizens (Harris 1996).

The disempowerment of citizens, found in traditional partnership models, is also to be found in some cross-sectoral partnerships. Even where the not-for-profit sector, or third sector, is included in partnerships, the power of professionals and/or 'experts', together with a bureaucratised policy-making process, is frequently to be observed (Sanderson 1999). Beyond voting in local elections, little or no input exists for local people, into the decisions that shape local community conditions. Where citizen input is sought, this often takes the form of consultation. Local people might be asked their views on a specific proposal and some slight amendments might even be possible but the purpose, budget, outcome etc. have generally been predetermined. As Arnstein argues, such consultation is usually little more than tokenism (1969).

Therefore, although cross-sectoral partnerships are now recognised as significant to modern policy-making (New Economics Foundation 1998), a more equitable approach is required at community level, one that transcends the inherently exclusive nature of traditional information society partnership models. Day describes the notion of 'tripartite collaboration' as an attempt to build on cross-sectoral partnership mechanisms (1998). Based on respect, equity and mutuality, tripartite collaboration recognises that each member contributes differently to a partnership but in that difference is the partnership's strength. Diversity of experience and knowledge and skills are therefore regarded as partnership assets.

Culturally, tripartite collaboration requires a directional shift from the dominant techno-economic model of current information society policy. It embraces the social economy as a significant element of local community life and requires changes to the societal roles and perspectives of formal organisations and agencies. Fresh and open minds are requisite to addressing the needs of local communities and the challenges of collaboration.

Partnerships developed through tripartite collaboration can promote a more democratic approach to societal changes. However, to be successful they must be based on equity and encourage participation, so that joint purpose, common values and mutual understanding can develop. Enabling local communities to engage in the shaping and utilisation of technologies in the information society is an important step towards a more inclusive society.

Research

However, the shaping of a more inclusive society requires policy-makers to extend their current focus on the community services approach of community practice (Day and Harris 1997) to include community development and community action approaches (Glen 1993). Glen argues that community practitioners should 'not be captive to any one of these methods over and above the other' and the same applies to policy-makers seeking to address social exclusion in local communities.

Despite evidence that the government recognises the importance of addressing social exclusion, its cultural ethos remains entrenched in a service-delivery mentality and economic competitiveness. This observation should not be construed as an argument to reject service mechanisms; on the contrary, public services remain an important component of our social lives. However, there is a need to expand the policy-making arena so that it encourages and benefits from active citizenship. It is here that research is urgently needed, if the 'digital divide' is indeed to be bridged.

PAT 15 highlights the lack of community informatics based research and urges the collection of 'comprehensive data' about attitudes to ICTs in 'deprived neighbourhoods so that a clear picture of the current situation can be obtained' (2000). It also suggests that the mapping of existing and potential neighbourhood capabilities is required to provide a national overview, which can in turn be fed into the implementation and development of local plans. Whilst this would provide interesting and useful datasets there is also a clear need for methodological research.

The development of a national methodological knowledge base of design, implementation and development strategies that can be exploited by communities would go a long way to releasing the community development and community action potential of ICTs. This is not to advocate methodological 'best practice', or a rule book for developing community-ICT initiatives, concepts at odds with the valorisation of diversity. Instead it promotes the development of a collaborative resource from which communities can, after reflection, select methods appropriate to their specific needs, or be inspired to develop their own. Such a knowledge base highlights the social-shaping potential of ICTs.

In a related area, PAT 15 raises the issue of local content. Whilst much of the focus here is on ICT-based training to promote greater literacy that might lead to other 'education, enterprise and employment programmes', there is a recognition that community-ICT initiatives should offer access to other activities that might 'be of greater interest to local people'. The argument is that the use of ICTs 'needs to be more relevant to people's lives'. To emphasise this point the report highlights the content of Knowsley Metropolitan Borough Council's local history and Rotherham Library's virtual-community magazine sites, both of which are examples of community service partnerships (PAT 15 2000). However, as observed earlier, if partnerships are to encourage active citizenship then community development and community action approaches also need to be encouraged.

Glen explains that community action involves communities in making demands of policy-makers to acknowledge their interests, whilst community development aims for communities 'to define their own needs and make provision for them' by 'fostering creative and co-operative networks of people and groups in communities' (1993). Ostensibly, both community action and community development relate to the social shaping of community life. Just as ICTs were earlier seen to be potentially useful tools in the development of a methodological knowledge base, so too can it be argued that they can be utilised to underpin existing social networks within local communities for information sharing and communicative activities (Schuler 1994).

However, this raises issues of how communities might determine their information and communication needs. How might they engage in knowl-edge-sharing and community campaigning? What forms will these creative and co-operative networks take? Again, these are methodological questions requiring urgent research before 'knowledge-economy' policies lock com-munities into one best way of local development. From the perspective of a government wishing to address social exclusion, the central question in this context should be: how can people shape their local communities as active citizens of the information society? It is here that the discourse is drawn back to Butcher's community values of solidarity, coherence and participation (1993), with participation holding the key.

There are, however, barriers to participation. It has already been contested that the 'bureaucratisation of authority, professional power and expertise' often prevent active participation (Sanderson 1999). In addition to these obstacles, Day and Harris have shown how organisational cultures and practices can also have a detrimental effect (1997). Bearing these points in mind, the decision to entrust the 'needs of citizens in the information age' to thirty-six senior civil servants as 'Champions of the Information Age' hardly inspires confidence that such consultation will be anything more than top-down tokenism (Arnstein 1969). It certainly suggests a continuation of a paternalistic approach to public services.

The design, implementation and development of community-ICT initiatives should not be left to professionals, experts and consultants in the hope that they can address local information and communication need. A wealth of participatory tools for involving people in shaping their communities exists today (New Economics Foundation 1998). Encouraging communities to design, develop and implement community-ICT initiatives that address the specific needs of the community will go a long way towards encouraging community development and community action.

Information and communication needs analyses can be conducted using tools such as scenario workshops (Street 1997), community appraisals (New Economics Foundation 1998), focus groups (Straw and Marks 1995) or the neighbourhood online game (Mackie and Wilcox 1999) to develop rich pictures of needs that can be fed into the policy process. By matching the results of research to identify needs with investigations outlined by PAT 15, a more meaningful and representative picture of local communities in the information society will emerge.

Citizen participation – issues for consideration

Indeed, there is growing evidence that participatory methods are being increasingly utilised at local level government. A study of public participation in English local authorities revealed that 47 per cent of local authorities had used focus groups, 26 per cent visioning exercises, 18 per cent citizens' panels and 5 per cent citizens' juries (Wilson 1999). Emphasising the costs in terms of time and money of public involvement in the policy process, Wilson identifies tensions between the government's aim of increasing public participation and its Best Value agenda of economy, efficiency and effectiveness. He also highlights the fears of many local councillors, who see public participation as a threat to their role in representative democracy.

However, participation should be viewed not as a replacement for representative democracy but as a method of enhancing it. As Wilson argues, it is the context of participation that is important and, despite the growing number of participatory exercises, little knowledge exists as to their social usefulness. Research is therefore required to develop an overview and evaluation of participatory techniques, in terms of process and outcomes.

Such research is necessary because evidence is emerging that suggests that public participation can sometimes be used as a tool to legitimise the knowledge of 'experts' and defend the existing social order (Street 1997). That is to say that such exercises give the appearance of openness without engaging in proper dialogue. This is especially true of traditional consultation exercises. To counter such trends it is important to ensure that the needs and understanding of citizens are seen as the starting point for participatory initiatives and that the authority, scope and implementation powers of participatory exercises are clarified from the outset. Participation needs to be seen to amount to more than a simple listening exercise. In other words, the involvement of local citizens in the policy-making process must lead to real policy change to avoid the risk of raising expectations that are subsequently frustrated through lack of action.

However, this is an area fraught with difficulty for local government. As was seen earlier, the values in local communities are often contested, and a danger exists that groups or third-sector 'experts' familiar with the process of local government will dominate participation. Wilson points to a study where significant numbers of socially excluded people felt deterred by a perception that the process was dominated by established groups (1999). Contested values can also lead to conflict, which can also deter the involvement of those new to forms of civic engagement. This conflict can also be used as an excuse for inaction by local authorities. Qualitative research investigating the reasons why people do and do not engage in local government participation initiatives could reveal some useful insights into local democracy.

Higgins proposes that active participation is related to issues of social rights and empowerment. That is to say, that where people feel valued by policy-makers as equal citizens and are able to act on this sense of worth, then they are more likely to contribute to, and participate in, shaping their local community. Local authorities therefore have obligations to citizens to respect and respond to collective contributions, needs and aspirations (Higgins 1999).

However, understanding participation is not simply a question of finding the right tools and techniques. The final area recommended for research within the context of social inclusion in the information society relates to the way local government functions.

The involvement of citizens in the policy process also requires a re-examination of assumptions and practices relating to the power of administrators. Without changes to the way bureaucracies function, authentic participation will be limited to experiments of academic interest only. Research from the US suggests that such changes are possible (King *et al.* 1998), but enabling administrators to become co-operative participants in the information society discourse requires a significant shift in values of the role of administrators and the organisational cultures of many local authorities. The development of more participatory and inclusive information society policies requires research not only into ways of empowering and educating citizens but also into ways of re-educating administrators and enabling administrative structures and processes to facilitate an effective dialogue between citizens, administrators and policy-makers (King *et al.* 1998).

Conclusion

The purpose of this chapter has been to raise issues pertinent to the community informatics agenda of addressing social exclusion in the information society. Many areas of relevance to this debate, such as community economic development (CED) (Gurstein 1998), have not been included and this should not be seen as diminishing their importance. However, the 'knowledge-economy' policy agenda lacks broad social analysis, and this chapter seeks to redress the policy imbalance in some small way. Powerful techno-economic interests currently shape information society developments. 'Knowledge economy' policy-makers regard people in terms of their market potential rather than as citizens. This consumerist discourse is divisive and fundamentally anti-democratic.

The customary approach to governance, that is informed by 'experts' and managed by professionals, also acts as a barrier to effective participation. In contrast, Agenda 21 highlights the need to broaden social dialogue by indicating that partnerships for sustainable development require the participation of all groups and organisations in the decision-making process (UNCED 1992).

In the UK, the government has expressed a desire to involve citizens in the policy-making process; however, the scale and nature of this consultation and participation is crucial. Despite a commitment to addressing social exclusion through the use of ICTs, the government remains rooted in a community-services approach and fails to appreciate the community development and community action potential of ICTs.

If the community informatics movement is to shape information society policy development, it faces significant challenges. Central to these challenges is the need to establish a framework of methodological tools that informs policy of more inclusive and collaborative pathways to the information society. However, community informatics is more than the development of a participatory approach to the design, implementation and development of community technologies. It is also about promoting policies that enable citizens to use ICTs as tools to determine and shape their conditions of existence in their local communities – what J. K. Galbraith would call the 'good society' (1994).

Chapter 19

Communities and community e-gateways

Networking for social inclusion

Sonia Liff and Fred Steward

Introduction

The concept of the 'digital divide' – a gap between those sections of the population with access to computers and the Internet and those without – has been documented and articulated most clearly by the National Telecommunications and Information Administration (NTIA) of the US Department of Commerce. A series of reports, collectively entitled *Falling Through the Net*, have documented the changing pattern of Internet use. While the reports themselves do not articulate explicit policy measures to address the divide, they do make a clear case for policy intervention. For example the summary of the most recent report says: 'increasing the number of Americans using the technology tools of the digital age is a vitally important national goal' (NTIA 2000: xv). Similar 'digital divides' and associated policy concerns are being identified within other developed nations, and international bodies such as the World Bank are drawing attention to the divide in connectivity between the western nations and those of the developing world.

The importance of widespread access and use of computers and the Internet is often expressed in rather vague terms as the danger of sections of the population being 'left behind'. It is becoming increasingly clear that this does not simply mean not having access to some *additional* opportunities for information and leisure activities. Instead the concern is that communication and information exchange will become ever more dependent on the use of computers and the Internet, and without such access and skills it will become difficult to get a job, gain an education, use government services or buy a good range of competitively priced goods. This is likely to cause problems not just for individuals but also for communities already left socially isolated by previous waves of technological development such as the motor car and telephone which have led shops to relocate to out-of-town sites and service provision to be concentrated in remote call centres.

In this way concern about access to ICT provision becomes part of broader debates about the decline of community, the economic regeneration of deprived areas and social exclusion. The UK government, which has initiated a range of broad policies to promote 'e-citizenship' and 'e-government', has recognised this specific dimension by establishing a Policy Action Team (hereafter referred to as PAT 15) within its Social Exclusion Unit to report on policies to promote the use of information and communication technologies in deprived areas. This team, which was made up primarily of civil servants and representatives from the voluntary sector, produced a report, *Closing the Digital Divide*, in March 2000. This report gave a key role to the provision of public access to computers and the Internet from sites within deprived areas (hereafter known as community e-gateways). As such it reflected concerns and approaches apparent in a series of other reports which stemmed mainly from the voluntary sector and which focused on ICT provision in local communities (National Working Party on Social Inclusion 1997, Day and Harris 1997, Shearman 1999).

While such reports draw on demographic data and some academic research, they are primarily attempts to draw inductively on practitioner experience to provide guidance on good practice and identify the ways in which the public sector and businesses can provide support. The focus of this chapter is on understanding both the advice given and the actual operation of successful public-access provision in a more analytical way. The intention is not an academic exercise of reconfiguring policy documents into sociological jargon. Instead it will argue that such an approach provides a better understanding of the strengths, and in some cases weaknesses, of policy prescription in this area and importantly provides a way to analyse the operation of existing community technology provision. The chapter draws on wider research on the provision of public access to computers and the Internet in the UK, the Los Angeles area of the USA and in Finland. A range of different types of facilities were studied, including cybercafes,[1] and these are referred to collectively in what follows as e-gateways. One of the UK case studies is reported in detail.

UK community-based ICT access: recommendations for success

The report from the PAT 15 team and earlier UK studies on information technology and social inclusion stress the need for community centres to support the uptake of ICTs, particularly in deprived areas. They make a range of suggestions about the characteristics of such centres; their relationships with other bodies and the communities of which they are part and the type of activities they should engage in to achieve this. Their suggestions are broadly complementary, although inevitably with differences in emphasis. They focus on two themes: that centres should be well connected to their local communities, well linked to and supported by local public agencies, and strongly led; and that they should provide a route into the use of technology based on local needs and interests, and work with users to develop the type of skills which will allow them to be content-creators and interact with others. Brief quotations from the main reports illustrate these concerns.

> [there is a need to focus on the ability of] people to be able to exploit information once they have it, and to generate and publish their own material . . . Policy makers have a role in helping to establish such initiatives (community networks and community resource centres) and supporting them . . . Community resource centres must have some form of public funding . . . The nature of partnerships in community networks is critical. They must be equal and all agencies need to examine their roles in this context . . . Community development strategies are still needed in local areas . . . empowerment will not come about without strategies for community involvement and basic capacity building among community groups.
>
> (National Working Party on Social Inclusion 1997: 64–5)

Community resource centres, and other community based IT initiatives, require:
* Skilled communicative workers and animators
* Relevant content and the opportunities and skills to generate their own content
* Systems that allow interaction and communication, not just one-way transmission
* Human networks, for support
* A non-threatening, community-managed public place to go.
                                                (based on Day and Harris 1997: 16)

Common success factors [of flagship projects are that]
* Technology is used as . . . a tool to achieve wider social, economic and/or community objective
* Each project started as small scale and local
* They are either community owned or deeply involved with the local community
* Each has been driven by one or two key individuals or local project champions
* They all have developed links and partnerships with local agencies
* They all have diversified their range of activities
* They have developed wider links beyond the local community.
                                                (based on Shearman 1999: 24)

Each deprived neighbourhood should have at least one publicly accessible community based facility . . . the number and location . . . should be determined locally . . . consideration should be given to providing ICT support to other community based activities, which can then provide an indirect introduction to ICTs . . . The local facility must also provide:

- Support for new and existing users
- Leadership to drive the facility forward
- Appropriate content to interest and meet the needs of local users
- Opportunities and support for local people to develop their own content
- Local promotion and outreach activities to encourage usage and the involvement of local people
- A strategy for being sustainable.

(based on PAT 15 2000: 57)

Such advice is likely to be uncontentious to community activists and those who have studied community IT provision. However, describing a centre as 'well connected' leaves many questions unanswered. For example, which type of bodies or individuals is it particularly important to be connected to? What sort of ties are needed? What specifically do such connections contribute to social inclusion or successful ICT use? Nor does it suggest a means for measuring relative levels, or forms, of connectiveness. Similar points can be made in relation to the other theme. In particular, what forms of training or context for learning are important for the type of skill acquisition advocated and what forms of public support are likely to sustain such an approach?

Being well connected

In social network terms the call for a centre to be well connected with its wider environment can be understood in terms of the scale and type of ties the centre, or key individuals within it, have with the wider community within which they are located. In general terms such ties can be described in terms of various characteristics such as their degree of intimacy, the number of different bases for interaction (for example friendship as well as shared professional interests) and degree of mutuality (whether the relationship is one-way or two-way, the types of support or benefit it provides) (Wellman and Wortley 1990). Relationships that score highly on these measures are described as strong ties (in contrast to weak ties which have low scores on these measures) and are generally seen as characteristics of kinship and traditional community ties. Similarly the extent to which people in a network have relationships with each other (network density) is also indicative of the social integration thought to be characteristic of traditional communities. Strong ties are generally seen as valuable because those with whom a person is connected in this way have been shown to be reliable providers of a range of resources in times of need.

It seems likely that these are the types of ties that the cited reports have in mind when they stress that community-based organisations providing ICT access should be well connected. Apart from the identified benefits that such ties bring in terms of integration and social support, the association with the characteristics thought to be indicative of traditional communities suggest that community e-gateways might contribute in a broader way to regeneration of deprived areas. Perhaps because being well connected seems to be a straightforward 'common-sense' concept, there has been little attempt to spell out how it is achieved, or how such links might help a community e-gateway to achieve its aims.

The community e-gateways and the other community or public organisations referred to can be thought of as social networks in their own right. The question then is how links are made between these groups. In network terms, connections are made by boundary-spanning between distinct social networks (Aldrich and Herker 1977). This can occur when an individual is a member of two otherwise distinct networks, where members of two distinct networks have a direct relationship or where this type of relationship occurs through a third party (Conway 1997). In the context under discussion this could be achieved by, say, a trainer in the community e-gateway also being a member of a mother-and-toddlers group or by the centre manager being a close neighbour of a person who runs the local youth club, or alternatively via a worker in a funding body who provides support to the centre and other community groups. The value of such boundary-spanning for an organisation is that it provides the means by which the organisation learns about the external environment and seeks to influence it. Studies suggest that such benefits are not achieved simply because the link exists. Instead certain skills are needed on the part of those who fulfil boundary-spanning or gatekeeper roles. These have been variously defined (and may provide some clues as to part of what is meant by the advice that centres should have strong and effective leadership) but focus on the ability to communicate effectively within and between networks (Tushman and Katz 1980, Katz and Allen 1982). These communication skills may involve the ability to move between social groups with different 'languages' (which could include the jargon associated with computer use) and norms of behaviour and helping others also to do so.

One key objective that can be supported by such boundary-spanning activities is that of attracting new users. They provide a route by which people get to know about the existence of a community e-gateway and what it offers and for the centre to learn about what the community might want. Such information is not simply the type that could be conveyed by a leaflet put through one's door or a survey of local residents. So in relation to the examples given above someone from the mothers-and-toddlers group might attend a training course because she knew the trainer in that context and trusted that she would be able and prepared to explain about the Internet in a comprehensible way. The centre manager in conversation with the youth worker might come to understand what would attract young people to come and use the computers and explain what they had to offer. From this they might jointly develop some targeted activities for youth-club members to be run by the community e-gateway. The worker from the funding body might find out about the need for computer training in one of the groups he or she works with and convey this to the community e-gateway and/or recommend the centre as a good source of appropriate training. As can be seen, such links are not simply about the neutral transmission of information but include the basis for building trust, pursuing shared values and understanding needs.

Learning based on interest and interaction

The other main area of recommendations centres on the need to start from people's interest and to create skills which allow them to be active users. Again the rationale for this is not strongly developed, nor is it clear what context or approaches for teaching or learning would facilitate it. Where it is discussed, the contrast is usually made between learning approaches based on formal course materials which start from the basics and build up the user's knowledge and those which take a more 'project' based approach where one identifies an area of interest and learns through pursuing this. It is usually argued that the latter is more likely to motivate those without a strong desire to learn. However, some people may not feel confident about this style of learning and it may lead to a rather fragmented understanding of the use of computers. In terms of the operation of e-gateways these are clearly significant choices (although the two are not incompatible). But behind such specific questions there are broader issues about the way people learn in a social context.

Lave and Wenger (1991) argue that learning is less about acquiring the skills to carry out specific tasks or activities and more about what they term becoming a full participant in a community of practice. They argue that all learning is situated – that is, it occurs in a specific social context – but further that it occurs through participation in a set of social practices. Of course learning specific things is important but in their view:

> activities, tasks, functions, and understandings do not exist in isolation; they are part of broader systems of relations in which they have meaning. These systems of relations arise out of and reproduced and developed within social communities, which are in part systems of relations among persons . . . Learning thus implies becoming a different person with respect to the possibilities enabled by these systems of relations.
>
> (Lave and Wenger 1991: 53)

So in this view learning about ICTs involves, for example, learning about new forms of communicating with persons known and unknown as much as it does the mastering the mechanics of a particular e-mail package. This may have significant implications for the learning process necessary to create users who are able to use the technology in creative ways.

Lave and Wenger (1991) describe various formal and informal 'apprentice-ship' systems through which such learning occurs. These vary in the degree to which they are structured but to be successful need to include not only opportunities to observe members of the community of practice but also opportunities for participation which help to make sense of the activities being undertaken. What they are describing could be understood as a social network where the actors are heterogeneous with respect to their levels of understanding and use of a particular area of practice – in this case the creative and interactive use of ICTs. If such social networks are to be not only effective learning mechanisms but also ways of promoting socially inclusive ICT use, then it is vital that they should have low barriers to entry. To a large extent this is dependent on the norms of the social network itself. However, some writers suggest that certain types of social place can facilitate the creation of inclusive social networks.

Oldenberg's (1991) account of the importance of third places (social space that is neither home nor work) where people can go and feel part of the community is particularly relevant in the context of community e-gateways. Such places function, he argues, as the core settings for an informal public life. Oldenberg says that the essential elements of an effective third place are that it is a neutral place where people feel comfortable and can come and go at will (as opposed to an interaction based on being the host or the guest), is socially inclusive in terms of the criterion for membership, stimulates good conversation, is accessible in terms of hours and location, is frequented by regulars and it is the possibility of meeting such friends that provides a primary motive for visiting it, is unpretentious in style and in mood, and has many of the characteristics of home without being one's home. Collectively one can see these characteristics as underlining the centrality of social interaction and the development of new social networks and describing a context that will facilitate. This includes the provision of opportunities for non-directed activities involving experimentation, and for creating a sense of identity which promotes inclusion by reducing barriers between people at different levels. Interestingly most of the specific types of third place Oldenburg describes are private-sector organisations such as pubs or coffee houses. However he acknowledges that they come to serve as third places often in spite of their formal designation: they 'are not constructed as such. Rather, establishments built for other purposes are commandeered by those seeking a place where they can linger in good company' (1991: 36). In this sense community centres may be a more conducive environment for the creation of this type of space.

Organisations characterised as e-gateways here are known under a number of hybrid names such as cybercafé, tele-cottage, community technology centre and electronic village hall. It is interesting in the light of Oldenburg's work that the non-computer part of their names tends to draw on types of organisation with third-place connotations. The café, the rural cottage, the community centre and the village hall are all social places which stress interaction as a key feature and do not tie participants down to narrow areas of activities. Interaction may well cross traditional organisational boundaries between work and leisure; learning and using; acquiring and giving information and so on. So for example in a community centre people may be used to going in to ask for advice on issues ranging from childcare problems, posting or responding to small ads for goods and services, through to work opportunities. At the same time the 'tele' or 'cyber' parts of e-gateways' names imply that there is something new here which may take one into new territory. This draws attention to the role such organisations are attempting to play in boundary-spanning between social networks of users and non-users (or partial or full participants in Lave and Wenger's terms).

There is another aspect of this interaction between new and old activities (such as drinking coffee and using computers) which is worth noting. Castells (1996) argues that the breakdown of boundaries between traditionally separate areas of activity is a key feature of information and communication technology. The same technology (the personal computer) and often very similar software allows one to do a range of activities that were previously distinct. Thus with a computer and a modem one can do the family accounts, play games, contact a friend in Australia, produce a community newsletter, do one's paid work from a remote location and order the shopping. While this observation relates to the potential of the technology to converge and integrate activities, it seems likely that some social locations will be better than others at helping users to understand and explore this potential. This provides one way of understanding the distinctive character of community-based technology access in contrast to similar technical provision within say libraries and colleges (Liff et al. 1999).

Network-mapping as a way to analyse links with resource providers and users

The practitioner literature on community e-gateways and studies of actual practice share views about importance of networking and embeddness within communities. By drawing on various social-science literatures, this account has tried to clarify why certain features are likely to be important and to draw attention to some of the limitations of the advice. The aim of the next section of the chapter is to demonstrate the way these ideas can be applied to a particular organisation. It uses a network-mapping approach (Steward and Conway 1998) to provide a visual representation of the relationships the organisation has with its resource providers and its users. This approach has some similarities with the technique of community-mapping which has developed in the US from the work of Kretzmann and McKnight (1993). They have stressed the importance of looking at what assets a community has rather than just understanding it in terms of 'needs' or 'deficits'. The

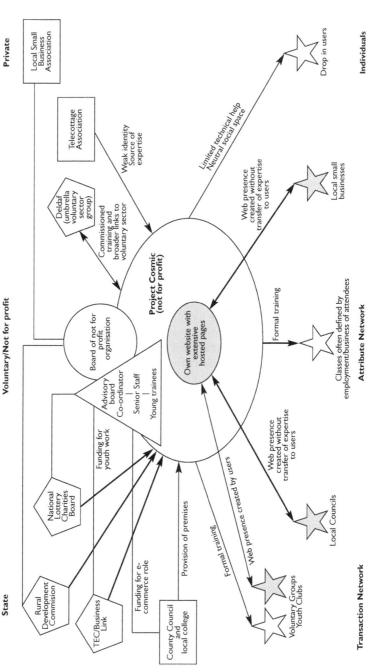

Figure 19.1 Network diagram for Project Cosmic

approach developed below also aims to map an organisation's assets but to do so in a way that is informed by the social-science understanding of different types of networks and forms of learning. Such an analysis might prove useful to centres themselves in identifying areas for future development. More broadly, sustainability for many community e-gateways depends on the provision of public funds (a factor acknowledged in the policy advice referred to earlier). This type of analysis can help to show the ways in which the current forms or terms of provision can support or constrain the achievement of goals of social inclusion and sustainability.

Analysing a community e-gateway

A small number of UK e-gateways were studied in depth as part of the broader research drawn on in this article. Case-study research involved observation, questionnaires to users and non-users, and interviews with staff and those in funding or other relationships with the centre. Case-study organisations were chosen following a broadly based survey and a number of shorter visits as providing a range of types of facility and location and as successful in attracting a significant number and range of users. One of these is the basis for this analysis.

Project Cosmic is a community-based facility at Ottery St Mary in Devon, UK. Ottery is a small town in a very rural area characterised by tourism and a large number of very small businesses. There is relatively little to attract young people in the area either in terms of work or leisure, and its population is ageing. The area also has a diverse and relatively vibrant voluntary sector. Project Cosmic is housed in an old railway-station building on the edge of town. The premises are owned by one of the local councils and other parts of the building are used by a local further education college for vocational and non-vocational adult courses. The youth service also runs regular evening youth clubs for different age groups. At the time of the study (early 1999) the building also housed a branch of the East Devon Volunteer Association.

Project Cosmic was established as a youth-orientated project with grants mainly from two sources: the National Lottery Charities Board and the Rural Development Commission (RDC). This funding was coming towards the end of its life and the organisation had begun to develop other sources of revenue by running training courses and designing web pages, often for local councils. They had had another grant from the local Training and Enterprise Council and Business Link to do outreach work to local businesses in the area of e-commerce. There were six people employed in various capacities.

Figure 19.1 provides a network map of Project Cosmic's links with resource-providers and with users. The central oval represents the organis-ation and the shaded oval contained within it is its website. The organisation is run as a not-for-profit company and has a board of directors and an advisory board. As can be seen, some but not all staff are directors and all senior, but not junior, staff are on the advisory board. Other members of the board of directors and advisory board are shown by the links to other bodies. It can be seen that these are mainly from the public sector but do also include people from the small business sector. It should also be noted that several of those who are members of Cosmic's management bodies come from organisations that are also providing funds to Cosmic (as indicated by links directly from, for example, the RDC to the organisation as well as from the RDC to the board of directors). In all these cases the people were there in a personal capacity and not as representatives of the funding body or as a condition of the funding. There were many more members of the advisory board but it is not possible to show them all on this scale of diagram. In terms of funding or resource-giving bodies the content of the link is briefly described on the diagram. Organisations shown by pentagons are those providing direct funding and the thicker lines represent the principal sources of funding at the time of the study.

The bottom half of Figure 19.1 shows relations with users. Users may come to the centre as individuals, as members say of a class where they are present with other people with whom they have shared interests but do not have strong existing ties (attribute network) or they may come as part of a functioning group (transaction network) who want to learn together or to use the technology for some shared purpose. In this case Cosmic had a small number of individual users who dropped in for specific purposes (such as web searching, emailing or advice on computer problems); it ran a significant number of courses, some focused around a particular computer application, others targeted on occupational groups such as hotel owners; and it also provided classes and less structured facilities for groups including local voluntary associations and the town's youth clubs. The thickness of the lines indicates those links which accounted for a major part of the organisation's activities. Shaded users are those whose link with Cosmic involved the creation of web material.

The account below highlights three areas where this analysis, drawing on the concepts developed above, can highlight the strengths and limitations of their activities.

Links to wider community for resources, users and identifying needs

As is clear from Figure 19.1 Cosmic used its advisory-board structure to establish connections with both funders and a range of people in the community, particularly those with links to education, youth work or local councils. This appeared to be a deliberate strategy aimed at getting as wide a range of knowledge and interest as possible. These people provide bridges into other communities, articulating their needs to Cosmic and transmitting information about Cosmic's facilities to their own networks. So for example a local headmaster who was on the advisory board provided information about training opportunities which might be associated with the national grid for learning and encouraged them to offer such provision for his staff.

In general these relationships were not 'strong' in terms of levels of intimacy but in a number of cases they did demonstrate other aspects of strong ties such as informality, multiple bases for interaction and mutuality. So for example contact with members of the advisory board often occurred outside formal meetings, through phone calls for example. A member of the advisory board who also ran a hotel had a website designed for him by Cosmic and so dropped in regularly to have it updated. Information was passed on that people thought would be of interest to Cosmic as well as advice and services being sought. In a rather different example the woman who ran the Volunteer Bureau passed on anything which looked as though it might fund computer-related activities which she received as part of her central role in the voluntary sector information networks. She also referred on any requests from people who wanted to get computer access. Cosmic reciprocated by sorting out any computer problems her office had and providing advice on computer-related purchases.

In some cases friendships or higher levels of familiarity strengthened the ties. One of the staff at Cosmic was a former council employee and had retained a friendship with the person who had taken over her job and with other people there. Her previous experience of the organisation helped her to gauge what they would want in terms of approach and services effectively, but the fact that she was still known by many people in the Council also meant that she had a credibility to them that someone else offering training or web design services would have been unlikely to have. Ties were also strengthened by shared values. A central figure in the local voluntary sector had obtained funds to provide training for voluntary groups in computers and the Internet. He assessed what was offered by a range of providers and chose Cosmic not only because they were good value for money but also because they were a not-for-profit organisation and so he felt that the money would stay in the voluntary sector and support an organisation with a commitment to social goals.

Attracting users

The links described above were clearly one-way links in which users found out about Cosmic's services and were encouraged to try them. There were also lots of other mechanisms in place, some drawing on strong, others on weak, links. The youth club operating in the same building as Cosmic demonstrated links of both kinds. One of the staff members at Cosmic had originally been a youth worker (and indeed this was the origin of the project). He retained his involvement with the local club, working there on some occasions. He was in a position through this to develop relationships with the children and the other youth workers. These relationships provided a basis for engaging the young people's interest in learning about and using computers for a range of purposes. These included web page design, Internet searching and chat rooms. At other times the computer room would just be open with one of the younger staff in place. He took no active part in the main activities of the youth club but the facilities were there as one of the things that they could do and young people drifted in and out as their interest was engaged without any commitment to follow a course of study or undertake any other formal activity.

Other strong ties that attracted users were the friendship networks of the young people who worked at Cosmic. They were employed as trainees mainly undertaking web design and creation for commercial clients. Their friends dropped in regularly after school and this created a group of casual users of the computers, a potential pool from whom new employees might arise, and created an environment that was attractive to other young people. The way the facilities were arranged helped these ties to develop. Junior staff worked from the computer room which provided drop-in facilities when it was not needed for formal training. This meant that some support could be provided without it tying up someone completely and they were able to develop their own culture away from the senior staff (who normally worked in another room). Less successfully exploited were the opportunities to make links with those visiting the building for adult education or recreation classes. In fact the opportunities for these weak links to be used were actively minimised by, for example, making efforts to ensure that those taking training courses at Cosmic did not take their coffee breaks at the same times as the adult learners.

Learning skills, buying services or participating in the information society

Project Cosmic had a very extensive website of its own and also hosted websites for a range of small businesses, local councils and voluntary groups. It regularly ran introduction to the Internet courses for a range of participants and had run week-long website design courses for voluntary groups. It had completed a project which had introduced a significant number of local small businesses to the potential of the Internet, including establishing a web presence for them. As such Cosmic had been highly successful at raising awareness of the scope and potential of ICTs in its local community.

Looked at from the perspective of communities of practice, there are reasons for being more cautious. The councils that had become customers for website design, and in particular the small businesses, showed little evidence of having engaged with the creative potential of the Internet. During the period of fieldwork a major commercial job being undertaken was the translation of one authority's brochure into web pages. The brief was that it should be as close as possible to their current printed version. Many of the small businesses who by formal measures (such as having a web page and an email address) would be seen as at the forefront of e-commerce in practice may not even have owned a computer – certainly few had their own Internet connection. They were provided with a service whereby any emails sent to them were picked up by Cosmic who then forwarded them on by fax. The reasons for this limited engagement were probably a combination of the companies' lack of understanding of e-commerce potential, their inability or unwillingness to commit funds or time to finding out, the terms of the funding which generated this area of work and Cosmic's limited expertise at that time in identifying businesses for whom such a development would be appropriate. As important are the consequences that these organisations are not participating in any real practice in relation to the information society and are likely at best to be developing only a limited understanding of its potential or significance for their activities.

The situation in relation to the voluntary groups was more positive in that they had designed their own web pages during a week-long course and as such had been forced to think through their own identity in this new medium. However, few seemed to be actively maintaining their pages or seeing them as anything other than an advertisement for their activities. Again this is likely to be in part a function of the nature of the funding which provided them only with the initial opportunity to create the site. It highlights the limitations of approaches which provide only one-off training opportunities or which subsidise the purchase of a service without facilitating any longer-term opportunities to become participants in a community of practice.

Reflections on the policy prescription and social practice

It was argued that understanding the prescriptions contained in the policies promoting ICT use in socially excluded communities in a more analytical way would highlight their rationale, or lack of it, and provide a stronger basis for assessing practice. The analysis has shown that much of what is recommended and practised has a sound basis as a way of engaging new users in the 'information society'. These aspects were identified in the earlier sections. However there are a number of areas where there are contradictory elements or where the full implications of what is proposed is either not recognised or not fully supported. Three are highlighted below. Attention to these issues is not intended to displace the main body of the advice given but rather to supplement it or occasionally temper it.

The underestimation of the contribution of weak ties to social inclusion

In stressing the importance of 'well connectedness', policy and practitioner advice were seen, implicitly at least, to be thinking of strong ties. There is undoubtedly a rationale for this, particularly in deprived areas where there are low levels of trust and an alienation from public institutions. Such ties can be vital in establishing the legitimacy of a centre with its community. However, there is evidence that weak ties can also be important in resource terms. Best known is Granovetter's 1973 study of job-search experiences, which demonstrates that weak ties (for example, friend of a friend) are valuable sources of information because they connect the person into networks with which they would not otherwise have contact. This suggests that an over-dependence on highly dense strong ties may also imply social isolation from wider society. Perri 6 makes this link explicit by defining social exclusion as 'network poverty' (1997: 16). While not denying the significance of strong ties, particularly for the young and old, he suggests that what most adults need is a network configuration 'rich in weak ties which span holes in social networks'. The practical value of weak ties to community e-gateways can be seen in Cosmic's advisory-board structure whose diverse, weakly linked members contributed knowledge about funding opportunities, work that could be tendered for, related activities by councils or other community or commercial groups and so on. This approach can be contrasted with another community e-gateway studied where the management committee was made up for the most part of those running and regularly using the facility. In some senses the latter draws on stronger ties and may be easier to manage since the basis of commitment to the centre is clearer and there are likely to be more shared values. However the range of information provided is likely to be greatly reduced.

Our wider research identified a type of e-gateway which was using weak ties as its primary way to attract new users. These gateways had prominent, attractive locations, and we refer to them collectively as shop-front e-gateways. Users tended to come in because they had seen the facility in passing, had seen some advertising or had been told about it by someone they knew. Shop-front e-gateway users tended to be more instrumental than those using community e-gateways in that their use was determined by factors such as the range of equipment, convenience of location and opening hours, and cost. None the less, many developed a strong network of regulars and a defining culture which was valued by users. Community e-gateways are often located in rather run-down buildings in out-of-the-way locations and may feel this shop-front approach is not open to them. However many did have opportunities which were under-utilised. For example premises are often shared with other community facilities. In such a context one would expect this to act as a bridge between different social networks. Users of other facilities in the building (such as community centre, location for adult education, primary health clinic) who might not define themselves as interested in computers are likely to pass by and potentially come into contact with those using the computer centre. Such casual passers-by could be targeted in an active way, for example by open days, taster sessions, putting a computer out in the corridor, inviting other groups to have meetings in the computer centre and so on. This could attract people who may not be part of any strong social network into which the community e-gateway is linked and could be appealing to those who might find a centre based on strong ties too cliquey. These types of devices did not seem to be being used, or used effectively, in the community e-gateways studied. At Project Cosmic and another similarly located centre in south-west Scotland, those using other community or adult-education facilities in the same building as the community e-gateways were surveyed, and while 85 per cent said they knew of the computer facility only 6 per cent had used it.

Boundary-spanning as a two-way process: the limitations of seeing technology only as a means to an end

A recurrent theme in the advice to those providing computer access in the community is to work from people's interests rather than from the technology. In network terms what is being suggested is that boundary-spanning between providers of computer access and current non-users is facilitated by participating in their language and practices. This reduces the barriers to entering the social network of users by making links to the current activities of non-users and discussing use in terms which makes sense to them. It can also be seen to link to Lave and Wenger's ideas about social learning since it stresses learning through practice rather than via the acquisition of an abstracted body of knowledge. Users surveyed for this research provided support for the view that learning can occur in this way without the presence of formal teaching. Most said that visiting the e-gateway had increased their knowledge and ability in relation to computers and that they felt more positively both about their ability to learn and about IT in general.

In the light of the prevalence of such well-grounded advice, it is surprising that the main activity of community e-gateways with respect to new users is the provision of relatively formal learning opportunities. In the case of Cosmic this took the form of classes introducing participants to various software packages or to the Internet. In other community e-gateways studied, the emphasis was more on supporting individuals to follow self-learning packages. In neither case were these strongly tailored to the particular interests or current practices of the participants. Learning through following self-identified interests with support from a more experienced user was much more commonly observed in the shop-front e-gateways studied (normally commercial or semi-commercial Internet cafés). This may in part reflect differences in users, with those going to shop-front e-gateways already being more clearly motivated to use the technology (as evidenced by their accessing the facility without the benefit of strong ties). However it is also a consequence of the approach taken by government and other funding regimes which have yet to catch up with the advice that they themselves are giving. So, for example, it is invariably a condition of funding that centres process large numbers of people through formal courses with clearly defined learning outcomes – the latter usually measured in terms of completion of a course rather than the learners' perceptions of what they have gained.

Even if funders were to be more flexible in their assessment of teaching and learning approaches in line with their own recommendations, there are still questions to be raised about the one-directional nature of the boundary-spanning that is being encouraged. The practitioner and policy literature also stresses the importance of communities using technology creatively and to its full potential. When new technologies are first developed, it is common to try to understand their potential in terms of what they might take the place of in existing technologies or how they might do the same things differently (for example television as an alternative to the cinema or the telephone as an alternative form of communication to mail). But a common characteristic of radical developments in technology is that they create new uses and patterns of social interaction that were not at all obvious at an early stage and which may be overlooked by those who argue just by analogy from old technologies (Williams 1974 discusses this in relation to television). This suggests a danger in just accepting non-users' current interests and activities as the framework for introducing them to the Internet which can be illustrated by the small businesses and local authorities for whom Cosmic was creating web pages. It was clear that such users were not learning to use the Internet in creative ways or understanding its full potential. The funding regimes and the nature of the commercial interactions were reinforcing the problem by supporting short-term engagement with clearly defined ends on the users' terms.

Drawing attention to this problem should not be taken as a demand to return to technology-focused forms of teaching materials. Rather it implies the need for a clearer articulation of the new community of practice being developed by users within e-gateways. This may require the creation of materials which support forms of boundary-spanning which focus on allowing non-users to understand more of the world of this particular group of users, opportunities for interactions over a longer period between new users and those who are more experienced, and perhaps the development of a stronger sense of collective self-identity among those running and promoting e-gateways.

The resource intensive nature of creating and sustaining social networks

This chapter has stressed the importance of social networks to the successful operation of e-gateways in terms of attracting new users and helping them to learn about and participate in the 'information society'. It has shown that such an approach is implicitly recognised in much policy advice although its full implications are not always drawn out and are contradicted by some funding regimes. In making the role of social networks explicit this analysis shows that what is important in creating effective e-gateways is not simply a set of activities but rather the social relations that sustain them. These social networks may not be consciously sought after or deliberately created but they would not function effectively without considerable effort by key individuals. The creation and maintenance of such relationships needs time and, as Oldenburg's writing on third places shows, can be facilitated by certain types of space and opportunities for non-directed interaction between people who might otherwise not come into contact with each other. Without a better recognition of the role of networking on the part of those funding and assessing e-gateways, the provision of inviting public space and facilities and time for informal interaction can seem an indulgence rather than the necessity this analysis suggests it is. Where such facilities and ways of working were observed their continued existence seemed precarious because of a lack of recognition and support by funding bodies. In the organisations studied, networking by those running the centres was often sustained at high personal cost to the individuals concerned in terms of hours of work and/or low levels of pay and yet can be shown to be vital to the centre's successful operation. Such issues are not only relevant to those running the facility; they relate also to the way people learn. So learning contexts and materials need to build in opportunities for people to get to know each other, to identify links and shared interests and to encourage opportunities for collaboration or mutual help rather than just working through pre-defined courses in isolation. In understanding the importance of this way of learning, it is also necessary to recognise that the role of the 'teacher' also changes. As well as being able to convey knowledge in ways which make sense to the learner, teachers are drawing upon existing relationships and building new ones. All such facilities and approaches are resource-intensive in comparison with, say, the purchase of an extra suite of computers equipped with online learning packages for a pre-existing library or college. However this analysis suggests that the former is much more likely to deliver the goals identified in policy documents of social inclusion and creative use of information and communication technology.

Note

1 The research project entitled 'Gateways to the Virtual Society: Innovation for Social Inclusion' was funded by the ESRC as part of the 'Virtual Society?' programme (L132251022). It was carried by the authors with Peter Watts, now of Canterbury Christ Church University College.

Glossary

Bandwidth   The amount of data, typically expressed as kilobits per second (Kbps), that can pass through a network connection.

Baud   A unit of data transmission speed, or the maximum speed at which data can be sent down a channel.

BBSs (Bulletin Board Services)   A shared file where users can enter information for other users to read or download. Many bulletin boards are set up according to general topics and are accessible throughout a network.

Bit   A contraction of binary digit. A bit is the smallest unit of information a computer can hold. The speed at which bits are transmitted or bit rate is usually expressed as bits per second or bps.

Browser   The program that finds and displays Web pages. Microsoft Internet Explorer, Netscape Navigator, Opera, Mosaic and Mozilla are browsers.

Byte   This is a number of bits used to represent a character. Eight bits is equivalent of a byte.

CCTV   Closed-circuit television, used to monitor activities.

CD-ROM   Read-only data on a compact disc.

Client   A computer or computer program that is one side of the client–server communication.

CMC   Computer-mediated communication.

CSCW   Computer-supported co-operative working.

Cookies   When you connect your Internet browser to a server to get a web page, each time you do this it is a totally separate connection, i.e. the browser and the server have no memory that they have just been connected a few seconds earlier. In order that the server can keep track of which users are doing what on the site, it copies some information to the user's machine which it can look at to remind itself that this is the same person. This is a cookie.

Cyberspace   A term coined by William Gibson, a science-fiction writer, to refer to a near-future computer network where users mentally travel through matrices of data. The term is now usually used to describe the Internet and other computer networks.

FAQ   Frequently Asked Questions.

Flame   An abusive message which, when placed publicly in a newsgroup, can provoke a flame war as people trade insults.

FTP   File Transfer Protocol is a protocol that allows the transfer of files from one computer to another. FTP is also the verb used to describe the act of transferring files from one computer to another.

Gopher   A distributed information system similar to the World Wide Web, but less versatile and generally used only for text files.

Home page   This term is used loosely. It can refer to the top or main page of an organisation, company or personal page for an individual.

HTML   An acronym for Hypertext Transfer Protocol, a protocol used to transfer documents on the World Wide Web.

ICTs   Information and communications technologies.

Information superhighway   A future symmetrical switched broadband network, which the Internet may evolve into. Not today's Internet.

Internet   The collection of networks and gateways that use the IP Protocol suite and function as a single, co-operative virtual network. The Internet reaches many universities, government research labs and military installations.

ISDN   Integrated Services Digital Network: a set of standards for high-speed transmission of simultaneous voice, data and video information over fewer channels than would otherwise be needed, through the use of out-of-band signalling.

ISP (Internet Service Provider)   A company that provides personal or business access to the Internet.

MUDS (Multi-User Dungeons)   Imaginary world in computer databases where people interact to improvise melodramas, build worlds and all the objects in them, and play games.

Netiquette   A corruption of network etiquette, that is, a generally accepted guide to 'good manners' when talking to other people on the Internet. Abuses of netiquette will generally result in you being flamed.

Netscape   A graphical Web browser.

Plug-in   A type of software that adds a specific capability to a program already on your computer. For instance, your browser probably requires a plug-in to see certain types of animation.

Protocol   An agreed-upon format for transmitting data between two devices. The protocol determines: (1) the type of error-checking to be used; (2) the data-compression method; (3) the method for discussion between the sending and receiving device.

Proxy   A server that sits between a client and a server. The proxy intercepts requests to see if it can fulfil the requests itself. In the digital media world, proxies are used to improve end-user experience and reduce bandwidth.

RAM   (Random Access Memory), needed for running programs.

Server   A computer or computer program that manages and delivers information for client computers.

Streaming media   An Internet data-transfer technique that allows the user to see and hear audio and video files without lengthy download times. The host or source 'streams' small packets of information over the Internet to the user, who can access the content as it is received.

TCP/IP   The basic protocols controlling communication on the Internet.

URL   (Uniform Resource Locator) the addressing system used in the World Wide Web and other Internet resources. The URL contains information about the method of access, the server to be accessed and the path of any file to be accessed.

VR   Virtual reality: a system that creates an alternate representation of data in a dynamic form. Data-representation is in the form of an interactive system that models in three dimensions and allows the participant to move about in an unrestricted manner to examine it from any perspective. Images are generated by a computer and projected in any number of fashions. VR systems range from aircraft flight simulators to Web browsers.

WAIS   The abbreviation for Wide Area Information Service, WAIS is a Net-wide system for looking up specific information in Internet databases.

Webcast   The broadcasting of streaming content over the Internet. Typically refers to a live broadcast.

Web page   An HTML document that is accessible on the Web.

World Wide Web   Also known as WWW, or W3, a way that information is moved around the Internet, the worldwide network of computer networks, providing text, files, graphics, sounds and moving pictures. It is a hypertext-based Internet service used for browsing Internet resources.

Bibliography

[RCM]
  http://www.retecivica.milano.it
[Tesoro00]
  http://fc.retecivica.milano.it/rcmweb/tesoro/tesoro99/frame1.htm
[Tesoro01]
  http://www.retecivica.milano.it/tesoro
Abbott. V. P. (2000) 'Web page quality: can we measure it and what do we find? A report of exploratory findings', *Journal of Public Health Medicine*, Vol. 22, No. 2, pp. 191–7.
Adam, A. (1998) *Artificial Knowing: Gender and the Thinking Machine*, London: Routledge.
Adam, A. and Green, E. (1998) 'Gender, agency, location and the new information society', in Loader, B. (ed.) *Cyberspace Divide: Equality, Agency and Policy in the Information Society*, London: Routledge.
Adamsen, L., Fisker, J. and Jørgensen, K. (1990) *Forsøgsstrategi – samfundsmæssige konsekvenser og fremtidsperspektiver*, Copenhagen: AKF Forlaget.
Adamsen, L. and Fisker, J. (1991) *Forsøgsstrategi – Samfundsmæssige konsekvenser og fremtidsperspektiver*, Copenhagen: AKF Forlaget.
Akrich, M. (1992) 'The de-scription of technical objects', in Bijker, W. E. and Law, L. (eds) *Shaping Technology/Building Society*, Cambridge, MA: MIT Press.
Albrecht, L. and Brewer, R. M. (1990) *Bridges of Power, Women's Multicultural Alliances*, Philadelphia: New Society Publishers.
Albrow, M., Eade, J., Dürrschmidt, J. and Washbourne, N. (1997) 'The impact of globalization on sociological concepts: community, culture and milieu', in Eade, J. (ed.) *Living the Global City: Globalization as Local Process*, London: Routledge.
Aldrich, H. and Herker, D. (1977) 'Boundary spanning roles and organisational structure', *Academy of Management Review*, April, pp. 217–30.
Alexander, C., Ishikawa, S. and Silverstein, M. (1977) *A Pattern Language: Towns, Building, Construction*, New York: Oxford.
Alkalimat, A. and Associates (1986) *Introduction to Afro-American Studies*, Chicago: Twenty First Century Books, on the Web at http://www.eblackstudies.net/intro.
Alkalimat, A., Gills, D. and Williams, K. (eds) (1995), *Job? Tech: The Technological Revolution and Its Impact on Society*, Chicago: Twenty First Century Books.
Alshejni, L. (1999) 'Unveiling the Arab woman's voice through the net', in Harcourt, W. (ed.) *Women@Internet: Creating New Cultures in Cyberspace*, London: Zed.

AMA (Association of Metropolitan Authorities) (1989) *Community Development, the Local Authority Role*, London: Association of Metropolitan Authorities.

Amnå, E. (1999) 'IT for democratic purposes' ('IT i demokratins tjänst', in Swedish), *Statens offentliga utredningar*, Vol. 117, Stockholm.

Andersen, H. S., Jensen, L., Jæger, B., Sehested, K. and Sørensen, E. (1999b) *Digitale byer i København og Europa*, Working Paper, Vol. 7, Roskilde University, Denmark.

Andersen, I.-E. and Jæger, B. (1999a) 'Multimedia in Denmark, an overview', *Science and Public Policy*, Vol. 26, pp. 331–40.

Anzaldúa, G. (1987) *Borderlands/La Frontera: The New Mestiza*, San Francisco: Aunt Lute Books.

Arnot, C. (1999) 'We've all been framed', *The Guardian*, 8 December.

Arnstein, S. R. (1969) 'A ladder of citizen participation', *Journal of the American Institute of Planners*, Vol. 35, No. 4, pp. 216–24.

Aurigi, A. (2000) 'Digital city or "Urban simulator"?', in Ishida, T. and Isbister, K. (eds) *Digital Cities: Technologies, Experiences and Future Perspectives – Lecture Notes in Computer Science*, Berlin: Springer-Verlag.

Aurigi, A. and Graham, S. (1998) 'The "crisis" in the urban public realm', in Loader, B. (ed.) *Cyberspace Divide: Equality, Agency and Policy in the Information Society*, London: Routledge.

Balbo, L. (1987) 'Crazy quilts: rethinking the welfare state debate from a woman's point of view', Showstack Sassoon, A. (ed.) *Women and the State*, London: Routledge.

Banse, R. (1999) 'Automatic evaluation of self and others: affective priming in close relationships', *Journal of Social and Personal Relationships*, Vol. 16, No. 6 (December).

Baran, S. J. and Davis, D. K. (2000) *Mass Communication Theory: Foundations, Ferment and Future*, 2nd edition, Belmont, CA: Wadsworth/Thomson Learning.

Barker, J. (1999) *Street-Level Democracy: Political Settings at the Margins of Global Power*, West Hartford, CT: Kumarian Press.

Barlow, J. P. (1996) 'Thinking locally, acting globally', *Cyber-Rights Electronic List*, 15 January.

Barthélmy, D. and Contamine, P. (1985) [1988] 'The use of private space', in Duby, G. (ed.) *A History of Private Life*, Cambridge, MA: Belknap Press.

Basalla, G. (1988) *The Evolution of Technology*, Cambridge: Cambridge University Press.

Bastani, S. (2000) 'Muslim women on-line', *Arab World Geographer,* Vol. 3, No. 1.

Bauer, R. A. (1984) 'The obstinate audience', *American Psychologist*, Vol. 19, pp. 319–28.

BBC (2000) *CCTV For 180 More Sites*, BBC UK News Site, 17 January, http://news2.thls.bbc.co.uk/hi/english/uk/newsid%5F607000/607000.stm.

BBC Online (2000) 'Blair's five-year Internet pledge', 7 March 2000, www.news.bbc.co.uk/english/newsid_6680001668759.

Beaud, P. (1980) *Community Media? Local Radio and Television and Audio-visual Animation Experiments in Europe*, Strasbourg: Council of Europe.

Belenky M., Clinchy, B. M., Goldberger, N. R. and Tarule, J. M. (1986) *Women's Ways of Knowing: The Development of Self, Voice and Mind*, New York: Basic Books.

Bell, C. and Newby, H. (eds) (1974) *The Sociology of Community: A Selection of Readings*, London: Frank Cass & Co.

Bell, D. (1973) *The Coming of Post-Industrial Society: A Venture in Social Forecasting*, Harmondsworth: Penguin, Peregrine Books.

Bennet, T. and Gelsthorpe, L. (1996) 'Public attitudes towards CCTV in public places', *Studies in Crime and Crime Prevention*, Vol. 5, No. 1, pp. 72–90.

Benson, T. W. (1996) 'Rhetoric, civility, and community: political debate on computer bulletin boards', *Communication Quarterly*, Vol. 44, No. 3, pp. 359–78.

Benton Foundation. http://www.digitaldividenetwork.org.

Bergman, S. and van Zoonen, L. (1999) 'Fishing with false teeth: women, gender and the Internet', in Downey, J. and McGuigan, J. (eds) *Technocities*, London: Sage.

Berkowitz, S. D. (1982) *An Introduction to Structural Analysis: The Network Approach to Social Research*, Toronto: Butterworth.

Bertot, J. C. and McClure, C. (2000) 'Public libraries and the Internet 2000: summary findings and data tables, NCLIS Web release version', on the Web at http://www.nclis.gov/statsurv/2000plo.pdf.

Besselaar, P., Van Der Melis, I. and Beckers, D. (2000) 'Digital cities: organisation, content, and use', in Ishida, T. and Isbister, K. (eds) *Digital Cities: Experiences, Technologies and Future Perspectives – Lecture Notes in Computer Science* 1765, Berlin: Springer-Verlag.

Bijker, W. E., Hughes, P. and Pinch, T. (1987) *The Social Construction of Technological Systems*, Cambridge, MA: MIT Press.

Bijker, W. E. (1995) *Of Bicycles, Bakelites, and Bulbs: Towards a Theory of Sociotechnical Change*, Cambridge, MA: The MIT Press.

Bion, W. R. (1961) *Experiences in Groups*, London: Tavistock.

Bishop, A. P. (2000) 'Communities for the new century', *Journal of Adolescent and Adult Literacy*, Vol. 43, February, on the Web at http://www.readingonline.org/electronic/jaal/2-00_Column.html.

Blair, T. (1999) *Libraries Entering the Information Age*, http://www.number-10.gov.uk/.

Blair, T. (2000) Speech by the UK Prime Minister to the *Knowledge 2000 Conference* – 7 March, http://www.number-10.gov.uk/news.asp?NewsId=637&SectionId=32.

Blanchard, A. and Horan, T. (1998) 'Virtual communities and social capital', *Social Science Computer Review*, Vol. 16, pp. 293–307.

Bloomberg News (2000) 'Internet not as connected as thought', *Utah Online (Salt Lake City Tribune)*, 12 May. Website: wysiwyg://93/http://www.sltrib.com/05122000/business/48507.htm.

Boberg, E. W., Gustafson, D. H., Hawkins, R. P., Chan, C. L., Bricker, E., Pingree, S., Berhe, H. and Peressini, A. (1995) 'Development, acceptance, and use patterns of a computer based education and social support system for people living with AIDS/HIV infection', in *Computers in Human Behaviour*, Vol. 11, No. 2, pp. 289–311.

Bodemann, Y. M. (1988) 'Relations of production and class rule: the hidden basis of patron-clientage', Wellman, B. and Berkowitz, S. D. (eds) *Social Structures: A Network Approach*, Cambridge: Cambridge University Press.

Bodker, S. and Gronbeck, K. (1991) 'Co-operative prototyping: users and designers in mutual activity', *The International Journal of Man-Machine Studies*, Vol. 34.

Bodker, S. and Greenbaum, J. (1993) 'Design of information systems: things versus people', in Green, E., Owen, J. and Pain, D. (eds) *Gendered by Design? Information Technology and Office Systems*, London: Taylor and Francis.

Bogason, P. (1996) *New Modes of Local Political Organizing: Local Government Fragmentation in Scandinavia*, Commack: Nova Science Publishers.

Booz-Allen and Hamilton Associates (2000) *Achieving Universal Access*, London: Booz-Allen & Hamilton Associates, also available http://www.number-10.gov.uk/.

Bornat, J., Pereira, C., Pilgrim, D. and Williams, F. (ed.) (1993) *Community Care: A Reader*, Basingstoke: Macmillan Press Ltd.

Bostock, S. and Seifert, J. (1987) 'The effects of learning environment and gender on the attainment of computer literacy', *Studies in the Education of Adults*, Vol. 19, No. 1, pp. 37–45.

Bott, E. (1957) *Family and Social Network*, London: Tavistock.

Bottoms, A. E. and Wiles, P. (1994) 'Crime and insecurity in the city', paper presented at Changes in Society, Crime and Criminal Justice in Europe international conference in Leuven, Belgium.

Bourdieu, P. (1986) *Distinction: A Social Critique of the Judgement of Taste*, London: Routledge.

Bowles, S. (1999) *Social Capital and Community Governance*, 31 July, on the Web at http://www-unix.oit.umass.edu/~bowles/papers/Socap.PDF.

Bradner, E. (2000) *Understanding Groupware Adoption: The Social Affordances of Computer-mediated Communication among Distributed Groups*, Working Paper, Department of Information and Computer Science, University of California, Irvine (February).

Brail, S. (1996) 'The price of admission: harassment and free speech in the wild, wild, west', in Cherny, L. and Weise, E. R. (eds) *Wired Women: Gender and New Realities in Cyberspace*, Seattle: Seal Press.

Braverman, H. (1974) *Labour and Monopoly Capital*, New York, Monthly Review.

Braverman, H. (1998) *Labor and Monopoly Capitalism*, New York: Monthly Review Press.

Breeden, L., Cisler, S., Guilfoy, V., Roberts, M. and Stone, A. (1998) *Computer and Communications Use in Low-income Communities: Models for the Neighborhood Transformation and Family Development Initiative*, December, on the Web at http://www.ctcnet.org/casey/.

Brothers, R. (1999) 'The computer-mediated public sphere and the cosmopolitan ideal', in *Proceedings of ETHICOMP '99: Look to the Future of the Information Society*, 5–7 October, Rome: Luiss Guido Carli University/De Montfort University.

Brown, B. (1995) *CCTV in Town Centres: Three Case Studies*, Crime Detention and Prevention Series, Paper No. 68. Home Office Police Department, London: Home Office.

Brown, M. and Smith, H. (1993) 'Women caring for people: the mismatch between rhetoric and women's reality', *Policy and Politics*, Vol. 21, No. 3, pp. 185–93.

Brown, S. (1998) 'What's the problem girls?: CCTV and the gendering of public safety', in Norris, C., Moran, J. and Armstrong, G. (eds), *Surveillance, Closed Circuit Television and Social Control*, Aldershot: Ashgate.

Bruckner, E. and Knaup, K. (1993) 'Women's and men's friendships in comparative perspective', *European Sociological Review*, Vol. 9, No. 3, pp. 249–66.

Buchstein, H. (1997) 'Bytes that bite: the Internet and deliberative democracy', *Constellations*, Vol. 4, No. 2, pp. 248–63.

Bulos, M. and Sarno, C. (1994) *Closed Circuit Television and Local Authority Initiatives: The First Survey*, School of Land Management and Urban Policy, London: South Bank University.

Bunton, R. and Peterson, A. (1997) 'Popular health, advanced liberalism and Good Housekeeping Magazine', in Bunton, R. and Peterson, A. (eds) *Foucault, Health and Medicine*, London: Routledge.

Burgess, J (1998) ' "But is it worth taking the risk?" How women negotiate access to urban woodland: a case study', in Ainley, R (ed.) *New Frontiers of Space, Bodies and Gender*, London: Routledge.

Burgess, R. G. (1984) *In the Field: An Introduction to Field Research*, London: George Allen & Unwin.

Burrows, R. and Nettleton, S. (2000) 'Reflexive modernisation and the emergence of wired self-help', in Renniger, K. and Shumar, W. (eds) *Building Virtual Communities: Learning and Change in Cyberspace,* New York: Cambridge University Press.

Burrows, R., Nettleton, S., Pleace, N., Loader, B. D. and Muncer, S. (2000) 'Virtual community care? Social policy and the emergence of computer mediated social support', *Information, Communication & Society*, Vol. 3, No. 1.

Butcher, H. (1993) 'Introduction: some examples and definitions', in Butcher, H., Glen, A., Henderson, P. and Smith, J., *Community and Public Policy*, London: Pluto.

Butler, S. and Wintram, C. (1991) *Feminist Groupwork*, London: Sage.

Buxton, B. (1992) 'Telepresence: integrating shared task and person spaces', paper presented to the Graphics Interface Conference, Vancouver, May.

Cabinet Office (1998) *People's Panel – A Quick Summary*, http://www.cabinet-office. gov.uk/servicefirst/1998/panel/ppsummary.htm.

Cabinet Office (1999) *Modernising Government*, London: Stationery Office, also available at http://www.cabinet-office.gov.uk.

Cabinet Office (2000) *E-government – A Strategic Framework for Public Services in the Information Age*, http://www.iagechampions.gov.uk/strategy.htm.

Calhoun, C. (ed.) (1992), *Habermas and the Public Sphere*, Cambridge, MA: MIT Press.

Callaghan, P. and Morrissey, J. (1993) 'Social support and health: a review', *Journal of Advanced Nursing,* No. 18, pp. 203–13.

Callon, M. (1991) 'Techno-economic networks and irreversibility', in Law, J. (ed.) *A Sociology of Monsters: Essays on Power, Technology and Domination*, London: Routledge.

Carey, J. (1989) *Communication as Culture*, Boston, MA: Unwin-Hyman.

Carnie, J. K. (1995) *The Safer Cities Programme in Scotland – Evaluation of Safe Greater Easterhouse*, Scottish Office Central Research Unit, Edinburgh: Scottish Office.

Casapulla G., De Cindio, F. and Gentile, O. (1995) 'The Milan civic network experience and its roots in the town', in *Proceedings of the 2nd International Workshop on Community Networking Integrated Multimedia Services to the Home*, IEEE Comm. Soc., ACM SIGCOMM, Princeton, NJ.

Casapulla G., De Cindio, F., Gentile, O. and Sonnante, L. (1998) 'A citizen-driven civic network as stimulating context for designing on-line public services', in *Proceedings of the Fifth Biennial Participatory Design Conference Broadening Participation*, PDC98, Seattle.

Castells, M. (1972) *The Urban Question*. London: Edward Arnold.

Castells, M. (1996) *The Information Age: Economy, Society and Culture*, Vol. I, *The Rise of the Network Society*, Oxford and Malden: Blackwell.

Castells, M. (1997) *The Information Age: Economy, Society and Culture*, Vol. II, *The Power of Identity*, Oxford and Malden: Blackwell.

Castells, M. (1998) *The Information Age: Economy, Society and Culture*, Vol. III, *End of Millennium* Oxford and Malden: Blackwell.

Castells, M. (1999) 'The informational city is a dual city: can it be reversed?', in Schon, D. A., Sanyal, B. and Mitchell, W. J. (eds) *High Technology and Low-income Communities*, Cambridge, MA: MIT Press.

CATNeT, http://uac.rdp.utoledo.edu/docs/catnet/catnethome.htm.

CCTA (1994) *Information Superhighways: Opportunities for Public Sector Applications*, London: CCTA.

CCTA (1995) *Report on the Information Superhighway*, London: CCTA.

CEC (1994a) *Growth, Competitiveness, Employment: The Challenges and Ways Forward into the 21st Century – White Paper*, Luxembourg: Office for Official Publications of the European Communities, pp. 107–15. http://www.ispo.cec.be/infosoc/backg/whitpaper/ch5a_1.html.

CEC (1994b) *Europe and the Global Information Society: Recommendations to the European Council*, CD-84-94-290-EN, http://www.ispo.cec.be./infosoc/backg/bangeman.html.

CEC (1994c) *Europe's Way to the Information Society: An Action Plan*, Brussels: CEC COM (94) 347 final, 19/7/94, http://www.ispo.cec.be/infosoc/backg/action.html.

CEC (1995a) *Introduction to the Information Society the European Way*, http://www.ispo.cec.be/infosoc/backg/brochure.html.

CEC (1995b) *The European Information Society in Action*, http://www.ispo.cec.be/infosoc/backg/action95.html.

CEC (1995c) *Statement: Towards the Information Society*, http://www.ispo.cec.be/infosoc/backg/statemnt.html.

CEC (1995d) *Information Society Forum Theme Paper*, http://www.ispo.cec.be/infoforum/pub/themepap.html.

Central Office of Information (1998) *Our Information Age: The Government's Vision*, London: Central Office of Information.

Centre for Environmental Studies (CES) (1984) *Interim Report: Preliminary Comparison of Four Outer Estates*, London: CES.

Centre for Environmental Studies (CES) (1985) *Outer Estates in Britain: Greater Easterhouse*, London: CES.

Chanan, G. (1989), *Social Change and Local Action: Coping With Disadvantage in Urban Areas*, Dublin: European Foundation for the Improvement of Living and Working Conditions.

Chanan, G. (1992) *Out of the Shadows: Local Community Action in the European Community*, Dublin: European Foundation for the Improvement of Living and Working Conditions.

Chanan, G. (1999), *Local Community Involvement: A Handbook for Good Practice*, Dublin: European Foundation for the Improvement of Living and Working Conditions.

Chanan, G., West, A., Garratt, C. and Humm, J. (1999), *Regeneration and Sustainable Communities*, London: CDF.

Chaney, D. (1978) 'Communication and community', *Communication,* Vol. 7, No. 1, pp. 1–32.

Chmielewski, T. and Wellman, B. (2000) 'Tracking Geekus Unixus: an explorers' report from the National Geographic Website', *SIGGROUP Bulletin*, Vol. 21, No. 1.

Chow, C., Ellis, J., Mark, J. and Wise, B. (1998) *Impact of CTCNet Affiliates: Findings from a National Survey of Users of Community Technology Centers*, Educational Development Center, Inc., on the Web at http://www.ctcnet.org/impact98.htm.

Chow, C., Ellis, J., Walker G. and Wise, B. (2000) *Who Goes There? Longitudinal Case Studies of Twelve Users of Community Technology Centers*, Educational Development Center, Inc., on the Web at http://www.ctcnet.org/publics.html.

CITU (1996) *Government.direct: Green Paper on the Electronic Delivery of Government Services*, November, London: Stationery Office, also available at http://www.citu.gov.uk/greenpaper.htm.

Civille, R. (1995) 'The Internet and the poor', in Kahin, B. and Keller, J. (eds), *Public Access to the Internet*, Cambridge, MA: MIT Press.

Clark, K. (1989) *Dark Ghetto: Dilemmas of Social Power*, Middletown, CT: Wesleyan University Press.

Cleaver, H. (1998) 'The Zapatista effect: the Internet and the rise of an alternative political fabric', *Journal of International Affairs*, Vol. 51, No. 2, on the Web 24 September 2000 at http://www.eco.utexas.edu/faculty/Cleaver/zapeffect.html.

Cleaver, H. (1999) 'Computer-linked social movements and the global threat to capitalism', January, on the Web at http://www.eco.utexas.edu/faculty/Cleaver/polnet.html.

Clement, A. and Shade, L. R. (2000) 'The access rainbow: conceptualizating universal access to the information/communications infrastructure', in Gurstein, M. (ed.), *Community Informatics: Enabling Communities with Information and Communications Technologies*, Hershey, PA: Idea Group.

Cockburn, C. (1981) 'The material of male power', *Feminist Review*, Vol. 9, pp. 41–58.

Cockburn, C. (1983) *Brothers: Male Dominance and Technological Change*, London: Pluto.

Cockburn, C. (1985) *Machinery of Dominance: Women, Men and Technical Know-how*, London: Pluto.

Cockburn, C. (1992) 'The circuit of technology: gender, identity and power', in Silverstone, R. and Hirsch, E. (eds) *Consuming Technologies: Media and Information In Domestic Spaces*, London: Routledge.

Cockburn, C. and Ormrod, S. (1993) *Gender and Technology in the Making*, London: Sage.

Cockburn, C. and Fürst-Dilic, R. (eds) (1994) *Bringing Technology Home: Gender and Technology in a Changing Europe*, Buckingham: Open University Press.

Cockburn, C. (1998) *The Space Between Us: Negotiating Gender and National Identities in Conflict*, London: Zed.

Cockburn, C. (1999) 'Crossing borders: ways of handling conflictual differences', *Soundings*, Vol. 12, pp. 99–114.

Code, L. (1991) *What Can She Know? Feminist Theory and the Construction of Knowledge*, Ithaca: Cornell University Press.

Code, L. (1995) *Rhetorical Spaces: Essays on Gendered Locations*, London: Routledge.

Cohen, A. (1985) *The Symbolic Construction of Community*, London: Tavistock.

Cohen, J. (2000) 'Love, honor, cherish. But reveal my password?', *New York Times*, 17 February.

Cohen, S. and Willis, T. (1985) 'Stress, social support and the buffering hypothesis', *Psychological Bulletin*, Vol. 98, pp. 310–57.

Cohen, S., Kaplan, G. A. and Salonen, J. T. (1999) 'The role of psychological characteristics in the relation between socio-economic status and perceived health', *Journal of Applied Social Psychology*, Vol. 29, No. 3, pp. 445–68.

Coleman, J. S. (1990) *Foundations of Social Theory*, Cambridge, MA: Harvard University Press.

Coleman, R. and Sim, J. (1998) 'From the docklands to the Disney store: surveillance, risk and security in Liverpool city centre', *International Review of Law, Computers and Technology*, Vol. 12, No. 1, pp. 27–45.

Coleman, S. (1999) 'Cutting out the middle man: from virtual representation to direct deliberation', in Hague, B. H. and Loader, B. D. (eds) *Digital Democracy. Discourse and Decision Making in the Information Age*, London and New York: Routledge.

Community Connector, http://www.si.umich.edu/Community.

Conroy, J. (2000) 'Up for it', *New Internationalist*, Vol. 327, September, pp. 20–1.

Contractor, N. S., Zink, D. and Chan. M. (1998) 'IKNOW: a tool to assist and study the creation, maintenance, and dissolution of knowledge networks', paper presented to the Sunbelt Social Networks Conference, Sitges, Spain, May.

Conway, S. (1997) 'Strategic personal links in successful innovation: link-pins, bridges and liaisons', *Creativity and Innovation Management*, Vol. 6, No. 4, pp. 226–33.

Cooley, C. (1987) *Architect or Bee? The Human Role of Technologies*, London: Hogarth Press.

Crawshaw, P. and Seabrook, T (2000) 'Gender, space and place: cultural geographies of risk', paper presented at Youth, Risk and Leisure Conference, University of Teesside, February.

Cronberg, T. (1990) *Fremtidsforsøg*, Copenhagen: Akademisk Forlag.

Cronberg, T. (1991) 'Experiments into the future', in Cronberg, T., Duelund, P., Jensen, O. M. and Qvortrup, L. (eds) *Danish Experiments – Social Constructions of Technology*, Copenhagen: New Social Science Monographs.

Cronberg, T., Duelund, P., Jensen, O. M. and Qvortrup, L. (eds) (1991) *Danish Experiments – Social Constructions of Technology*, Copenhagen: New Social Science Monographs.

Crow, G. and Allan, G. (1994) *Community Life: An Introduction to Local Social Relations*, London: Harvester.

CTCNet, http://www.ctcnet.org.

Curno, A. (1982) *Women and Collective Action*, Newcastle: Association of Community Workers.

Dahl, R. (1989) *Democracy and its Critics*, New Haven, CT: Yale University Press.

Dalmiya, V. and Alcoff, L. (1993) 'Are "old wives' tales" justified?', in Alcoff, L. and Potter, E. (eds) *Feminist Epistemologies*, London: Routledge.

Danet, B., Ruedenberg, L. and Rosenbaum-Tamari, Y. (1998) ' "Hmmm . . . Where's that smoke coming from?" Writing, play and performance on Internet relay chat', in Sudweeks, F., McLaughlin, M. and Sheizaf, R. (eds) *Network and Netplay: Virtual Groups on the Internet*, Cambridge, MA: MIT Press

Darke, J. (1996) 'The man-shaped city', in Booth, C., Darke, J. and Yeandle, S. (eds), *Changing Places: Women's Lives in the City*, London: Paul Chapman Publishing.

Darkwa, O. and Mazibuko, F. (2000) 'Creating virtual learning communities in Africa: challenges and prospects', *First Monday*, Vol. 5, No. 5, website http://firstmonday. org/issues/issue5_5/darkwa/index.html.

Davies, S. (1996) *Big Brother: Britain's Web of Surveillance and the New Technological Order*, London: Pan Books.

Davis, M. (1990), *City of Quartz: Excavating the Future in Los Angeles*, London: Verso.

Davis, N. Z. (1983) *The Return of Martin Guerre*. Cambridge, MA: Harvard University Press.

Dawson, M. (1994) 'A black counterpublic? Economic earthquakes, racial agenda(s), and black politics', *Public Culture*, Vol. 7, No. 1.

Day, P. and Horner, D. (1995) 'Policies for the information society: social innovation and rural communities', in *Proceedings, European Conference on Management of Technology, Technological Innovation and Global Challenges*, Birmingham, International Association for Management of Technology (IAMOT), July, pp. 408–15.

Day, P. (1996a) 'Information communication technology and society: A community-based approach', in Gill, K. S. (ed.) *Information Society: New Media, Ethics and Postmodernism*, London: Springer-Verlag.

Day, P. (1996b) 'The human-centred information society: a community-based approach', *AI & Society*, Vol. 10, No. 6, pp. 181–98.

Day, P. and Harris, K. (1997) *Down-to-Earth Vision: Community Based IT Initiatives and Social Inclusion*, London: IBM/CDF, http://www.uk.ibm.com/community/ uk171.html.

Day, P. (1998) 'Community development in the information society: a European perspective of community networks', position paper presented to the Designing Across Borders: the Community Design of Community Networks joint workshop of the PDC98 & CSCW 98 Conferences, Seattle, 12–14 November, http://www.scn.org/ tech/the_network/Projects/CSCW-PDC-ws-98/day-pp.html.

Day, P. (1999) 'Informing policy and promoting active communities in the information society', position paper presented to the Broadening our Understanding: Community Networks and Other Forms of Computer Supported Community Work workshop of the ECSCW '99 Conference, Copenhagen, 12 September, http://www. scn.org/tech/the_network/Proj/ws99/day-pp.html.

De Cindio, F. and Simone, C. (1993) 'The universes of discourse for education and action research', in Green, E., Owen, J. and Pain, D. (eds) *Gendered by Design? Information Technology and Office Systems*, London: Taylor and Francis.

De Cindio, F. (1999) 'Community networks: a learning community for networking and groupware', *ACM SIGGROUP Bulletin*, Vol. 20, No. 2.

De Cindio, F. (2000) 'Community networks for reinventing citizenship and democracy', in Gurstein, M. (ed.) *Community Informatics: Enabling Communities with Information and Communications Technologies*, Hershey, PA: Idea Group·

Dear, M. J., Schockman, H. E. and Hise, G. (eds) (1996) *Rethinking Los Angeles*, Thousand Oaks, CA: Sage.

DEE (2000) *ICT Learning Centres Initiative Pack*, London: Department for Education and Employment.

Denzin. N. (1998) 'In search of the inner child: co-dependency and gender in a cyberspace community', in Bendelow, G. and Williams, S. (eds) *Emotions in Social Life*, London: Routledge.

Department of Commerce [US] (2000) *Technology Opportunities Program: Research and Evaluation*, on the Web at http://www.ntia.doc.gov/otiahome/top/research/research.htm.

Department of Culture, Media and Sport (1999) *Appraisal of Annual Library Plans*, Croydon: IPF

DETR (1998) *Modern Local Government: In Touch with the People*, http://www.local-regions.detr.gov.uk/lswp/index.htm.

DETR (2000) *Indices of Deprivation 2000*, http://www.regeneration.detr.gov.uk.

Dibbell, J. (1996) 'A rape in cyberspace; or how an evil clown, a Haitian trickster Spirit, two wizards and a cast of dozens turned a database into a society', in Goodwin, M. (ed.) *High Noon on the Electronic Frontier*, Cambridge MA: MIT Press.

Dienes, B. and Gurstein, M. (1998) 'Remote management of a province-wide summer employment program using Internet/Intranet technologies', in *Annals of Cases on Technology Applications and Management in Organizations, 1*, Hershey, PA: Idea Group.

Dienes, B. and Gurstein, M. (1999) 'A "community informatics" approach to health care for rural Africa', The African Telemedicine Project: Conference '99, The Role of Low-cost Technology for Improved Access to Public Health Care Programs Throughout Africa, Economic Commission for Africa/UN, Invited plenary presentation, Nairobi, Kenya, 19–21 February.

Ditton, J. (1998), 'Public support for town centre CCTV schemes: myth or reality', in Norris, C., Moran J. and Armstrong, G. (eds) *Surveillance, Closed Circuit Television and Social Control*, Aldershot: Ashgate.

Ditton, J. and Short, E. (1998) 'Evaluating Scotland's first town centre CCTV scheme', in Norris, C., Moran, J. and Armstrong, G. (eds) Surveillance, *Closed Circuit Television and Social Control*, Aldershot: Ashgate.

Ditton, J., Short, E., Phillips, S., Norris, C. and Armstrong, G. (1999) *The Effects of Closed Circuit Television on Recorded Crime Rates and Public Concern About Crime in Glasgow*, The Scottish Office Central Research Unit, Edinburgh: Scottish Office.

Docter, S. and Dutton, W. H. (1998) 'The First Amendment online: Santa Monica's public electronic network', in Tsagarousianou, R., Tambini, D. and Bryan, C. (eds) *Cyberdemocracy. Technology, Cities and Civic Networks*, London and New York: Routledge.

Dominelli, L. (1990) *Women and Community Action*, Birmingham: Venture Press.

Donath J. S. (1999) Identity and deception in the virtual community', in Kollock, P. and Smith M. (eds) *Communities in Cyberspace*, Berkeley: University of California Press.

DTI (1994) *Creating the Superhighways of the Future: Developing Broadband Communications in the UK*, London: HMSO.

DTI (1995) *Competitiveness: Forging Ahead*, London: HMSO.

DTI (1996a) 'Lang launches information society initiative', *European Focus*, issue 7, March.

DTI (1996b) *Building the Information Society: A National Strategy*, London: DTI.

DTI (1996c). *Welcome to ISI IT for All: Make the Most of IT*, London: DTI.

Dutton, W. H. (1997) 'Multimedia visions and realities' in Kubicek, H., Dutton, W. H. and Williams, R. (eds) *The Social Shaping of Information Superhighways: European and American Roads to the Information Society*, Frankfurt: Campus Verlag.

Dybkjær, L. and Lindegaard, J. (1999) *The Digital Denmark* (*Det digitale Danmark*, in Danish), in *Ministry of Research (1999) Det digitale Danmark* Copenhagen: Forskningsministeriet.

Dyer-Witheford, N. (1999) *Cyber Marx: Cycles and Circuits of Struggle in High-technology Capitalism*, Urbana, IL: University of Illinois Press.

Dyson, C. (2000) *An Evaluation of Women-only Provision in IT Training*, unpublished Master's Thesis.

Ellis, J. (1989) *Breaking New Ground: Community Development with Asian Communities*, London: NVCO: Bedford Square Press.

Espinoza, V. (1999) 'Social networks among the urban poor: inequality and integration in a Latin American city', in Wellman, B. (ed.) *Networks in the Global Village*, Boulder, CO: Westview Press.

ETHOS (1998) *Use of IT by the UK Government, the Story So Far*. http://www.tagish.co.uk/ethosub/lit6/f6e6.htm.

Everts, S. (1998) *Gender & Technology: Empowering Women, Engendering Development*, London: Zed.

Eysenbach, G., Sa, E. R. and Diepgen, T. L. (1999) 'Shopping around the Internet today and tomorrow: towards the millennium of cybermedicine', *British Medical Journal*, Vol. 319, p. 1294.

Federal Trust (1995) *Network Europe and the Information Society*, London: Federal Trust.

Feldman, T. R. and Assaf, S. (1999) 'Social capital: conceptual frameworks and empirical evidence', in *Social Capital Initiative Working Paper No. 5*, The World Bank, on the Web at http://www.worldbank.org/poverty/scapital/wkrppr/sciwp5.pdf.

Felsentein, L. (1993) 'The commons of information', in *Dr Dobbs' Journal*, May, Interval Research Corp.

Ferrand, A., Mounier, L. and Degenne, A. (1999) 'The diversity of personal networks in France: social stratification and relational structures', in Wellman, B. (ed.) *Networks in the Global Village*, Boulder, CO: Westview Press.

Ferris, S. (1996) 'Women online: cultural and relational aspects of women's communication in online discussion groups', *Interpersonal Computing and Technology* Vol. 4, pp. 29–40, online at: http://www.helsinki.fi/science/optek/1996/n3/ferris.txt (17 January 1999).

Finch, J. (1989) *Family Obligation and Social Change*, Cambridge: Polity Press.

Finn, J. (1999) 'An exploration of helping processes in an online self-help group focussing on the issues of disability', *Health and Social Work*, Vol. 24, No. 3, pp. 220–31.

Fischer, C. (1982) *To Dwell Among Friends*, Berkeley: University of California Press.

Fischer, C. (1992) *America Calling: A Social History of the Telephone to 1940*, Berkeley: University of California Press.

Fiske, J. (1998) 'Videotech', in Mirzoeff, N. (ed.) *Visual Culture Reader*, London, Routledge.

Fiske, J. (1995) *Forsøgsprojekter og offentlige organisationer*, Copenhagen: AKF Forlaget.

Fleck, J. (1988) *Innofusion or Diffusation? The Nature of Technological Development in Robotics*, Edinburgh: Edinburgh University.

Fletcher, J. (1998) 'Relational practice, a feminist reconstruction of work', *Journal of Management Inquiry*, Vol. 7, No. 2, pp. 163–86.

Flex, K. and Koch-Nielsen, I. (1992) *Kommunerne og SUM-programmet*, Copenhagen: Social Forsknings Instituttet.

Flusty, S. (1994), 'Building paranoia: the proliferation of interdictory space and the erosion of spatial justice', *Los Angeles Forum for Architecture and Urban Design*.

Foley, M. W. and Edwards, B. (1999) 'Is it time to disinvest in social capital?', *Journal of Public Policy*, Vol. 19, No. 2, pp. 141–73.

Foner, L. N. (1997) 'Yenta: a multi-agent, referral-based matchmaking system', paper presented at International Conference on Autonomous Agents ('Agents '97'), Marina del Rey, California.

Formaper (ed.) (2000) 'Analysis of the ICT demand for SMEs', *ADAPT Project Report*, Formaper-Chamber of Commerce of Milan (in Italian).

Forster, E. M. (1909) 'The machine stops', in *The Eternal Moment and Other Stories*, New York: Harcourt, Brace.

Foucault, M. (1974) *The Archaeology of Knowledge*, London: Tavistock.

Foucault, M. (1977) *Discipline and Punish: The Birth of the Prison*, London: Penguin.

Francissen, L. and Brants, K. (1998) 'Virtually going places: square-hopping in Amsterdam's digital city', in Tsagarousianou, R., Tambini D. and Bryan, C. (eds) *Cyberdemocracy: Technology, Cities and Civic Networks*, London and New York: Routledge.

Freeman, L. (1992) 'The sociological concept of group: an empirical test of two models', *American Journal of Sociology*, Vol. 98, pp. 152–66.

Freire, P. (1992) *Pedagogy of Hope: Reliving Pedagogy of the Oppressed*, New York: Continuum.

Friedman, A. and Cornforth, D. (1989) *Computer Systems Development: History, Organisation and Implementation*, London: Wiley.

Frye, M. (1983) *The Politics of Reality: Essays in Feminist Theory*, Trumansburg, NY: Crossing Press.

Fulford, R. (2000) *The TEDCity Conference, National Post*, Toronto, 10 June.

Furger, R. (2000) 'Who's watching you on the Web?', *PC World*, March, pp. 33–4.

Fyfe, N. R. and Bannister, J. (1996) 'City watching: closed circuit television surveillance in public spaces', *Area*, Vol. 28, No. 1, pp. 37–46.

Galbraith, J. K. (1994) 'The good society considered: the economic dimension', *Journal of Law and Society*, Annual Lecture – St David's Hall, Cardiff, 26 January, Cardiff: Cardiff Law School.

Gans, H. (1962) *The Urban Villagers*, New York: Free Press.

Garber, M., Matlock, J. and Walkowitz. R. (eds) (1993) *Media Spectacles*, New York: Routledge.

Garnham, N. (1994) 'Whatever happened to the information society?', in Mansell, R. (ed.), *The Management of Information and Communication Technologies*, London: Aslib.

Gaver, W. (1996) 'Affordances for Interaction: the social is material for design', in *Ecological Psychology*, Vol. 8, pp. 111–29.

Giddens, A. (1994) *Beyond Left and Right: The Future of Radical Politics*, Cambridge: Polity Press.

Gilchrist, A. (1998) *Community Development and Networking*, London: CDF.

Gill, K. S. (1990) *Summary of Human-centred Systems Research in Europe*, Working Paper, Brighton: Seake Centre, Brighton Polytechnic.

Gittler, A. (1999) 'Mapping women's global communications and networking', in Harcourt, W. (ed.) *Women@Internet Creating New Cultures in Cyberspace*, London: Zed Books.

Glen, A. (1993) 'Methods and themes in community practice', in Butcher, H., Glen, A., Henderson, P. and Smith, J. (eds.) *Community and Public Policy*, London: Pluto.

Goede, P., de Hollander, E. and van der Linden, C. (eds) (1996) 'Lokale media en lokaal bestuur: achtergronden, moeilijkheden en mogelijkheden', Houten/Diegem: Bohn Stafleu van Loghem.

Goffman, E. (1963) *Behavior in Public Places*, New York: Free Press.

Goodwin, M., Johnstone, C. and Williams, K. (1998) 'New spaces of law enforcement: closed circuit television, public behaviour and the policing of public space', paper presented to the Association of American Geographers Annual Conference, Boston, MA, March.

Gordon, M. *et al.* (1980) 'Crime, women and the quality of urban life', *Signs*, Vol. 5, pp. 44–66.

Gore, A. (1993) *Speech to the Press Club*, http://www.hpcc.gov./white-house/gore.nii.html.

Graham, S. (1996) 'CCTV – Big brother or friendly eye in the sky?', *Town and Country Planning*, Vol. 65, No. 2, pp. 57–60.

Graham, S., Brooks, J. and Heery, D. (1996) 'Towns on television: closed circuit television surveillance in British towns and cities', *Local Government Studies*, Vol. 22, No. 3, pp. 1–27.

Graham, S. and Marvin, S. (1996) *Telecommunications and the City: Electronic Spaces, Urban Places*, Routledge: London.

Graham, S. (1998) 'Spaces of surveillant simulation: new technologies, digital representations, and material geographies', *Environment and Planning D: Society and Space*, Vol. 6, pp. 483–504.

Granovetter, M. (1973) 'The strength of weak ties', *American Journal of Sociology*, Vol. 78, pp. 1360–80.

Green, E. and Keeble, L. (2000) 'The technological story of a women's centre: a feminist model of user centred design', paper presented at University of Teesside: CIRA – Community Informatics Conference, April.

Green, E., Owen, J. and Pain, D. (1993) *Gendered by Design? Information Technology and Office Systems*, London: Taylor & Francis.

Green, E. and Adam, A. (eds) (2001) *Virtual Gender: Technology, consumption and identity*, Routledge: London.

Greenwood, D. J. and Levin, M. (1998) *Introduction to Action Research: Social Research for Social Change*, London: Sage.

Greider, W. (1993) *Who Will Tell the People?*, New York: Simon and Schuster.

Grint, K. and Gill, R. (eds) (1995) *The Gender-technology Relation: Contemporary Theory and Research*, London: Taylor and Francis.

Groombridge, N. and Murji, K. (1994) 'As easy as A B and CCTV?', *Policing*, Vol. 10, No. 4, pp. 283–90.

Guardian (5 December 1999) 'Cure for your ills at NHS online: computer doctor lets patients diagnose themselves at home'.

Gurstein, M. (1996) 'Managing technology for community economic development in a non-metropolitan environment', in *International Conference on Technology Management: University/Industry/Government Collaboration*, Istanbul, Turkey, UNIG: UNESCO.

Gurstein, M. (1998) 'Information and communications technologies and local economic development', in MacIntyre, G. (ed.) *A Roundtable on Community Economic Development*, Sydney, Nova Scotia: University College of Cape Breton Press.

Gurstein, M. and Dienes, B. (1998) 'Community enterprise networks: partnerships for local economic development', paper presented at the Libraries as Leaders in Community Economic Development Conference, Victoria, BC.

Gurstein, M. (1999) 'Community access and flexible networking', in Funston, A. (ed.) *Community Networking: Networking Communities*, Melbourne: Victoria University of Technology Press.

Gurstein, M. (1999a) 'Flexible networking, information and communications technology and local economic development', *First Monday*, February <http://firstmonday.dk/issues/issue4_2/index.html>.

Gurstein, M. (ed.) (2000) *Community Informatics: Enabling Communities with Information and Communications Technologies*, Hershey, PA: Idea Group.

Gurstein, M. (2000a) *Burying Coal: An Experiment in Community Research Using Information and Communications Technology for Local Economic Development*, Vancouver, BC: Collective Press.

Gurstein, M. (2000b) 'Introduction', in Gurstein, M. (ed.) *Community Informatics: Enabling Community Uses of Information and Communications Technology*, Hershey, PA: Idea Group.

Gurstein, M. (2000c) 'E-commerce and community economic development enemy or ally?', conference paper presented at DIAC 2000, Shaping the Network Society: The Future of the Public Sphere in Cyberspace, Seattle, 20 May.

Gurstein, M. (2000d) *Forging Community Innovation with Information and Communications Technology: Universities, Research, and Economic Development in a Remote and Rural Community; The University College of Cape Breton Chair in the Management of Technological Change as a Catalyst for Change in a Lagging Region*, Sydney, Nova Scotia: University College of Cape Breton Press.

Habermas, J. (1989) *The Structural Transformation of the Public Sphere: An Inquiry into a Category of Bourgeois Society*, Cambridge: Polity.

Hague, B. and Keeble, L. (1999) 'Good technology? Information and communications technologies and cultural change in the voluntary and community sector', paper presented to the fifth NCVO Researching the Voluntary Sector conference, 7–8 September.

Hague, B. and Loader, B. D. (eds) (1999) *Digital Democracy: Discourse and Decision Making in the Information Age*, London and New York: Routledge.

Hale, M., Musso, J. and Weare, C. (1999) 'Developing digital democracy: evidence from Californian municipal web pages', in Hague, B. N. and Loader, B. D. (eds.) *Digital Democracy. Discourse and Decision Making in the Information Age*, London and New York: Routledge.

Hall, P. (1997) 'Regeneration policies for peripheral housing estates', *Urban Studies*, Vol. 34, No 5, pp. 873–81.

Halloran, J. (1977) *Communication and Community: The Evaluation of an Experiment*, Strasbourg: Council of Europe.

Hampton, K. N. and Wellman, B. (2000) 'Examining community in the digital neighborhood: early results from Canada's wired suburb', in Ishida, T. and Isbister, K. (eds) *Digital Cities: Technologies, Experiences and Future Perspectives*, Berlin: Springer-Verlag.

Hanmer, J. and Saunders, S. (1984) *Well Founded Fear*, London: Hutchinson.

Haraway, D. (1985) 'A manifesto for cyborgs: science, technology and socialist feminism in the 1980s', *Socialist Review*, Vol. 80, pp. 65–107.

Haraway, D. (1986) 'Primatology is politics by other means', in Bleier, R. (ed.) *Feminist Approaches to Science*, London: Pergamon Press.

Haraway, D. (1991) 'Situated knowledges: the science question in feminism and the privilege of partial perspective', in *Simions, Cyborgs and Women*, London: Free Association Books

Harcourt, W. (1999) 'The politics of cyberspace: women and the new ICTs', paper presented at From Social Exclusion to Social Change on the Information Superhighway: Women Connect, CDF, London, DTI: 22 November.

Hardey, M (1999) 'Doctor in the house: the Internet as a source of lay health knowledge and the challenge to expertise', *Sociology of Health and Illness*, Vol. 21, No. 6, pp. 820–35.

Hardey, M (2000) 'The story of my illness: personal accounts of illness on the Internet', paper presented at the ESRC Virtual Society? conference 'Virtual Society? Get Real!', Ashbridge Management Centre, 5 May.

Harding, S. (1991) *Whose Science? Whose Knowledge? Thinking From Women's Lives*, Milton Keynes: Open University Press.

Harris, K. (1996) 'Social inclusion in the information society', in *Inventing the Future: Partnerships for Tomorrow*, Brighton: Partnership Books, http://panizzi.shef.ac.uk/community/socinc.html.

Harris, V. (ed.) (1994) *Community Work Skills Manual*, Newcastle: Association of Community Workers.

Harrison, T. and Stephen, T. (1999) 'Researching and creating community networks', in Jones, S. (ed.) *Doing Internet Research. Critical Issues and Methods for Examining the Net*, Thousand Oaks, CA: Sage.

Haythornthwaite, C. and Wellman, B. (1998) 'Work, friendship and media use for information exchange in a networked organization', *Journal of the American Society for Information Science*, Vol. 49, No 12, pp. 1101–14.

Haywood, T. (1998) 'Global networks and the myth of equality: trickle down or trickle away?', in Loader, B. D. (ed.) *Cyberspace Divide: Equality, Agency and Policy in the Information Society*, London: Routledge.

Hegland, T. J. (1990) Sum-programmet-en historisk sociologisk baggrtundsanalyse in *SUMma Summarum*, Vol. 1, pp. 8–23.

Henshall, S. (2000) 'The COMsumer manifesto: empowering communities of consumers through the Internet', *First Monday*, Vol. 5 (May), http://firstmonday.org/issues/issue5_5/henshall.index.html.

Henwood, F. (1993) 'Establishing gender perspectives on information technology; problems, issues and opportunities', in Green, E., Owen, J. and Pain, D. (eds) *Gendered by Design? Information Technology and Office Systems*, London: Taylor & Francis.

Herman, C. (1999) 'Women and the Internet', in Liberty (ed.) *Liberating Cyberspace: Civil Liberties, Human Rights and the Internet*, London: Pluto.

Herring, S. (1994) 'Politeness in computer culture: why women thank and men flame', in Bucholtz, *et al.* (eds.) *Cultural Performances: Proceedings of the Third Berkeley Women and Language Conference*, Berkeley: University of California.

Hick, S., Halpin, E. F. and Hoskins, E. (2000) *Human Rights and the Internet*, Basingstoke: Macmillan.

Higgins, J. (1999) 'Citizenship and empowerment: a remedy for citizen participation in health reform', *Community Development Journal*, Vol. 34, No. 4, pp. 287–307.

Hillery Jr, G. (1955) 'Definitions of community: areas of agreement', *Rural Sociology*, Vol. 20, pp. 111–22.

Hine, C. (2000) *Virtual Ethnography*, London: Sage.

Hirscheim, R. (1985) *Office Automation: A Social and Organisational Perspective*, Chichester: Wiley

HM Treasury (2000) 'Spending review 2000', in *Cross Departmental Review of the Knowledge Economy file:///B/chap35.html*.

Hoggett, P. (1997a) 'Contested communities', in Hoggett, P. (ed.) *Contested Communities: Experiences, Struggles, Policies*, Bristol: Policy Press.

Hoggett, P. (1997b) *Contested Communities: Experiences, Struggles, Policies*, Bristol: Policy Press.

Holderness, M. (1998) 'Who are the world's information poor?', in Loader, B. (ed.) *Cyberspace Divide*, London: Routledge.

Hollander, E. (1982) *Kleinschalige massacommunicatie: lokale omroepvormen in West Europa*, The Hague: State Publishing Co.

Hollander, E. (1988) *Lokale communicatie en lokale openbaarheid. Openbaarheid als communicatiewetenschappelijk concept*, Ph.D. dissertation, Department of Communication, University of Nijmegen.

Hollander, E. and Stappers, J. G. (1992) 'Community media and community communication', in Jankowski, N. W., Prehn, O. and Stappers J. G. (eds), *The People's Voice: Local Radio and Television in Europe*, London: John Libbey.

Hollander, E., Vergeer, M. and Verschuren, P. (1993) 'Het publiek van lokale en regionale media' in *Massacommunicatie*, Vol. 21, No. 1, pp. 22–45.

Hollander, E. (1998) 'Informatie- en communicatietechnologie in de lokale context', in Hanssen, L., Jankowski, N. and van Dijk, J. (eds) *Toegang tot en kwaliteit van het elektronisch debat*, Utrecht/Nijmegen: Stichting Wetenschap en Techniek Nederland.

Hollander, E. (forthcoming 2001) 'Community media and online communities: toward a theoretical and methodological framework', in Jankowski, N. and Prehn, O. (eds) *Community Media in the Information Age: Perspectives and Prospects*, Cresskill, NJ: Hampton Press.

Home Office (1994) *Closed Circuit Television: Looking Out For You*, London: HMSO.

Home Office (2000a) *Crime Reduction: CCTV*, Home Office, Department of the Environment, Transport and the Regions and Office of the Welsh Assembly Press Release, 31 March, London: Home Office.

Home Office (2000b) *Crime Reduction Programme: CCTV Initiative. Application Prospectus: Crime Reduction – CCTV*, March, London: Home Office.

Honess, T. and Charman, E. (1992) *Closed Circuit Television in Public Places: Its Acceptability and Perceived Effectiveness*, Home Office Police Research Group, Crime Prevention Unit Series, Paper No. 35, London: Home Office.

hooks, B. (1990) *Yearning: Race, Gender and Cultural Politics*, Boston: South End Press.

House of Lords Select Committee on Science and Technology (1996) *The Information Society: Agenda for Action in the UK*, HL Paper 77, London: Stationery Office, http://www.parliament.the-stationery-office.co.uk/pa/ld199596/ldselect/inforsoc/inforsoc.htm.

Hudson, H. E. (2000) 'Designing research for telecentre evaluation', International Development Research Centre, Canada, on the Web at http://www.idrc.ca/telecentre/evaluation/nn/20_Des.html/.

Hyland, A. (2000) 'Girls' night out on the net', *Guardian*, 27 April, www.guardianunlimited.co.uk/archive/article/0,4273,4011995,00.

IBM (1997) *The Net Result: Social Inclusion in the Information Society – Report of the National Working Party on Social Inclusion*, available online at http://www-5.ibm.com/uk/community/uk117.html.

IITF (1993) 'Information Infrastructure Task Force', in *National Information Infrastructure: Agenda for Action*, Washington, DC: National Telecommunications and Information Administration, http://nii.nist.gov.

INSINC (1997) *The Net Result: Social Inclusion in the Information Society: Report of the National Working Party on Social Inclusion*, London: IBM UK. www.uk.ibm.com/comm/community/uk117.html.

Jacobs, J. (1967) *The Death and Life of Great American Cities*, New York: Penguin.

Jæger, B., Manniche, J. and Rieper, O. (1990) *Computere, lokalsamfund og virksomheder: evaluering af Egvad Teknologiforsøg og Erhvervsprojektet i Ringkøbing Amt*, Copenhagen: AKF Forlaget.

Jæger, B. and Qvortrup, L. (1991) 'Danish experiments – social constructions of technology', in Cronberg, T., Duelund, P., Jensen, O. M. and Qvortrup, L. (eds) *New Social Science Monographs*, Copenhagen, pp. 27–41.

Jæger, B. and Rieper, O. (1991) *Local Public Service as Self Service – Evaluation of an Experiment with Videotex*, Copenhagen: AKF Forlaget.

Jæger, B. (1992) *Formidling på krys og tværs – evaluering af SUM-programmets formidlingsenheder*, Copenhagen: AKF Forlaget.

Jæger, B. (1997) In Jæger, B. and Storgaard, K. (eds) *Telematics and Rural Development*, Proceedings from an International Workshop on the Danish Island of Bornholm, Research Centre of Bornholm, Nexø, Denmark, pp. 94–104.

Jæger, B. (1999) 'Digitale byer i København og Europa (Digital Cities in Copenhagen and Europe)', in Andersen, K. V., Friis, C. S., Hoff, J. and Nicolajsen, H. W. (eds) *Informationsteknologi, organisation og forandring – den offenlige sektor under forvandling*, Copenhagen: Jurist- og Økonomomforbundets Forlag.

Jæger, B. and Hansen, F. J. S. (1999) 'Multimedia in Denmark, an overview', in Willliams, R. and Slack, R. S. (eds) *Europe Appropriates Multimedia: A Study of the National Uptake of Multimedia in Eight European Countries and Japan*, Vol. Report No. 42, Trondheim, Norway: Norway University of Science and Technology, pp. 83–121.

Jæger, B., Slack, R. and Williams, R. (2000) 'Europe experiments with multimedia: an overview of social experiments and trials', *The Information Society*, Vol. 16, No. 4, pp. 277–301.

Jankowski, N. W. (1988) *Community Television in Amsterdam: Access to, Participation in and Use of the 'Locale Omroep Bijlmermeer*, Ph.D. dissertation. Department of Communication, University of Amsterdam.

Jankowski, N. W. (1991) 'Qualitative research and community media', in Jensen, K. B. and Jankowski, N. W. (eds) *A Handbook of Qualitative Methodologies for Mass Communication Research*, London: Routledge.

Jankowski, N. W. and Wester, F. (1991) 'The qualitative tradition in social science inquiry: contributions to mass communication research', in Jensen, K. B. and Jankowski, N. W. (eds) *A Handbook of Qualitative Methodologies for Mass Communication Research,* London: Routledge.

Jankowski, N. W., Prehn, O. and Stappers, J. (1992) *The People's Voice. Local Radio and Television in Europe*, London: John Libbey.

Jankowski, N. W. and Prehn, O. (eds) (2001) *Community Media in the Information Age: Perspectives and Prospects*, Cresskill, NJ: Hampton Press.

Janlert, L.-E. and Stolterman, E. (1997) 'The character of things', *Design Studies*, Vol. 18, No 3 (July), pp. 297–314.

Janowitz, M. (1952) *The Community Press in an Urban Setting*, Glencoe, IL: Free Press.

Jensen, M. K. (1992) *Slut-SUM: en sammenfatning af projekterfaringerne fra Socialministeriets Udviklingsprogram*, Copenhagen: Social Forsknings Instituttet.

Jhunjhunwala, A. (2000) 'Bytes for all', paper presented at Affordable Telecom & IT Solutions for Developing Countries conference, Chennai, India, February–March.

Jones, S. (1995) 'Understanding community in the information age', in Jones, S. (ed.) *CyberSociety: Computer Mediated Communication and Community*, London: Sage.

Jones, S. (1999) *Doing Internet Research: Critical Issues and Methods for Examining the Net*, Thousand Oaks, CA: Sage Publications.

Jordan, B. (1996) *A Theory of Poverty and Social Exclusion*, Cambridge: Polity.

Jordan, T. (1999) *Cyberpower: The Culture and Politics of Cyberspace and the Internet*, London: Routledge.

Joy, B. (2000) 'The future doesn't need us', *Wired*, April, http://www.wired.com/wired/archive/8.04/joy_pr.html.

Jungk, R. (1977) *The Everyman Project: Resources for a Humane Future*, New York: Liveright.

Kalil, T. A. (1997) 'The Clinton–Gore national information infrastructure initiative', in Kubicek, H., Dutton, W. H. and Williams, R. (eds) *The Social Shaping of Information Superhighways: European and American Roots to the Information Society*, Frankfurt: Campus Verlag.

Karl, T. and Trenberth, K. (1999) 'The human impact on climate', *Scientific American*, December, pp. 100–5.

Katz, R. and Allen, T. (1982) 'Investigating the not invented here syndrome: a look at the performance, tenure, and communication patterns of 50 R&D projects', *R&D Management*, Vol. 12, No. 1, pp. 7–19.

Keating, M. (1988) *The City That Refused to Die*, Aberdeen: Aberdeen University Press.

Keck, M. and Sikkink, K. (1998) *Activists Beyond Borders: Advocacy Networks in International Politics*, Ithaca: Cornell University Press.

Keeble, L. and Loader, B. D. (2000) 'Electronic community networks: women's place, women's space?', *CPSR Newsletter*, Vol. 18, No. 3.

Kelly, L. and Radford, J. (1996) 'Nothing really happened: the invalidation of women's experiences of sexual violence', in Hester, M., Kelly, L. and Radford, J. (eds) *Women, Violence and Male Power*, Buckingham: Open University Press.

Kim, J., Wyatt, R. and Katz, E. (1999) 'News, talk, opinion participation: the part played by conversation in deliberative democracy', *Political Communication*, Vol. 16, pp. 361–85.

King, C. S., Felty, K. M. and O'Neill, Susel B. (1998) 'The question of participation: towards authentic public participation in public administration', *Public Administration Review*, Vol. 58, No. 4, pp. 317–26.

King, M. and Herring, D. (2000), 'Monitoring Earth's vital signs', *Scientific American*, April, pp. 72–7.

King, S. (1994) 'Analysis of electronic support groups for recovering addicts', *Interpersonal Computing and Technology*, Vol. 2, No. 3, pp. 47–56.

Kling, R. and Iacono, S. (1984) 'Computing as an occasion for social control', *Journal of Social Issues* Vol. 40, No. 3, pp. 77–96.

Kochen, M. (ed.) (1975) *Information for Action: From Knowledge to Wisdom*, San Diego: Academic Press.

Kochen, M. (1989) *The Small World*, Norwood, NJ: Ablex.

Koku, E., Nazer, N. and Wellman, B. (2001 forthcoming) 'Netting scholars: online and offline', *American Behavioral Scientist*, Vol. 43.

Korten, D. (1990) 'NGO strategic networks: from community projects to global transformations', paper prepared for the Asian Regional Workshop on Strategic Networking for Sustainable Development and Environmental Action, 24 November.

Kramarae, C. (ed.) (1988) *Technology and Women's Voices*, London: Routledge & Kegan Paul.

Kramarae, C. and Taylor H. J. (1993) 'Women and men on electronic networks: a conversation or a monologue', in Taylor, H. J., Kramarae, C. and Ebben, M. (eds) *Women, Information Technology and Scholarship*, Urban Centre for Advanced Study.

Kraut, R., Patterson, M., Lundmark, V., Kiesler, S., Mukopadhyay, T. and Scherlis, W. (1998) 'Internet paradox: a social technology that reduces social involvement and psychological well being?', *American Psychologist*, September 1998, pp. 1017–31. http://www.apa.org.journals/amp/amp5391017.html.

Kretzmann, J. P. and McKnight, J. L. (1993) *Building Communities from the Inside Out*, Chicago: ACTA Publications.

Kretzmann, J. P. (1993) *Building Communities from the Inside Out: A Path Toward Finding and Mobilizing a Community's Assets*, Chicago: Institute for Policy Research, Northwestern University.

Krouk, D., Pitkin, B. and Richman, N. (2000) 'Internet-based neighborhood information systems', in Gurstein, M. (ed.) *Community Informatics: Enabling Communities with Information and Communications Technologies*, Hershey, PA: Idea Group.

Kubicek, H., Dutton, W. H. and Williams, R. (1997) *The Social Shaping of Information Superhighways: European and American Roads to the Information Society*, Frankfurt: Campus Verlag.

Kubicek, H. and Dutton, W. H. (1997) 'The social shaping of information superhighways: an introduction', in Kubicek, H., Dutton, W. H. and Williams, R. (eds)

The Social Shaping of Information Superhighways: European and American Roads to the Information Society, Frankfurt: Campus Verlag.

Labour Party (1995) *Communicating Britain's Future*, London: The Labour Party.

Labour Party (1997) *General Election Manifesto*, London: The Labour Party.

Landry, B. (1987) *The New Black Middle Class*, Berkeley, CA: University of California Press.

Latané, B. and Darley, J. (1976) *Help in a Crisis: Bystander Response to an Emergency*, Morristown, NJ: General Learning Press.

Latour, B. (1993) *We Have Never Been Modern*, Cambridge, MA: Harvard University Press.

Latour, B. (1999) *Pandora's Hope – Essays on the Reality of Science Studies*, Cambridge, MA: Harvard University Press.

Lave, J. and Wenger, E. (1991) *Situated Learning: Legitimate Peripheral Participation*, Cambridge: Cambridge University Press.

Lee, G. B. (1996) 'Addressing anonymous messages in cyberspace', *Journal of Computer-Mediated Communication*, Vol. 2, No. 1, available at: http://www.ascusc.org/jcmc/vol2/issue1/anon.html.

Leebaert, D. (ed.) (1999) *The Future of the Electronic Marketplace*, Cambridge, MA: MIT Press.

Lentz, B., Straubhaar, J., LaPastina, A., Main, S. and Taylor, J. (2000) 'Structuring access: the role of public access centers in the "digital divide"', on the Web at http://www.utexas.edu/research/tipi/reports/joe_ICA.pdf.

Lerg, W. (1981) 'Verdrängen oder Ergänzen die Medien einander?', *Publizistik*, Vol. 26, No. 2, pp. 193–201.

Lévi-Strauss, C. (1962) *The Savage Mind*, Chicago: The University of Chicago Press.

Levitt, B. and March, J. G. (1988) 'Organizational learning', *Annual Review of Sociology*, No. 14, pp. 319–40.

LIC (1998) *New Library: The People's Network*, London: LIC.

Liff, S., Steward, F. and Watts, P. (1999) 'Public access to the Internet: new approaches from internet cafes and community technology centres and their implications for libraries', *The New Review of Information Networking*, Vol. 5, pp. 27–41.

Lindblom and Cohen (1979) *Usable Knowledge: Social Science and Social Problem Solving* New Haven, CT: Yale University Press.

Lippman, W. (1925) *The Phantom Public*, New York: Harcourt, Brace and Company.

Loader, B. D. (1998) (ed.) *Cyberspace Divide: Equality, Agency, and Policy in the Information Society*, London: Routledge.

Loader, B. D., Hague, B. N. and Eagle, D. (2000) 'Embedding the Net: community development in the age of information', in Gurstein, M. (ed.) *Community Informatics: Enabling Communities with Information and Communications Technologies*, Hershey, PA: Idea Group.

Loader, B. D., Ellison, N., Pleace, N. and Schuler, D. (2002) *Key Concepts in Cyberculture*, London: Routledge.

Lofland, L. H. (1998) *The Public Realm: Exploring the City's Quintessential Social Territory*. New York: Aldine de Gruyter.

Lomnitz, L. A. (1977) *Networks and Marginality: Life in a Mexican Shantytown*, New York: Academic Press.

Longhi, I. (2000) *A Suite of Parameters and Tools for Monitoring Virtual Communities*, Master Degree in Computer Science, A. A. 1999–2000, to appear.

Lorde, A. (1984) 'The master's tools will never dismantle the master's house' [1979], reprinted in *Sister Outsider*, Freedom, CA: Crossing Press.

Lovell, T. (ed.) (1990) *British Feminist Thought: A Reader*, Oxford: Basil Blackwell.

Lugones, M. (1997) 'Playfulness, "world"-travelling, and loving perception' [1987], reprinted in Meyers, D. T. (ed.) *Feminist Social Thought: A Reader*, London: Routledge.

Lyon, D. (1994), *The Electronic Eye: The Rise Of Surveillance Society*, Cambridge: Polity Press.

McAdam, D. (1999) *Political Process and the Development of Black Insurgency 1930–1970*, Chicago: University of Chicago Press.

McAuley, C. (2000) 'CCTV extension plan hit by funding crisis', *The Glaswegian*, 2 March, p. 7.

McCahill, M. (1998) 'Beyond Foucault: towards a contemporary theory of surveillance', in Norris, C., Moran J. and Armstrong, G. (eds) *Surveillance, Closed Circuit Television and Social Control*, Aldershot: Ashgate.

Macey, M. and Beckett, C. (2001 forthcoming) 'Race, gender and sexuality: the oppression of multiculturalism', *Women's Studies International Forum*.

McGill, I. and Beaty, L. (1992) *Action Learning: A Practitioner's Guide*, London: Kogan Page.

McGivney, V. (1994) 'Women, education and training', *Adults Learning: A Research Report*, Vol. 5, No. 5, pp. 118–20.

McGivney, V. (1999) *Returning Women: Their Training and Employment Choices and Needs*, Leicester: NIACE.

McKibben, B. (2000) 'Muggles in the ozone', *Mother Jones*, March/April, p. 13.

Mackie, A. (2000) 'Lack of cash is a real turn off', *The Extra*, letters page, 9 March, p. 18.

Mackie, D. and Wilcox, D. (1999) *Neighbourhood Online Game*, http://www. partnerships.org.uk/nolgame/index.htm.

McLeish, H. (1998) 'Scottish Office CCTV challenge competition – 1998', *The Herald*, 28 February, p. 11.

McQuail, D. (2000) *McQuail's Mass Communication Theory*, London: Sage.

Mann, C. and Stewart, F. (2000) *Internet Communication and Qualitative Research: A Handbook for Researching Online*, London: Sage.

Marcelle, G. M. (1998) 'Strategies for including a gender perspective in African information and communications technologies (ICTs) policy', paper presented to the ECA International Conference on African Women and Economic Development, Addis Ababa, April.

Mark, J., Cornebise, J. and Wahl, E. (1997) *Community Technology Centers: Impact on Individual Participants and Their Communities*, Education Development Center, Inc. on the Web at http://www.ctcnet.org/eval.html.

Marling, G. (1991) 'Local Television and Development', in Cronberg, T., Duelund, P., Jensen, O. M. and Qvortrup, L. (eds) *Danish Experiments – Social Constructions of Technology*, Copenhagen: New Social Science Monographs.

Marshall, A. (2000) *ICTs for Health Promotion in the Community: A Participative Approach*, unpublished MA dissertation in Information Management, University of Brighton.

Massey, D. (1994) *Space, Place and Gender*, Cambridge: Polity Press.

Masuda, Y. (1981) *The Information Society as Post-industrial Society*, Bethesda, MD: World Futures Society.

Mayo, M. (1994) *Communities and Caring: The Mixed Economy of Welfare*, Basingstoke: Macmillan.

Meier, R. (1962) *A Communications Theory of Urban Growth*, Cambridge, MA: MIT Press.

Mele, C. (1999) 'Cyberspace and disadvantaged communities: The Internet as a tool for collective action', in Smith M. A. and Kollock, P. (eds) *Communities in Cyberspace*, London: Routledge.

Mellor, M. (1992) *Breaking the Boundaries: Towards a Feminist Green Socialism*, London: Virago.

Merton, R. K. (1949) 'Patterns of influence: a study in interpersonal influence and communication behaviour in a local community', in Lazersfeld, P. F. and Stanton,F. N. (eds) *Communication Research 1948–1949*, New York: Harper & Brothers.

Merz, M. (1998) 'Nobody can force you when you are across the ocean – face to face and e-mail exchanges between theoretical physicists', in Smith, C. and Agar, J. (eds) *Making Space for Science: Territorial Themes in the Shaping of Knowledge*, London: Macmillan.

Meyers, D. (1997) *Feminist Social Thought: A Reader*, London: Routledge.

Miller, P. (2000) 'CTCNet, the community technology movement and the prospects for democracy in America', in Gurstein, M. (ed.) *Community Informatics: Enabling Communities with Information and Communications Technologies*, Hershey, PA: Idea Group.

Miller, S. (1996) *Civilizing Cyberspace: Policy, Power, and the Information Superhighway*, Reading, MA: Addison-Wesley.

Ministry of Research and Information Technology (1994) *Info-samfundet år 2000* (Infor-Society Year 2000), Copenhagen: MRIT.

Moggridge, A. (1999) *Evaluation of Women Connect Phase 1*, Bristol: University of the West of England, Community Information Systems Centre.

Moore, G. (1990) 'Structural determinants of men's and women's personal networks', *American Sociological Review*, Vol. 55 (October), pp. 726–35.

Morahan-Martin, J. (1998) 'Women and girls last: females and the Internet', paper presented to the IRISS 1998 Conference.

Morgan, D. (1996) *Family Connections*, Cambridge: Polity.

Morris, A. D. (1984) *The Origins of the Civil Rights Movement: Black Communities Organizing for Change*, New York: Free Press.

Mortberg, C. (ed) (2000) *Where Do We Go From Here? Feminist Challenges of Information Technology*, Lulea, Sweden: Lulea University of Technology.

Moss, G. (2000) 'Enough of boys' toys, women say', *The Guardian*, 2 December, www.guardianunlimited.co.uk/archive/article/0,42734099323,00.

Mousand, J. (1997) 'Sanctuary: social support on the Internet', in Behar, J. (ed.) *Mapping Cyberspace*, New York: Dowling College Press.

Mulholland, M. and Patel, P. (1999) 'Inclusive movements, movements for inclusion', *Soundings*, Vol. 12, pp. 127–44.

Mullard, M. and Spicker, P. (1998) *Social Policy in a Changing Society*, London: Routledge.

Muncer, S., Burrows, R., Pleace, N., Loader, B. and Nettleton, S. (2000) 'Births, deaths, sex and marriage but very few presents? A case study of social support in cyberspace', *Critical Public Health*, Vol. 10, No. 1.

Murchison Center, http://www.murchisoncenter.org.

Murray, F. and Woolgar, S. (1990) 'Social perspectives on software', report produced for the *ESRC Programme on Information and Communication Technologies*, University of Manchester Institute of Science and Technology: PICT.

Musso, J. A., Weare, C. and Hale, M. C. (1999) *Designing Web Technologies for Local Governance Reform: Good Management or Good Democracy?*, http://www.usc.edu/dept/LAS/SC2/junior_publications.html.

Narayan, U. (1988) 'Working together across difference: some considerations on emotion and political practice', *Hypatia*, Vol. 3, No. 2, pp. 31–47.

National Association of Local Authorities in Denmark (1996) *Midtvejsrapport om spydspidskommunerne* (Midway Report about the Spearhead Municipalities), Copenhagen: NALAD.

National Association of Local Authorities in Denmark (1997) *Kom med I front* (Join Us in the Front), copenhagen: NALAD.

National Working Party on Social Inclusion (1997) *The Net Result: Social Inclusion in the Information Society*, London: IBM.

Negroponte, N. (1995) *Being Digital*, London: Coronet, Hodder Stoughton.

Negt, O. and Kluge, A. (1993) *Public Sphere and Experience: Toward an Analysis of the Bourgeois and Proletarian Public Sphere*, Minneapolis: University of Minnesota.

Nelson, L. H. (1993) 'Epistemological communities', in Alcoff, L. and Potter E. (eds) *Feminist Epistemologies*, London: Routledge.

Net-Life Research Group at Department of Informatics, Umea University, more information at: http://www.informatik.umu.se/nlrg/.

Nettleton, S., Burrows, R., Loader, B., Muncer, S. and Pleace, N. (2001 forthcoming) 'The reality of virtual social support', in Woolgar, S. (ed.) *Virtual Society? Get Real!*, Oxford: Oxford University Press.

New Economics Foundation (1998) *Participation Works! 21 Techniques of Community Participation for the 21st Century*, London: New Economics Foundation.

Newman, O. (1972) *Defensible Space: People and Design in the Violent City*, London: Architectural Press.

Neyland, D. (2000) 'Time and space reconfigured: CCTV, the "super follow" and the "impatient patient"', paper presented at the BSA Annual Conference, York University, 17–20 April.

Nie, N. and Erbring, L. (2000) *Study Offers Early Look at How Internet is Changing Daily Life Report*, Stanford University, Stanford CA, February, website: www.stanford.edu/group/siqss/Press_Release/press_release.html.

Niebel, M. (1997) 'The action plan of the European Commission', in Kubicek, H., Dutton, W. H. and Williams, R. (eds) *The Social Shaping of Information Superhighways: European and American Roads to the Information Society*, Frankfurt: Campus Verlag.

Norén, L. (2000) 'The influence of citizens on public markets' ('Offentliga marknader och brukarinflytande', in Swedish), *Kommunal ekonomi och politik*, Vol. 4, No. 1, pp. 7–29.

Norman, D. (1999) 'Affordance, conventions, and design', *Interactions*, May–June, pp. 38–44.

Norris, C. and Armstrong, G. (1999) *The Maximum Surveillance Society, the Rise of CCTV*, Oxford: Berg.

Nozawa, S. (1997) *Marital Relations and Personal Networks in Urban Japan*, Working Paper, Department of Sociology, Shizouka University, May.

NTIA (National Telecommunications and Information Administration) (2000) *Falling Through the Net: Toward Digital Inclusion*, Washington: Department of Commerce.

Oc, T. and Tiesdell, S. (1997) *Safer City Centres: Reviving the Public Realm*, London: Paul Chapman.

OCCCN, http://www.occcn.org.

Ogburn, W. F. (1950) 'Social evolution reconsidered', in Ogburn, W. F. (ed.) *Social Change*, New York: Viking.

Ohri, A. and Manning, B. (1982) *Community Work and Racism*, Newcastle: Association of Community Workers.

Oldenburg, R. (1991) *The Great Good Place: Cafes, Coffee Shops, Community Centres, Beauty Parlors, General Stores, Bars, Hangouts, and How They Get You Through the Day*, New York: Paragon House.

Olsen, L. (1998) *Viden, der gør forskel: erfaringsdannelse fra forsøg med videnscentre på handicapområdet*, Copenhagen: UCSF og Sociologisk Institut.

Ormrod, S. (1995) 'Feminist sociology and methodology: Leaky black boxes in gender/technology relations', in Grint, K. and Gill, R. (eds) *The Gender Technology Relation: Contemporary Theory and Research*, London: Taylor & Francis.

Orr, M. (1999) *Black Social Capital: The Politics of School Reform in Baltimore, 1986–1998*, Lawrence, KS: University Press of Kansas.

Otani, S. (1999) 'Personal community networks in contemporary Japan', in Wellman, B. (ed.) *Networks in the Global Village*, Boulder, CO: Westview Press.

Page, M. and Scott, M. (1999a) *Women Connect Phase 1 Report*, London: The Community Development Foundation.

Page, M. and Scott, M. (1999b) *Use and Shape the Internet, a Handbook for Women's and Other Voluntary and Community Organisations*, London: The Community Development Foundation.

Painter, K. (1992) 'Differential worlds: the spatial, temporal and social dimensions of female victimisation', in Evans, R., Fyfe, N. and Herbert, D. (eds), *Crime, Policing and Place: Essays in Environmental Criminology*, London: Routledge.

Parks, M. R. and Floyd, K. (1996) 'Making friends in Cyberspace', *Journal of Computer Mediated Communication*, Vol. 1, No. 4, http://www.ascusc.org/jcmc/.

PAT 15 (2000) *Closing the Digital Divide: Information and Communication Technologies in Deprived Areas – A Report by Policy Action Team 15*, London: DTI.

Pateman, C. (1970) *Participation and Democratic Theory*, Cambridge: Cambridge University Press.

Pearce, J. (1996) 'Urban youth cultures: gender and spatial forms', *Youth and Policy*, No. 52 (spring), pp. 1–11.

Pepper, K. and Clegg, C. (1999) 'On-line communities: issues for research', *Proceedings of Workshop: Broadening Our Understanding: Community Networks and Other Forms of Computer Supported Community Work. ECSCW 99*, Copenhagen: http://www.scn.org/tech/the_network/Proj/ws99/pepper-pp.html.

Perez, M. (1999) *Infoville Critical Success Factors (CSF)*, Internal Report, Spain: Oracle.

Perri 6 (1997) *Escaping Poverty: From Safety Nets to Networks of Opportunity*, London: Demos.

Pile, S. (1996) *The Body and the City*, London: Routledge.

Pinter, H. (2000) 'Cruel, inhuman, degrading', *New Internationalist*, September, p. 16.

Piore, M. and Sable, C. (1984) *The Second Industrial Divide: Possibilities for Prosperity*, New York: Basic Books.

Piven, F. F. and Cloward, R. A. (1979) *Poor People's Movements*, New York: Vintage Books.

Pleace, N., Burrows, R., Loader, B., Muncer, S. and Nettleton, S. (2000) 'On-line with the friends of Bill W: social support and the Net, *Sociological Research Online*, Vol. 5, No. 2.

Plumwood, V. (1993) *Feminism and the Mastery of Nature*, London: Routledge.

Putnam, R. (1993) 'The prosperous community: social capital and public life', *The American Prospect*, Vol. 13 (spring), http://epn.org/prospect/13/13putn.html.

Putnam, R., Leonardi, R. and Nanetti, R. Y. (1993) *Making Democracy Work: Civic Traditions in Modern Italy*, Princeton, NJ: Princeton University Press.

Putnam, R. (1995) 'Bowling alone: America's declining social capital', *Journal of Democracy*, Vol. 6, No. 1, pp. 65–78.

Putnam, R. (1996) 'The strange disappearance of civic America', *American Prospect*, Vol. 7, No. 24 (winter), pp. 34–48.

Putnam, R. (2000) *Bowling Alone: The Collapse and Revival of American Community*, New York: Simon & Schuster.

Quarterman, J. S. (1993) 'The global matrix of minds', in Harasim, L. (ed.) *Global Networks: Computers and International Communication*, London: MIT Press.

Rafensperger, L. (1997) 'Defining good science: a new approach to the environment and public health', in Murphy, D., Scammel, M. and Sclove, R. (eds) *Doing Community Based Research*, Amherst, MA: Loka Institute.

Ramazanoglu, C. (1989) *Feminism and the Contradictions of Oppression*, London: Routledge.

Ramrayka, L. (2000) 'Web line', *Guardian*, 12 September, www.guardianunlimited.co.uk/archive/article/0,4273,4062457,00.

Ranerup, A. (1998) 'Can Internet improve democracy in local government?', in Henderson-Chatfield, R., Kuhn, S. and Muller, M. (eds) *PDC 98: Proceedings of the Participatory Design Conference*, Seattle: CPSR and ACM.

Ranerup, A. (1999) 'Contradictions when Internet is used in local government', in Heeks, R. (ed.) *Reinventing Government in the Information Age*, London and New York: Routledge.

Ranerup, A. (2000a) 'On-line forums as an arena for political discussions', in Ishida, T. and Isbister, K. (eds) *Digital Cities: Technologies, Experiences, and Future Perspectives*, Berlin: Springer-Verlag.

Ranerup, A. (2000b) 'Do citizens "do politics with words"?', in Tjoa, A.-M., Wagner, R. R. and Al-Zobaidie, A. (eds) *Proceedings of the 11th International Workshop On Database & Expert Systems Applications*, Los Alamitos, CA: IEEE.

Reason, P. (ed.) (1994) *Participation in Human Inquiry*, London: Sage.

Reason, P. and Bradbury, H. (eds) (2000) *Handbook of Action Research: Participative Inquiry and Practice*, London: Sage.

Reeve, A. (1998), 'The panopticisation of shopping: CCTV and leisure consumption', in Norris, C., Moran, J. and Armstrong, G. (eds) *Surveillance, Closed Circuit Television and Social Control*, Aldershot: Ashgate.

Reid, E. M. (1994) 'Virtual worlds: culture and imagination', in Jones, S. G. (ed.) *CyberSociety: Computer-mediated Communication and Community*, Thousand Oaks, CA: Sage.

Reid, E. M. (1996) 'Text based virtual realities: identity and the cyborg body', in Goodwin, M. (ed.) *High Noon on the Electronic Frontier*, Cambridge, MA: MIT Press.

Reinke, W. (1999) 'The other World Wide Web: global public policy networks' *Foreign Policy*, winter, pp. 44–57.

Renckstorf, K., McQuail, D. and Jankowski, N. (eds) (1996) *Media Use as Social Action: A European Approach to Audience Studies*, London: John Libbey.

Resnick, P. (2000) *Beyond Bowling Together: Socio-technical Capital*, on the Web at http://faculty.si.umich.edu/~presnick/papers/stk/index.html.

Rheingold, H. (1993a) *The Virtual Community: Homesteading on the Electronic Frontier*, Reading, MA: Addison-Wesley, available online at http://www.rheingold. com/book/.

Rheingold, H. (1993b) 'A slice of life in my virtual community', in Harasim, L. (ed.) *Global Networks: Computers and International Communication*, London: MIT Press.

Rheingold, H. (1994) *The Virtual Community: Finding Connection in a Computerised World*, London: Secker and Warburg.

Rheingold, H. (1996) 'My slice of life in my virtual community', in Goodwin, M. (ed.) *High Noon on the Electronic Frontier*, Cambridge, MA: MIT Press.

Rheingold, H. (2000) *The Virtual Community*, revised edition. Cambridge, MA: MIT Press.

Rhodes, R. A. W. (1997) *Understanding Governance – Policy Networks, Governance, Reflexivity and Accountability*, Philadelphia: Open University Press.

Richard, R. (1999) 'Tools of governance?' in Hague, B. N. and Loader, B. D. (eds) *Digital Democracy: Discourse and Decision Making in the Information Age*, London and New York: Routledge.

Riedel, E., Dresel, L., Wagoner, M. J., Sullivan, J. L. and Borgida, E. (1998) 'Electric communities: assessing equality of access in a rural Minnesota community', *Social Science Computer Review*, Vol. 15, No. 4, pp. 370–90.

Riger, S. and Gordon, M. T. (1981) 'The fear of rape: a study in social control', *Journal of Social Issues*, Vol. 37, No. 4, pp. 71–92.

Riordan, S. (1999) *Women's Organisations in the Voluntary Sector: A Force for Change*, London: University of East London: Centre for Institutional Studies.

Risman, B., Tomaskovic-Devey, D. and Dimes, M. (2000). 'Utopian visions: engaged sociologies for the twenty-first century', *Contemporary Sociology*, Vol. 29, No. 1.

Robbins, B. (1993) (ed.) *The Phantom Public Sphere*, Minneapolis: University of Minnesota Press.

Roberts, B. (1978) *Cities of Peasants*, London: Edward Arnold.

Roeder, L. (1999) 'The global disaster information network', *ASIS Bulletin*, October/ November, http://www.asis.org/Bulletin/Oct/roeder.html.

Ronfeldt, D. and Martinez, A. (1997) 'A comment on the Zapatista netwar', in Arquilla, J. and Ronfeldt, D. (eds) *In Athena's Camp: Preparing for Conflict in the Information Age*, Santa Monica: RAND.

Rose, G. (1993) *Feminism and Geography: The Limits of Geographical Knowledge*, Cambridge, Polity.

Rosenbrock, H. (1989) *Designing Human-centred Technology: A Cross Disciplinary Project in Computer-aided Manufacture*, Amsterdam: Springer-Verlag.

Ross, D. and Hood, J. (1998) 'Closed circuit television (CCTV) – the Easterhouse case study', in Montanheiro, L., Haigh, B., Morris, D. and Hrovatin, N. (eds) *Public and Private Sector Partnerships: Fostering Enterprise*, Sheffield: Sheffield Hallam University Press.

Runyan, C. (1999) 'Action on the frontlines', *World Watch*, November/December, pp. 12–21.

Safe Greater Easterhouse (SGE) (1997) *Safe Greater Easterhouse: Recorded Crime in Greater Easterhouse, 1990–1996*, Glasgow: SGE.

Salaff, J., Wellman B. and Dimitrova, D. (1998) 'There is a time and place for teleworking', in Suomi, R., Jackson, P., Hollmén, L. and Aspnäs, M. (eds) *Teleworking Environments: Proceedings of the Third International Workshop on Telework*, 1–4 September, Turku, Finland: Turku Center for Computer Science, General Publication No. 8.

Sanderson, I. (1999) 'Participation and democratic Renewal: from "instrumental" to "communicative rationality"?', in *Policy & Politics*, Vol. 27, No. 3, pp. 325–41.

Sartre, J.-P. (1992) 'Intentionality' [1939]; reprinted in Crary, J. and Kwinter, S. (eds) *Incorporations*, New York: Zone.

Schiesel, S. (2000) 'Zagat survey gets investment for expansion', *New York Times on the Web*, 14 February. URL: http://www.nytimes.com/library/dining/021400zagat.html.

Schiller, H. (1996) *Information Inequality*, London: Routledge.

Schon, D. A., Sanyal, B. and Mitchell, W. J. (eds) (1999) *High Technology and Low-income Communities: Prospects for the Positive Use of Advanced Information Technology*, Cambridge, MA: MIT Press.

Schuler, D. and Namioka, A. (eds) (1993) *Participatory Design – Principles and Practices*, Hillsdale, NJ: LEA.

Schuler, D. (1994) *New Community Networks: Wired for Change*, Reading, MA: Addison-Wesley.

Schuler, D. (1996) *New Community Networks: Wired for Change – Second Edition*, Reading, MA: Addison-Wesley, on the Web at http://www.scn.org/civic/ncn/.

Schuler, D. (1997) 'Community computer networks: a critical opportunity for collaboration among democratic technology researchers and practitioners', in *Technology and Democracy: User Involvement in Information Technology*, Oslo: Center for Technology and Culture, University of Oslo.

Schuler, D. (2001) 'Part of the solution? Computer professionals and the next culture of democracy', *Communications of the ACM*, January, pp. 52–7.

Scientific and Technological Options Assessment Unit (STOA) (1998) *An Appraisal of Technologies of Political Control (Working Document)*, European Parliament, Directorate General of Research, PE 166 499, The STOA Programme, Luxembourg: European Parliament.

Sclove, R. (1995) *Democracy and Technology*, Guilford Press.

Scott, A., Semmens, L. and Willoughby, L. (1999) 'Women and the Internet: the natural history of a research project', *Information Communication and Society*, Vol. 2, No. 4.

Scottish Executive (2000) *More CCTV Cameras Mean More Protection and Better Detection*, press release, No. SE0730/2000, 17 March, Edinburgh: Scottish Executive.

Scottish Office (1998) *Government Cash Boost Puts Easterhouse CCTV Project in the Picture*, Scottish Office news release, No. 1818/98, 10 September, Edinburgh: Scottish Office.

SEU (2000) *The Social Exclusion Unit Leaflet*, http://www.cabinet-office.gov.uk/seu/index/leaflet.

Shade, L. (1998) 'A gendered perspective on access to the information infrastructure', *The Information Society*, Vol. 14, pp. 33–44.

Shearman, C. (1999) *Local Connections: Making the Net Work for Neighbourhood Renewal*, London: Communities on Line.

Short, E. and Ditton, J. (1995) 'Does CCTV affect crime?', *CCTV Today*, Vol. 2, No. 2, pp. 10–12.

Short, E. and Ditton, J. (1996) *Does CCTV Prevent Crime? An Evaluation of The Use of CCTV Surveillance Cameras in Airdrie Town Centre*, Edinburgh: Scottish Office Central Research Unit.

Short, E. and Ditton, J. (1998), 'Seen and now heard: talking to the targets of open street CCTV systems', *British Journal of Criminology*, Vol. 38, No. 3, pp. 404–28.

Showstack Sassoon, A. (1987) (ed.) *Women and the State*, London: Routledge.

SIFO, http://www.sifointeractive.com/index2.html.

Silver, D. (2000) *Cyberspace Under Construction: Design, Discourse, and Diversity in the Blacksburg Electronic Village and the Seattle Community Network*, Ph.D. dissertation, Department of American Studies, University of Maryland.

Silverstone, R. and Hirsch, E. (1992) 'Consuming technologies', in Silverstone, R. and Hirsch, E. (eds.) *Consuming Technologies: Media and Information In Domestic Spaces*, London and New York: Routledge.

Skeggs, B. (1997) *Formations of Class & Gender*, London: Sage.

Smit, E. Y. M. and van Boeschoten, R. M. (1998) *Deliverable 3: Forum Workshop. Impressions and results. Forum: A Workshop on Public Debates on the Internet*, ISPO 97066, Rotterdam: Commission of the European Communities.

Smith, M. (1999) 'Invisible crowds in cyberspace: mapping the social structure of the Usenet', in Smith, M. A. and Kollock, P. (eds) *Communities in Cyberspace*, London: Routledge.

Smith, M. and Kollock, P. (eds) (1999) *Communities in Cyberspace*, London: Routledge.

Smith, M. R. and Marx, L. (eds) (1994) *Does Technology Drive History? The Dilemma of Technological Determinism*, Cambridge, MA: MIT Press.

Smith, T. (1999) *The Emerging 21st Century American Family*, report, Chicago: National Opinion Research Center.

Snijder, E. J. and Flos, B. J. (2000) *Overheid oNLine: trendonderzoek naar gemeenten en provincies op internet*, Rotterdam: Deloitte & Touche.

Spender, D. (1995) *Nattering on the Net: Women, Power and Cyberspace*, Melbourne: Spinifex.

Stacey, M. (1974) 'The myth of community studies', in Bell, C. and Newby, H. (eds) *The Sociology of Community*, London: Frank Cass & Co.

Stamm, K. R. (1985) *Newspaper Use and Community Ties: Toward a Dynamic Theory*, Norwood, NJ: Ablex.

Stanko, E. (1985) *Intimate Intrusions: Women's Experiences of Male Violence*, London: Routledge.

Stanko, E. (1987) 'Typical violence, normal precaution: men, women and interpersonal violence in England, Wales, Scotland and the USA', in Hanmer, J. and Maynard M. (eds) *Women, Violence and Social Control*, London: Macmillan.

Stanko, E. (1990) *Everyday Violence: How Women and Men Experience Physical and Sexual Danger*, London: Pandora Press.

Stanko, E. (1991) 'When precaution is normal: a feminist critique of crime prevention', in Gelsthorpe, L. and Morris, A. (eds) *Feminist Perspectives in Criminology*, Buckingham: Open University Press.

Stanko, E. (1993) 'Ordinary fear: women, violence and personal safety', in Bart, P. and Moran, E. (eds) *Violence Against Women: The Bloody Footprints*, London: Sage.

Stanley, L. and Wise, S. (1993) *Breaking Out Again: Feminist Ontology and Epistemology*, London: Routledge.

Stappers, J., Hollander, E. and Manders, H. (1978) *Vier experimenten met lokale omroep*, research report, Nijmegen: Institute of Mass Communication, University of Nijmegen.

Stappers, J., Olderaan, F. and Wit, P. de (1992) 'The Netherlands: emergence of a new medium', in Jankowski, N. W., Prehn, O. and Stappers, J. (eds) *The People's Voice: Local Radio and Television in Europe*, London: John Libbey.

Star, S. L. (1991) 'Power, technology and the phenomenology of conventions: on being allergic to onions', in Law, J. (ed.) *A Sociology of Monsters: Essays on Power, Technology and Domination*, London: Routledge.

Steward, F. and Conway, S. (1998) 'Situating discourse in environmental innovation networks', in *Organization*, Vol. 5, No. 4, pp. 479–502.

Stoecker, R. and Stuber, A. C. S. (1997) 'Building an information superhighway of one's own: a comparison of two approaches', paper presented at the annual meeting of the Urban Affairs Association, Toronto, on the Web at http://www.murchisoncenter.org/catnetdraft/history.html.

Stolterman, E. (1998) 'Technology matters in virtual communities', positioning paper for the workshop 'Designing Across Borders: The Community Design of Community Networks', PDC '98/CSCW '98, Seattle, November, Seattle: CPSR/ACM.

Stolterman, E. (1999) 'The design of information systems – parti, formats and sketching', *Information Systems Journal*, Vol. 9, Issue 1, January.

Storgaard, K. (1991) In Cronberg, T., Duelund, P., Jensen, O. M. and ovortrup, L. (eds) *Danish Experiments – Social Constructions of Technology*, Copenhagen: New Social Science Monographs.

Storgaard, K., Jæger, B., Manniche, J., Marcussen, C. H., Hansen, J. and Johansen, S. (1997) *Bornholm på Nettet*, Nexø, Denmark: Bornholms Forskningscenter, AKF og SBI.

Straw, M. K. and Marks, K. (1995) 'Use of focus groups in program development', *Qualitative Health Research*, Vol. 5, No. 4, pp. 428–43.

Street, P. (1997) 'Scenario workshops: a participatory approach to sustainable urban living?', *Futures*, Vol. 29, No. 2, pp. 139–58.

Stringer, E. T. (1999) *Action research*, 2nd edition, London: Sage.

Stuber, A. (n.d.) 'The development of CATNeT – the Coalition to Access Technology and Networking in Toledo' , on the Web at http://www.murchisoncenter.org/catnetdraft/history.html.

Suchman, L. (1991) 'Closing remarks on the Fourth Conference on Women, Work and Computerization: Identities and Differences', in Eriksson, I.V., Kitchenham, B. A. and Tijdens, K. (eds) *Women, Work and Computerization: Understanding and Overcoming Bias in Work and Education*, Amsterdam: Elsevier/North Holland.

Suchman, L. (1994) 'Supporting articulation work: aspects of a feminist practice of technology production', in Adam, A., Emms, J., Green, E. and Owen, J. (eds) *Women, Work and Computerization: Breaking Old Boundaries, Building New Forms*, Amsterdam: North Holland.

Suttles, G. (1972) *The Social Construction of Communities*, Chicago: University of Chicago Press.

Tabb, W. K. (2000) 'After Seattle: understanding the politics of globalization', *Monthly Review*, Vol. 51, Issue 10.

Tambini, D. (1998) 'Civic networking and universal rights to connectivity: Bologna', in Tsagarousianou, R., Tambini, D. and Bryan, C. (eds) *Cyberdemocracy. Technology, Cities and Civic Networks*, London and New York: Routledge.

Tang, P. (1998) 'Managing the cyberspace divide: government investment in electronic information services', in Loader, B. (ed.) *Cyberspace Divide: Equality, Agency and Policy in the Information Society*, London: Routledge.

Taylor, I. (1995) 'Developing superhighways in the United Kingdom', *International Technology and Public Policy*, Vol. 13, No. 3, pp. 194–5.

Thébert, Y. (1985) [1987] 'Private life and domestic architecture in Roman Africa', in Veyne, P. (ed.) *A History of Private Life*, Cambridge, MA: Belknap Press.

Tilley, N. (1993) *Understanding Car Parks, Crime and CCTV*, Crime Prevention Unit Series paper 42, London: Home Office.

Tilly, C. (1973) 'Do communities act?', *Sociological Inquiry*, Vol. 43: pp. 209–40.

Tilly, C. (2000) *Spaces of Contention*, working paper, Columbia University, 21 January.

Toffler, A. (1980) *The Third Wave*, London: Pan.

Tsagarousianou, R., Tambini, D. and Bryan, C. (1998) (eds) *Cyberdemocracy. Technology, Cities and Civic Networks*, London and New York: Routledge.

Turk, A. and Trees, K. (2000) 'Facilitating community processes through culturally appropriate informatics: an Australian indigenous community information systems case study', in Gurstein, M. (ed.) *Community Informatics: Enabling Communities with Information and Communications Technologies*, Hershey, PA: Idea Group.

Tushman, M. and Katz, R. (1980) 'External communication and project performance: an investigation into the role of gatekeepers', *Management Science*, Vol. 26, No. 11, pp. 1071–85.

Twelvetrees, A. (1998) *Community Work*, London: Macmillan.

UNCED (1992) *Agenda 21*, New York: UN Publications.

Urban University and Neighborhood Network (1996) *Limited Access: The Information Superhighway and Ohio's Neighborhood-Based Organizations*, on the Web at http://www.murchisoncenter.org/catnetdraft/history.html.

US Department of Commerce, http://www.digitaldivide.gov.

Valentine, G. (1989) 'The geography of women's fear', *Area*, Vol. 21, pp. 385–90.

Valentine, G. (1992) 'Images of danger: women's sources of information about the spatial distribution of male violence', *Area*, Vol. 24, No. 4, pp. 22–9.

Van der Linden, C., Hollander, E. and Vergeer, M. (1994) 'Recent onderzoek naar en theorievorming over kleinschalige massacommunicatie', in van Raaij, F., Schuijt, G., Stappers, J., Wieten, J., van Woerkum, C. and van der Linden, C. (eds), *Communicatie en informatie: een stand van zaken*, Houten/Zaventem: Bohn Stafleu van Loghem.

Vari, D. (2000) 'How activists used the Internet to organize protests against the spring meetings of the International Monetary Fund, World Bank, and the World Trade Organization scheduled for April 16–17 in Washington, D.C.', student research paper written to fulfil the Virtual Community Research Project for Sociology and the Internet taught by Professor Robert E. Wood, Rutgers University, on the Web at http://camden-www.rutgers.edu/~wood/445/vari.htm.

Vehviläinen, M. (1986) 'A study circle approach as a method for women to develop their work and computer systems', paper presented at the Second IFIP Women, Work and Computerization conference, Dublin.

Vehviläinen, M. (2001) 'Gender and citizenship in the information society: women's information technology groups in North Karelia', in Green, E. and Adam, A. (eds) *Virtual Gender: Technology, Consumption and Identity*, London: Routledge.

Virilio, P. (2000) *Polar Inertia*, London: Sage.

Wacjman, J. (1991) *Feminism Confronts Technology*, Cambridge: Polity.

Wakeford, N. (1997) 'Networking women and grrrls with information/communication technology: surfing tales of the world wide web', in Terry, J. and Calvert, M. (eds) *Processed Lives: Gender and Technology in Everyday Life*, London: Routledge.

Wakeford, N. (1998) 'Urban cultures for virtual bodies: comments on lesbian "identity" and "community" in San Francisco Bay Area cyberspace', in Ainley, R. (ed.) *New Frontiers of Space, Bodies and Gender*, London: Routledge.

Walch, J. (1999) *In the Net: An Internet Guide for Activists*, London: Zed.

Walker, G. (2000) 'Editorial', *News on Community Networking in Newcastle upon Tyne and Beyond Online*, Issue 1, March.

Wallerstein, I. (1999) *The End of the World as We Know It*, Minneapolis: University of Minnesota Press.

Walther, J. B. (1995) 'Relational aspects of computer-mediated communication: experimental observations over time', *Organization Science*, Vol. 6, No. 2, pp. 186–203.

Ward, P. (1999) *A History of Domestic Space: Privacy and the Canadian Home*, Vancouver: UBC Press.

Webster, C. W. R. (1996) 'Closed circuit television and governance: the eve of a surveillance age', *Information Infrastructure and Policy*, Vol. 5, No. 4, pp. 253–63.

Webster, C. W. R. (1998a) 'Surveying the scene: geographic and spatial aspects of the closed circuit television surveillance revolution in the UK', paper presented to XIII meeting of the Permanent Study Group on Informatization in Public Administration, European Group of Public Administration annual conference, Paris, France, 14–17 September.

Webster, C. W. R. (1998b) 'Changing relationships between citizens and the state: the case of closed circuit television surveillance cameras', in Snellen, I. Th. M. and Donk, W. B. H. J. van de, *Public Administration in an Information Age: A Handbook*, Informatization Developments and the Public Sector Series, No. 6. Amsterdam: IOS Press, pp. 79–96.

Webster, C. W. R. (1999a) 'Cyber society or surveillance society? Findings from a national survey on closed circuit television in the UK', in Armitage, J. and Roberts, J. (eds) *Exploring Cyber Society: Social, Political and Cultural Issues, Proceedings of the Conference*, Vol. 2, 5–7 July, University of Northumbria at Newcastle.

Webster, C. W. R. (1999b) 'Closed circuit television and information age policy processes', in Hague, B. N. and Loader B. D. (eds) *Digital Democracy: Discourse and Decision Making in the Information Age*, London: Routledge.

Webster, F. (1995) *Theories of the Information Society*, London: Routledge.

Webster, J. (1990) *Office Automation: the Labour Process and Women's Work in Britain*, Hemel Hempstead: Harvester Wheatsheaf.

Weil, S. (1952) *The Needs for Roots: Prelude to a Declaration of Duties Towards Mankind*, London: Routledge and Kegan Paul.

Weinberg, N., Schmale, J., Uken, J. and Wessel, K. (1996) 'Online help: cancer patients participate in a computer mediated support group', *Health and Social Work*, Vol. 21, No. 1, pp. 24–9.

Wellman, B. (1979) 'The community question', *American Journal of Sociology*, Vol. 84, pp. 1201–31.

Wellman, B. and Leighton, B. (1979) 'Networks, neighborhoods and communities', *Urban Affairs Quarterly*, Vol. 14, pp. 363–90.

Wellman, B. (1985) 'Domestic work, paid work and net work', in Duck, S. and Perlman, S. (eds) *Understanding Personal Relationships*, London: Sage.

Wellman, B. (1988) 'Structural analysis: from method and metaphor to theory and substance', in Wellman, B. and Berkowitz, S. D. (eds) *Social Structures: A Network Approach*, Cambridge: Cambridge University Press.

Wellman, B. and Wortley, S. (1990) 'Different strokes from different folks: community ties and social support', *American Journal of Sociology*, Vol. 96, No. 3, pp. 558–88.

Wellman, B. and Wellman, B. (1992) 'Domestic affairs and network relations', *Journal of Social and Personal Relationships*, Vol. 9, pp. 385–409.

Wellman, B. (1992a) 'Men in networks: private communities, domestic friendships', in Nardi, P. (ed.) *Men's Friendships*, Newbury Park, CA: Sage.

Wellman, B. (1992b) 'Which types of ties and networks give what kinds of social support?', *Advances in Group Processes*, Vol. 9, pp. 207–35.

Wellman, B. (1997) 'An electronic group is virtually a social network', in Kiesler, S. (ed.) *Culture of the Internet*, Mahwah, NJ.: Lawrence Erlbaum.

Wellman, B. and Gulia, M. (1999) 'Net surfers don't ride alone', in Wellman, B. (ed.) *Networks in the Global Village*, Boulder, CO: Westview Press.

Wellman, B. and Hampton, K. (1999) 'Living networked on and offline', *Contemporary Sociology*, Vol. 28, No. 6, pp. 648–54.

Wellman, B. (1999a) 'The network community', in Wellman, B. (ed.) *Networks in the Global Village*, Boulder, CO: Westview.

Wellman, B. (1999b) 'Ties and Bonds', *Connections*, Vol. 22, No. 1.

Wellman, B. (2000a) 'Changing connectivity: a future history of Y2.03K', *Sociological Research Online*, Vol. 4, No. 4, February, website: http://www.socresonline.org.uk/4/.

Wellman, B. (2000b) 'Must community have a place?', in *An Online Discussion of the American Sociological Association's Community and Sociology section*, January–February, website: http://www.urbsoc.org/communityweb/.

Wells, H. G. (1971) *World Brain*, Freeport, NY: Books for Libraries Press.

Westerik, H. (2001 forthcoming) *Het gebruik van lokale en regionale media*, Ph.D. Dissertation, Department of Communication, University of Nijmegen.

Whitmore, E. (1994) 'To tell the truth: working with oppressed groups in participatory approaches to inquiry', in Reason, P. (ed.) *Participation in Human Inquiry*, London: Sage.

Wilhelm, A. G. (1999) 'Virtual sounding board: how deliberative is online political discussion?', in Hague, B. H. and Loader, B. D. (eds) *Digital Democracy: Discourse and Decision Making in the Information Age*, London and New York: Routledge.

William, R., Slack, R. and Stewart, J. (2000) *Social Learning in Multimedia Final Report*, Edinburgh: University of Edinburgh, Research Centre of Social Sciences/Technology Studies Unit.

Williams, F. (1993) 'Women and community', in Bornat, J., Pereira C., Pilgrim, D. and Williams, F. (eds) *Community Care: A Reader*, Basingstoke: Macmillan.

Williams, F. (1999) 'Good-enough principles for welfare', *Journal of Social Policy*, Vol. 28, No. 4, pp. 667–87.

Williams, K. and Alkalimat, A. (2001 forthcoming) 'A census of public computing in Toledo, Ohio', in Schuler, D. and Day, P. (eds) *Shaping the Network Society: The New Role of Civic Society in Cyberspace*, Cambridge, MA.: MIT Press.

Williams, K. (2000) 'Libraries as ISPs', *Ohio Libraries*.

Williams, R. (1974) *Television: Technology and Cultural Form*, London: Fontana.

Wilson, D. (1999) 'Exploring the limits of public participation in local government', *Parliamentary Affairs*, Vol. 52, No. 2, pp. 246–59.

Wilson, R. (2000) 'Crime camera cash blow', *The Extra*, News, 2 March, p. 7.

Wilson, W. J. (1987) *The Truly Disadvantaged: The Inner City, the Underclass, and Public Policy*, Chicago: University of Chicago Press.

Winner, L. (1985) 'Do artifacts have politics?', in MacKenzie, D. and Wajcman, J. (eds) *The Social Shaping of Technology*, Milton Keynes: Open University Press.

Wolf, E. (1966) 'Kinship, friendship and patron–client relations', in Banton, M. (ed.) *The Social Anthropology of Complex Societies*, London: Tavistock.

Women Connect (1999a) *Report on Women and Information Technology (ICTS)* to Social Exclusion Unit's Policy Action Team 15; copy posted on www.womenconnect.org.uk

Women Connect (1999b) Conference report, 'Social exclusion to social change on the information superhighway: Women Connect at CDF', London, DTI: 22 November, copy posted online, available at www.womenconnect.org.uk.

Wright, E. O. (1979) *Class, Crisis and the State*, London: Verso.

Wright, P. (1989) 'Gender differences in adults' same- and cross-gender friendships', in Adams, R. and Blieszner, R. (eds) *Older Adult Friendship*, Newbury Park, CA: Sage.

Wyatt, S. (1999) 'They came, they surfed, they went back to the beach: why some people stop using the Internet', presentation at the Society for Social Studies of Science Conference, October.

Yeandle, S. and Morrell, H. (1994) 'Evaluating policy interventions promoting women's safety: issues from research in progress', paper presented at the BSA Conference, University of Central Lancashire.

Yuval-Davis, N. (1997) *Gender and Nation*, London: Sage.

Yuval-Davis, N. (1999) 'What is transversal politics?', *Soundings*, Vol. 12, pp. 94–8.

Index